MEDICINE
FOR THE
OUTDOORS

MEDICINE
FOR THE
OUTDOORS

The Essential Guide to Emergency Medical Procedures and First Aid

REVISED AND
EXPANDED EDITION

Paul S. Auerbach, M.D.

Illustrations by Christine Gralapp and Alexandrine Bartlett

The Lyons Press

Revised and Expanded edition

Printed in the United States of America
Design and composition by G&H SOHO, Inc.

10 9 8 7 6 5 4 3 2 1

Library of Congress Cataloging-in-Publication Data

Auerbach, Paul S.
    Medicine for the outdoors: the essential guide to emergency medical
  procedures and first aid / Paul S. Auerbach: illustrations by
  Christine Gralapp and Alexander Bartlett.—Rev. and expanded ed.
      p.   cm.
  Includes index.
  ISBN 1-55821-723-1
    1. Outdoor medical emergencies.   2. First aid in illness and
  injury.   I.Title.
  RC88.9.095 A94   1999
  616.02'52—dc21   98-12402
                                             CIP

Publisher's Note:
This book is meant to provide authoritative emergency
medical and first-aid information to those venturing
outdoors. It should not be used as a substitute for professional
advice or training. The author and publisher disclaim any
responsibility for problems that may occur as a result of
following the information, procedures, or techniques
included in this work.

CONTENTS

PREFACE

The outdoor environment is beautiful, but it is ever changing and can become hostile in a moment. Good fortune favors the well prepared, and there are no more important considerations for a successful outdoor experience than safety and first aid. Severe weather, wild animals, rugged terrain, and equipment failure all conspire to create or complicate medical hardships that must be diagnosed swiftly and remedied with certainty. The therapies can be integral to survival. Medical education is thus as compelling as any other form of learning.

This revised and expanded edition of *Medicine for the Outdoors* has been updated and rewritten based upon suggestions from readers and reviewers of the previous edition. I am indebted to my family and friends, who have always supported me in my writing endeavors. Sherry, Brian, Lauren, and Dan the Mammal make it all worthwhile. For this edition, I thank Warren Bowman, Peter Hackett, Brownie Schoene, Roger Hubbard, Bob Norris, Lanny Johnson, Eric Johnson, Dan Danzl, Howard Backer, Howard Donner, Chris Moore, Hank Herrmann, Barbara Kennedy, Bob Mutch, Mel Otten, Eric Weiss, and all of the other people who dedicate their time to teaching others about wilderness medicine.

INTRODUCTION

The purpose of this book is to provide you with brief explanations of a wide variety of medical problems, and to offer practical solutions. The book is arranged to make information easy to retrieve. Part 1 outlines basic principles of health care that should be applied to all outdoor travel. Parts 2 and 3 describe medical situations, beginning with life threats and covering, in turn, major and minor medical problems you might encounter. Part 4 discusses disorders related to various wilderness settings. Part 5 covers additional practical information, such as evacuation guidelines and techniques, water disinfection, useful knots and hitches, drug injection techniques, and recommendations for immunization. Appendix 1 lists common medications and doses. Conversion tables for common measurements are found as Appendix 2. Appendix 3 outlines guidelines for prevention of hepatitis, AIDS, and other diseases transmitted by human body fluids. The glossary defines medical and technical terms. The index will guide you swiftly to any topic.

To keep the book to a manageable size, I have assumed that you have a basic understanding of how your body and organs are supposed to work. Thus, explanations are brief and to the point. This is neither a survival manual nor a sports medicine encyclopedia. Rather, the book is meant to be carried on a journey as a ready reference for a layperson who needs to medically rescue or aid an ill or injured victim. I have included information that is necessary to make simple, accurate diagnoses and to act on them.

This book does not transform a layperson into a physician, but unfortunately, there are times when medical help is miles or even days away. No intervention is completely without risk; however, some familiarity with diseases and injuries can minimize that risk. Although some of the techniques and drugs described could worsen a situation if misapplied or incorrectly administered, the treatments presented are current and well accepted. Still, *the recommendations should not be considered substitutes for prompt evaluation by a trained medical professional.* If at any time a diagnosis is uncertain, or a victim appears to be more than minimally ill, all efforts should be directed at seeking a professional medical opinion.

The basic therapies recommended are not those that could be rendered by a physician with sophisticated equipment and a large armamentarium of drugs. I have not described every infectious or tropical disease that could possibly be contracted during a journey abroad. However, the diagnosis and management of illnesses such as schistosomiasis, malaria, Lyme disease, ehrlichiosis, yellow fever, dengue fever, and Rocky Mountain spotted fever are relevant to many people who travel domestically and overseas in wilderness areas, and have therefore been included.

To use this or any medical reference to best advantage, review the pertinent sections prior to your expedition. Practice the manual skills, such as the application of splints and slings, until you are confident.

I have also provided information that is as important as medical knowledge. This includes such topics as how to avoid being struck by lightning, drowning prevention, and what to do if caught in a flood zone or near a forest fire.

I hope that you are enlightened, and that good luck prevails.

PART ONE

General Information

HOW TO USE THIS BOOK

In order to use this book to best advantage, read the appropriate sections *before* you embark on a trip. In this way, you'll remember where to find information in case of an emergency. Use the index to locate specific topics, such as bee stings, frostbite, or choking. When reading about different problems, you may be referred to general instructions for medical aid, which are presented in parts 1 and 2. All readers are encouraged to participate in formal first-aid courses, such as those offered by the National Ski Patrol, American Red Cross, Outward Bound, and National Outdoor Leadership School. CPR training that conforms to American Heart Association standards is available through multiple venues.

Many drugs recommended in the book are available only through prescriptions provided by physicians, who should explain each drug's use and side effects. All pregnant women should consult a physician prior to any expedition for current advice on the advisability of immunizations and the use of particular drugs.

For estimation of body weight, 1 kilogram (kg) equals 2.2 pounds (lb), so each pound equals 0.45 kilogram. For temperature conversion (when reading thermometers) between Fahrenheit and Centigrade (Celsius), use the following formula:

DEGREES FAHRENHEIT = (⅘ times degrees Centigrade) plus 32
   or
DEGREES CENTIGRADE = ⅚ times (degrees Fahrenheit minus 32)

A temperature conversion table is found on page 459. Volume and weight conversion tables are found on pages 461 and 462. For most practical purposes, 1 liter of liquid can be used interchangeably with 1 quart. I have also provided metric equivalents (sometimes rough) for most of the measurements given.

Although most people do not have ready access to oxygen tanks and masks, I have sometimes recommended oxygen administration for the benefit of those who are so equipped. Information about oxygen administration is found on page 383.

When administering an injection, *never* share needles between people. Appendix 3 briefly discusses guidelines for prevention of hepatitis, AIDS, and other diseases transmitted via contact with human blood and other body fluids.

BEFORE YOU GO

Be Prepared

There is no substitute for preparedness. Adherence to this basic rule will prevent or ease the majority of mishaps that occur in the wild. Proper education prior to situations of risk allows you to cope in a purposeful fashion, rather than in a state of fear and panic. At least two, and preferably all, members of a wilderness expedition should understand first aid and medical rescue. On a casual family outing, one responsible adult should be skilled in first aid. Manual skills, such as mouth-to-mouth breathing, cardiopulmonary resuscitation (CPR), and the application of bandages and splints, should be practiced beforehand. Become familiar with technical rescue techniques pertinent to the environment you will be in (for example, high-angle rock, swift water, or avalanche-prone areas). Be certain to carry appropriate survival equipment, such as maps, a compass, waterproof matches, a knife, nonperishable food, a flashlight, and adequate first-aid supplies. Minimize the need for improvisation.

Prior to undertaking a trip where you will be far from formal medical assistance, it is wise to attend to any obvious medical problems. If you have not done so within the past 6 months, visit a dentist. Make certain that all of your immunizations are up to date (see page 397). If you have a significant medical problem, you should carry an information card or a Medic-Alert bracelet or tag; the latter has imprinted medical information and a phone number link to more detailed medical information.

A sexually active woman of childbearing age should have a test for early pregnancy detection prior to a wilderness expedition. Any pregnancy under 8 weeks' gestation has a 25% chance of miscarriage. Furthermore, it might be sensible to confirm that the fetus is properly situated within the uterus, and that there is not a risk for an ectopic (outside-the-uterus) pregnancy (see page 119), which might rupture and threaten the mother's life.

Common Sense

Many accidents occur because people ignore warning signs or don't anticipate problems. Swimmers are stung by jellyfish outside protective net enclosures; nonswimmers drown while participating in hazardous white-water rafting adventures. *Pay heed to rangers, posted warnings, weather reports, and the experience of seasoned guides.* Prepare for situations of risk by developing your skills in less challenging conditions. Wear recommended personal safety equipment, such as a flotation jacket, safety harness, or climbing helmet. Do not tolerate horseplay in dangerous settings.

Conditioning and Acclimatization

Many health hazards of wilderness travel, such as falls, can be avoided by a reasonable degree of strength and endurance—which can only be acquired by conditioning. Every expedition member should begin from a state of maximum fitness. Other health hazards, such as temperature extremes and high-altitude disorders, can in certain circumstances be avoided by acclimatization to the environment. Acclimatization is a physiological adaptation that is often different from, and may be unrelated to, physical fitness.

Equipment

Be prepared for foul-weather conditions. Always assume that you will be forced to spend an unexpected night outdoors. Carry warm clothing and waterproof rain gear. Break in all footwear, and take care to pad rough edges and exposed seams. Consider carrying a compact emergency position-indicating radio beacon (EPIRB).

All expedition leaders should carry safety and first-aid supplies for the most likely mishaps. Medical supplies must be arranged so that they can be rapidly located and deployed. Recommended first-aid items are listed in part 5.

Communication

Prepare a trip plan (itinerary) and record it in a location (trailhead, ranger station, marina, or the like) where someone will recognize when a person or party is overdue and potentially lost or in trouble. Similarly, determine beforehand a plan for getting help in an emergency, whether it involves radio communication, ground-to-air or ship-to-shore signals, cellular telephone, or knowing the location of the nearest pay telephone, ranger station, or first-aid facility. If mobile rescue-grade equipment is to be used, it should be checked and double-checked prior to departure, and regularly scheduled communications prepared. At least two members of any expedition should be able to fashion standard ground-to-air distress markers. Make sure that children wear an item of bright clothing and carry a whistle that they know to blow if they are frightened or lost. If you carry a radio, know how to tune in to a weather information channel. The National Weather Service issues a "watch" when conditions are right for the development of a particular weather pattern, and a "warning" when its arrival is imminent.

Trip Plans

In most stories of miraculous ocean or wildland survival, the first chapter includes the account of how the victim lost his way. All wilderness travelers should carry maps, be proficient with compass routing, and know in advance where they intend to explore. People with specific medical disabilities, such as chronic severe lung disease, may be advised by a physician to avoid certain stressful environments, such as high altitude. If you are traveling in snow country, you should know how to avoid being caught in an avalanche, and consider carrying an avalanche transceiver that operates on dual frequencies: 457 kilohertz (kHz) (new standard) and 2,275 hertz (Hz) (old standard).

Medicines

There is no need to carry a drugstore on a day hike. On the other hand, drugs necessary to treat established medical problems (such as nitroglycerin tablets for a person with angina) should always be on hand. It is the responsibility of the trip leader to be aware of any potential medical problems and to insist that people in obviously poor physical condition not undertake activities that might endanger themselves or others. Any person with allergies, diabetes, epilepsy, or special medical instructions should wear an identification bracelet or carry a medical information card. Anyone who takes medications should carry a list of drugs and doses. If you travel abroad, it is wise to carry an adequate supply of routine medications, as well as a note from a physician stating their necessity, should you be questioned or need refills. All people should receive adequate antitetanus and other locally required immunizations prior to the trip. Basic medical supplies are listed in Part 5.

Nutrition

Anyone who undertakes vigorous physical activity should consume adequate calories in a well-balanced diet. A debilitating weight-reduction program should not be continued in the wilderness, where a rescue might depend on extraordinary effort and endurance.

To avoid dehydration and exhaustion, take adequate time to eat, drink, and rest. Most adult males require 3,000 to 5,000 food calories each day in order to sustain heavy physical exertion. Women require 2,000 to 3,500 calories. A nutritious diet can easily be maintained with proper planning. Don't plan to live off the land unless you are a survival expert.

Consider carrying a supply of energy bars, such as the Clif Bar, Promax Bar, or PowerBar. For example, the Clif Bar weighs 68 g and delivers approximately 2 to 6 g fat, 45 to 52 g carbohydrates, and 4 to 12 g protein. For a less nutritive energy boost of carbohydrate, sodium, and potassium, carry Clif Shot Energy Gel (64 g tube).

Fluid Requirements

Fluid requirements have been well worked out for all levels of exercise. They are discussed in the section on heat illness (see page 281). Most people underestimate their fluid requirements. Encourage frequent rest stops and water breaks. If natural sources of drinkable water (springs, wells, ice-melt runoff) will not be encountered, you should carry at least a 48-hour supply. Carry supplies for water disinfection (see page 385).

GENERAL FIRST-AID PRINCIPLES

In all first-aid situations, the rescuer must remain calm. If you panic, you will lose control of the victim, as well as of yourself. To establish authority, speak and act calmly and purposefully. Allow the victim to discuss the incident, his situation, and his fears. If you can involve the victim in his rescue and treatment, it is often good for his morale. Save criticism for after the event, and try not to be judgmental. Avoid laying any blame on people; they may get hurt emotionally or become argumentative as a result.

Do not endanger additional inexperienced rescuers. If you cannot get to the victim easily, send for help. Approach all victims safely; don't allow the sense of urgency to transform a sensible rescue into a series of risky, or even foolhardy, maneuvers. If it appears that the victim is too ill to be moved, set up camp immediately. In all cases, protect the victim from above and below from the elements.

If you have paper and a writing instrument, record your observations. If you send someone for help, have him carry a piece of paper that states the victim's location, the nature of the emergency, the number of people needing help, the condition of the victim(s), what is being done to treat the victim(s), and any specific environmental conditions or physical obstacles. Accident report forms are available from organizations such as The Mountaineers.

Always assume the worst. Assume that each victim you encounter has a broken neck or a heart attack until proven otherwise. Always be conservative in your treatments and recommendations for further evaluation or rescue.

Never move a seriously injured victim unless he is in danger from the environment or needs to be moved for medical reasons. Don't encourage a victim to get up and "shake it off" until you have examined him for a potentially serious problem.

If you must remain in a wilderness location for a prolonged period of time caring for a victim, remember to attend to the basic survival requirements, which include air (oxygen) for breathing, shelter, water, food, psychological support, and human waste disposal.

Never administer medicines or perform procedures if you are not sure what you are doing. The good Samaritan has certain legal protections for his actions so long as he operates within prudent limits and takes reasonable care. This book will not make you a doctor. A good rule to follow is *primum non nocere:* "First of all, do no harm." If you are not certain what to do and the situation isn't worsening, don't interfere. Explain to the victim that you are not a physician, but will do your best to get him through whatever crisis he has encountered, to the best of your knowledge and ability. If you encounter a victim who may be seriously ill, seek an expert opinion as soon as possible. Even if your treatment seems successful, it is wise to consult a physician if you would have ordinarily done so.

Secure the Scene

Be certain that you, the victim, and other rescuers are protected from inclement weather, lightning, rockfall, avalanche hazard, and so on. Create a shelter or assign someone to this task as soon as you can. Retreat from a venomous snake, swarm of stinging insects, the edge of a swiftly flowing frigid river, or the like.

Evaluate the Victim

Immediately determine if the victim is breathing, if his heart is beating, and if he has any obvious major injuries. Techniques and procedures for treatment are covered in part 2.

Listen and feel for breathing. Put your ear close to the victim's mouth and nose, and try to detect if he is moving air into and out of his lungs. Watch for chest wall motion. In cold weather, look for a vapor cloud or feel for warm air moving across your hand. If the victim is not breathing well (or at all), you must manage the airway (see page 17) and begin to breathe for him (see page 24), *taking care to maintain the position of the neck if there is any chance of a cervical spine injury* (see page 31). Observe the number of breaths per minute; normal is 12 to 18 per minute for adults, 18 to 25 per minute for small children, and 25 to 50 per minute for infants.

Characterize the nature and effort of breathing. Look to see if breathing is effective—the chest expands and air movement is appreciated. Observe if the victim is laboring to breathe. In an adult, if the breathing rate is less than 10 or greater than 30, the skin color is blue, and/or the victim is confused or unconscious, be prepared to assist breathing (see page 24).

If the breathing is noisy, rattling, or "musical" and high pitched, suspect an airway obstruction (see page 17), particularly if the victim is lying on his back. If the victim has a loose denture or another dental appliance, remove it. If there is no chance of a cervical spine injury (see page 31) and it appears that the victim may vomit, position him on his side. If you are concerned about a neck injury, use the logrolling maneuver (see page 34).

Near the condition of death, a person may show "agonal respirations," characterized by infrequent mouth openings without any chest rise, sometimes accompanied by head lifting.

Feel for a pulse. Place the tips of your index and middle fingers (not your thumb, which can generate a "false" pulse—your own!) gently on the radial artery in the wrist (see figure 10C; page 27). If you cannot detect a pulse there (particularly if your fingers are cold), move your fingers to the brachial artery (this is particularly useful for infants) at the midpoint of the inside of the upper arm (see figure 10E; page 27), femoral artery in the groin (see figure 10B; page 26) or the carotid artery in the neck (see figure 10A; page 26). If no pulse is detected in any of these locations (and the victim is not breathing or verbalizing), begin chest compressions (see page 28). Observe the pulse rate; normal is 55 to 90 per minute for adults, 80 to 110 per minute for small children, and 100 to 130 per minute for infants. The pulse rate is faster with excitement or fear and slower in trained athletes. A rapid and weak ("thready") pulse is a sign of impending shock (see page 54), usually due to excessive bleeding, dehydration, or heart problems. An irregular pulse may indicate an abnormal heart rhythm.

Locate brisk bleeding. Quickly survey the victim to locate any obvious sources of brisk bleeding. Quickly apply firm pressure to these areas (see page 48).

Once you have dealt with these life-threatening problems, begin a careful, complete examination of the victim.

If an injury may be extensive, examine the whole victim. Particularly dangerous situations include falls; blows to the head, neck, chest, or abdomen; altered mental status; difficulty breathing or shortness of breath; and injuries to children. In these cases, or whenever the diagnosis is not readily apparent, evaluate the victim from head to toe. Weather and appropriate modesty permitting, be sure to undress the victim sufficiently to perform a proper examination. Look around the neck or on the wrist(s) for a medical alert (such as MedicAlert) tag, and in a wallet or pack for an information card.

Because most bodies are bilaterally symmetrical, if you are having difficulty determining if a body part is abnormal or deformed, compare it to the opposite side. Always ask a victim to move a body part before you do it for him; if he resists because of pain or weakness, you need to suspect a broken bone or spinal cord (nerve) injury. Do not "force" a motion.

Take as much time as you can afford to explain to a victim what you are going to do. This is usually reassuring. If the victim is a child, it is important to make eye contact, and to be continually supportive. If someone is doing or has done something with which you don't agree, make any argument or criticism out of earshot of the victim. If the examiner is opposite in gender to the victim, try to have a same-gender witness (chaperone).

1. Check the victim's mental status. If he is awake, determine if he is oriented to time, place, and person. ("What is the date? Where are you? Who are you?") If the answers are in any way abnormal, suspect a head injury, intoxication, stroke, central nervous system infection (such as meningitis), hyperthermia, hypothermia, severe altitude illness, low blood sugar, or hypoxia (insufficient oxygen to the brain). Maintain constant observation of the victim until all of his responses are appropriate.

2. Examine the neck. Without turning the victim's head, feel each cervical vertebra from behind and note tenderness or muscle spasm. The seventh vertebra will be the most prominent. Check for swelling. Feel the Adam's apple in the front of the neck for tenderness or a "crunching" sensation (noted by both the examiner and victim). If there is a chance of neck injury, immobilize the neck (see page 31).

3. Examine the spinal column. Run your fingers down the length of the spine to elicit any tenderness. Check for spinal cord injury by having the victim voluntarily move his arms and legs and report his sense of feeling. Ask the victim to squeeze your hand with each of his, and then to "press down on the gas pedal" with each foot against your hand. Pinch the skin on the back of the hand and top of the foot as a crude measure of sensation. If any response hand-to-hand or foot-to-foot is asymmetrical, suspect a spinal cord injury or stroke (see pages 31 and 129).

4. Examine the head—but try not to move it. Feel the entire scalp for raised areas or cuts. Look into the ears for drainage (clear [spinal] fluid, blood, or pus). Feel the nose for obvious malalignment or instability. Look up into the nostrils. If you have a flashlight, shine it into the eyes to see if the pupils constrict and are equal in size. If you don't have a flashlight, cover the eyes and then uncover them to see if the pupils constrict. Pinpoint (constricted) pupils may be a sign of brain injury or drug overdose. Unequal pupils may represent a direct injury to an eye or a brain injury. Nonreactive and bilaterally dilated pupils may represent a severe brain injury.

   Have the victim open and close his mouth to see if the teeth fit properly. Check the teeth for looseness or breaks, and the tongue for cuts. Ask the victim if he can swallow. Ask him to say "Ah" and see if you can get a glimpse of the back of his throat. Smell for any unusual odor on his breath.

5. Examine the skin. Look for sweating, skin color (normal may and pale does indicate inadequate circulation; dusky blue indicates hypothermia or shock; reddened indicates heat illness or sunburn; yellow indicates liver disease; mottled indicates low blood pressure, shock, or massive infection), bruises, rashes, burns, bites, and cuts. Note the skin temperature. Look inside the lower eyelids for a pale color that might indicate anemia or internal bleeding.

6. Examine the chest. Observe whether the chest expands fully and equally on both sides with breathing. Feel the chest wall for tenderness and inspect for deformation or embedded objects. Place your ear against each side of the chest to listen for breath sounds.

7. Examine the back and abdomen. Gently press in all areas to elicit tenderness. Examine the buttocks and genitals.

8. Examine all bones. Gently press on the chest, pelvis, arms, and legs to elicit any tenderness. Run your fingers down the length of the clavicles (collarbones) and press centrally where they join the sternum. Trace each rib with your fingers. Look for deformation or discoloration.

9. Take a temperature. Use a digital, mercury, or alcohol thermometer, if possible one that can detect hypothermia and/or hyperthermia, depending on the circumstance. Rectal temperature measurement is more reliable than oral or axillary (see page 151) measurement, but may be impractical in the field. Remember to shake down a mercury or oral thermometer, and to hold it in place for at least 3 minutes to obtain a reading.

Send for help early. As soon as you have determined that a situation will require extrication, rescue, and/or advanced life support, initiate your prearranged plan for communication and transportation. Don't assume that someone will call for help; you must assign this task to a specific individual.

If you are in a situation where you can access the emergency medical service (EMS) system (911 or other telephone number), be prepared to provide the following information: the victim's location, your phone number, the nature of the emergency, the number of people needing help, the condition of the victim(s), what is being done to treat the victim(s), and any specific environmental conditions or physical obstacles. Speak slowly and clearly, and don't hang up until the dispatcher tells you he has all the information he needs.

While you are waiting for help to arrive:

1. Take an adequate history. Listen carefully to the victim; in most cases, he will lead you to the affected organ system. Inquire about allergies (especially to medications), previous surgeries (for instance, if he has had his appendix out, he can't get appendicitis), previous illnesses, medications, and the current event.

2. Reassure the victim. Most disorders are not life threatening and will allow you plenty of time to formulate a treatment plan. Be sure to introduce yourself to the victim, and explain what you are doing in a direct fashion. Avoid making comments such as "Oh my God,"

"This is a hopeless situation," or "Whoops!" Let the victim know that you are capable and in charge. Accentuate the positive aspects of the situation, to build a climate of hope. Do not argue with other rescuers in the presence of the victim. Be particularly gentle, parental, and reassuring with children. Always warn the victim before you do anything that might cause him pain.

3. Keep the victim comfortable and warm. Do not feed a victim who cannot purposefully swallow. If he can eat and drink, offer water, clear soups, and clear juices. Use Oral Rehydration Salts (see page 185) or an electrolyte-containing sports beverage to maintain hydration. Avoid coffee, tea, and other caffeinated beverages.

4. Keep a written record of all medications given. If possible, also record symptoms and objective measurements (such as temperature) with times noted.

5. Remove all constrictive clothing or jewelry from any injured areas. If the victim has a hand wound, all watches and rings (see page 423) should be removed before swelling makes doing so impossible. In particular, rings left in place can become inadvertent tourniquets on swollen fingers.

Always remember to reexamine and reevaluate a victim at regular intervals. A person may not experience difficulties until after a time delay, particularly if the problem is related to a head injury or internal bleeding. If you are concerned enough about a person to examine him once, wait a while and then examine him again. The interval between examinations is determined by your level of concern. For instance, someone with possible internal bleeding (see page 53) should be examined every 10 to 15 minutes until you are confident that the severity of the situation has declined sufficiently to warrant less vigilance. *If someone has an altered mental status (particularly after a head injury), he requires your constant attention.*

MEDICAL DECISION MAKING

The art of outdoor medicine absolutely depends upon observation, anticipation, and resourcefulness. The cardinal rule is to act conservatively and not take unnecessary risks when making the decision to continue a journey or to postpone travel and seek formal medical attention. Similarly, you may need to decide whether to carry out a disabled victim, or to stay put and signal or send for help.

Although every situation is unique, all decisions begin with an accurate assessment of the victim's condition. The situation should be categorized as trivial (small cuts, insect sting without allergic reaction, a single episode of diarrhea); minor (sprained ankle, small burn wound, sore throat); moderately disabling (broken wrist, kidney stone, bronchitis); potentially severe (chest pain, severe abdominal pain, high fever); totally disabling (seizure, broken hip, severe high-altitude illness); or life and limb threatening (uncontrolled bleeding, extensive frostbite, venomous snakebite with symptoms). In all cases that are other than trivial or minor, it is proper to insist upon prompt evacuation or rescue for thorough evaluation. Never overestimate your abilities as a healer or count on good fortune. *The assumption under which you must operate is that a victim's clinical condition will deteriorate, particularly in a harsh environmental setting.* No adventure is worth a lost life or permanent disablement.

If more than one victim is injured, you must set priorities and attend to the most critically injured. Continually evaluate each victim to detect improvement or deterioration over time. Do not focus on situations that are beyond reasonable hope. For example, if a victim is near death from severe burns, decide if there is really anything you can do to save him, and if not, get busy with the people you can help. These are emotionally charged and extremely difficult decisions, even for those of us who have made them for years.

You may have to decide whether to evacuate a victim or wait for a rescue party. In some instances, this is an easy decision—when a victim must be carried to a lower altitude to treat severe mountain sickness, for instance, or when the transport route is short and easily negotiated. The judgment call is based on weather conditions, the nature and severity of the injury or illness, and the distance that needs to be covered.

PART TWO

Major Medical Problems

This section describes common disorders that may be life threatening. The problems are often present in combination and require prompt recognition and management.

AN APPROACH TO THE UNCONSCIOUS VICTIM

Any disorder that decreases the supply of oxygen or sugar to the brain or that causes brain swelling, bleeding into the brain, or alteration of critical body chemistries can lead to unconsciousness. Thus, virtually every major illness or injury can ultimately render a person unconscious. If you come upon someone who cannot be awakened, you must rapidly assess him for any treatable life-threatening conditions, then try to discover the cause of the altered mental state.

The victim should not be moved until you carefully perform the following examination in sequence. *Until you are absolutely certain that the victim does not have a neck injury, do not attempt to arouse him by vigorous shaking methods.*

1. Evaluate the airway (see below).
2. Evaluate breathing (see page 23).
3. Check for pulses (see page 26).
4. Protect the cervical spine (see page 31).
5. Control obvious bleeding (see page 48).
6. Examine the victim for chest injury (see page 35), broken bones (see page 61), and burns (see page 98).
7. Consider shock (see page 54), head injury (see page 55), seizure (see page 59), low blood sugar (see page 128), stroke (see page 129), fainting spell (see page 150), hypothermia (see page 269), heat illness (see page 281), high-altitude cerebral edema (see page 296), high-altitude pulmonary edema (see page 294), lightning strike (see page 350), poisoning, and alcohol (drug) intoxication.
8. Remove contact lenses (see page 165).
9. Transport the victim to medical attention (see page 405).

Airway

Airway obstruction is one of the leading causes of death in victims of head injury, and a frequent complication of vomiting in an unconscious person. Adequacy of the airway and breathing must be attained rapidly in every victim. In the absence of hypothermia, an interval of 4 minutes in which there is a failure to oxygenate the brain can lead to irreversible damage.

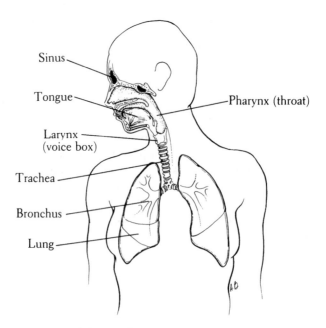

Figure 1. Anatomy of the respiratory system.

Figure 1 depicts the anatomy of the respiratory system. Air enters the mouth and nose (where it is humidified), traverses the pharynx (throat), passes through the trachea (windpipe) and bronchi, and normally proceeds into the smallest air sacs of the lungs, known as the alveoli. Within these distal air spaces, inspired oxygen is exchanged for carbon dioxide, one of the end products of human metabolism. During swallowing, the epiglottis and tongue cover the entrance (via the vocal cords) to the trachea, so that food and liquid enter the esophagus and not the airway.

Obstruction of the airway at any level can interfere with the passage of air, delivery of oxygen via the lungs to the blood, and exhalation of carbon dioxide. The mouth and pharynx may fill with blood, vomitus, or secretions. With facial injury, deformation of the jaw or nose may hinder breathing. In a supine (faceup) unconscious victim, the tongue may fall back into the pharynx and occlude the opening to the trachea. Inhalation of food can obstruct the opening between the vocal cords and cause rapid suffocation.

Symptoms of airway obstruction include sudden inability to speak, an appearance of panic with bulging eyes, blue skin discoloration (cyanosis),

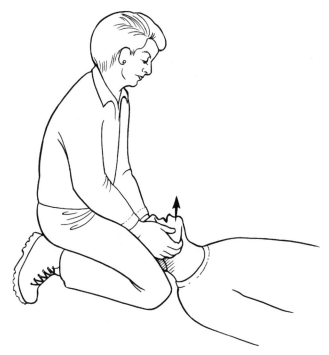

Figure 2. Jaw pull to open the airway.

choking gestures (hand held to the throat) (see figure 6), harsh and raspy or "musical" and high-pitched noise that comes from the throat during breathing (stridor), and difficulty with breathing as evidenced by struggling and profound agitation. Any person who collapses suddenly, particularly while eating, or who has been in an accident should be examined rapidly for airway obstruction.

1. *Under no circumstance should the neck be manipulated if there is a possibility of injury to the spine or spinal cord.* If a victim is unconscious and has suffered a fall or multiple injuries, it is safest to assume that his neck is broken. If this is the case, keep the airway open by gently but firmly lifting his jaw, either by grasping the lower teeth and jaw and pulling directly forward (away from the face), or by maintaining a forward pull on the angles of the jaw (figure 2). Do not bend the neck forward or backward. A modified jaw thrust (see figure 3) can be performed by a single rescuer while stabilizing the neck.

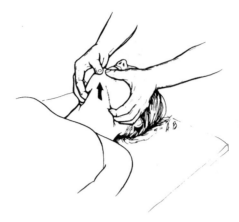

Figure 3. Jaw thrust to open the airway. Grasping the angles of the lower jaw firmly, the rescuer pulls forward to lift the tongue out of the throat.

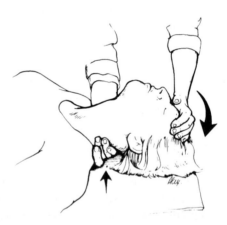

Figure 4. Positioning the head to control the airway. The forehead is gently pushed back while support is maintained under the neck. *Never* manipulate the head or neck if a broken neck is suspected.

2. *If there is no chance of a broken neck,* maintain the airway with the jaw lifts previously described or by tilting the head backward while gently lifting under the neck (figure 4).
3. Keep the airway clear of blood, vomitus, loose dentures, and debris. This can be accomplished by sweeping the mouth with two fingers or by continuous suction with a field suction apparatus powerful enough to extract chunks. Take care not to force objects deeper into the throat. If the tongue appears to be the problem, wrap the end of the

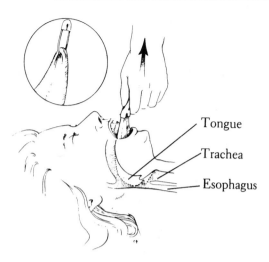

Figure 5. Manual tongue traction. With a cloth or safety pin (inset) to secure the grip, the tongue is lifted out of the mouth to clear the airway.

tongue in a cloth or gauze bandage, grasp firmly, and pull it out of the mouth (figure 5). If it cannot be held in this manner, a large safety pin or sharp-pointed wire may be passed through the tongue and used to improve the grip (figure 5); take care to avoid the large, visible blood vessels at the base of the tongue. To keep the tongue out of the mouth, a string can be tied to the safety pin and then secured to the victim's shirt button or jacket zipper. Fortunately, in most cases the jaw lift will carry the base of the tongue out of the airway.

4. If the victim is unconscious, and there is no chance of a broken neck or back, do not leave him lying flat on his back. Turn him on his side so that if vomiting occurs, the fluid can drain from his mouth and the victim won't choke or drown.

5. Choking is a life-threatening condition in which the upper airway (above the vocal cords) is obstructed by a foreign object (tongue, broken teeth, dentures, food). The choking person is profoundly agitated (until he becomes unconscious from lack of oxygen), may appear to be panicked with bulging eyes, may grasp at his throat in a choking gesture, cannot breathe, and is unable to speak. You must respond rapidly:

Sweep the mouth with one or two fingers to remove any foreign material. Take care not to force material farther into the throat. Quickly extract loose dentures.

Using an open hand, give the victim two to four rapid, sharp blows

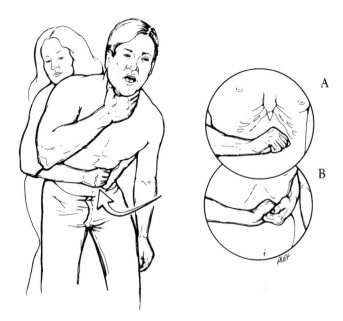

Figure 6. The Heimlich maneuver. (A) A hand is placed on the upper abdomen. (B) The second hand interlocks to create a tight grip. A sudden, forceful squeeze ("bear hug") causes the victim to cough.

on the back between the shoulder blades. This may be more effective if the victim is lying on his side or is bent forward at the waist. If a small child is choking, perform this maneuver while holding him facedown or upside down. If the victim is an infant, place him facedown on one of your forearms, with his head lower than his body. Support his head. Give five quick back blows, then turn the infant over and give five quick chest thrusts (similar to those given during CPR—see page 28).

Perform the Heimlich maneuver (figure 6). Position yourself behind the victim and encircle him with your arms, clasping your hands in a fist in the upper abdomen just below his ribs. Squeeze the victim suddenly and firmly ("bear hug") two or three times, in an attempt to produce a brisk exhalation (cough) and ejection of the foreign (choking) material. If your first attempt is unsuccessful, alternate back blows with the Heimlich maneuver. If you are the victim and no one is present to help during a choking episode, you can throw yourself against a log or table edge in an attempt to perform a self Heimlich maneuver.

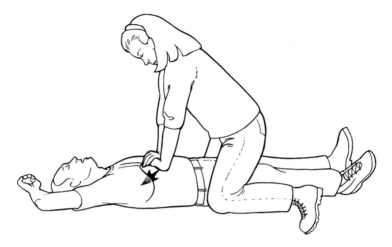

Figure 7. Heimlich maneuver with the victim lying down.

If the victim is lying on his back (supine), perform the Heimlich maneuver by sitting astride his thighs, facing his head (figure 7). Place the heel of one hand on his upper abdomen and cover it with your other hand. Press into the abdomen suddenly and firmly in a direction toward the chest. Do this a few times, then perform the chin lift (see step 1 on page 19) and sweep a finger deeply through the mouth to extract any foreign material forced up by your efforts. Take care not to push anything back into the throat.

For a child older than 1 year of age, keep him supine (because the child is too large to hold facedown or upside down) and place the heel of your hand well below his breastbone but above his navel.

If the victim is obese or pregnant, apply the force (with the victim sitting or lying down) to the center of the chest (breastbone), rather than the abdomen.

6. If necessary, begin mouth-to-mouth breathing (see page 24).

Breathing

The act of breathing delivers oxygen to the lungs during inhalation, exchanges oxygen for carbon dioxide in the lungs, transfers oxygen into the bloodstream, and removes carbon dioxide during exhalation. The rate and depth of breathing are controlled by the oxygen and carbon dioxide levels in the blood, by the body's oxygen demand, by the ability of the blood to unload oxygen to the tissues, by brain and brain stem regulatory sensory systems, and by emotional factors. If there is a head or spinal cord injury, however, the central nervous system stimulus for breathing may be lost. In many instances, this is only transient (lightning strike is a good example); thus, it is imperative to provide breathing assistance for a period of time before giving up hope. Exhaled air from a human contains 16% oxygen, which is enough to support life (via mouth-to-mouth or mouth-to-mask breathing) at low altitudes.

A direct chest injury (broken ribs, fractured breastbone, bruised or collapsed lung) may render respirations inadequate because of pain or mechanical dysfunction. The accumulation of fluid in the lungs because of inhalation (such as in a drowning or burn injury), heart failure, or constriction of the smaller branches of the airway (in asthma or an allergic reaction) may make the work of breathing overwhelming for the victim.

How to Assist Breathing (Mouth-to-Mouth)

1. Position the victim's head in the "sniffing position" by placing one hand under his neck and the other on his forehead, to lift behind the neck (gently) and tilt the head backward (see figure 4). If you suspect a broken neck, do not move the victim's neck; merely lift his jaw (see figure 3).

2. Quickly sweep two fingers through the victim's mouth to remove any foreign material. Remove loose dentures.

3. Pinch the victim's mouth closed and cover his mouth with your own (figure 8). If you have a barrier (pocket mask or mouth shield) to prevent transmission of infectious diseases, use it as directed. If you are using the jaw lift technique (see step 1 on page 19) to open the airway, press your cheek against the victim's nose to occlude it during mouth-to-mouth breathing. For mouth-to-nose breathing, close the victim's mouth and cover his nose with your mouth. For small children and infants, cover both the mouth and nose with your mouth (figure 9).

4. Blow air (for about 2 seconds) into the adult victim until you see his chest rise. Give two full breaths, pausing between them to inhale and see if the chest rises. With small children and infants, do not blow forcefully. If the chest does not rise, be certain the airway is open (proper head position, tongue and mouth clear—see pages 19–20). If the positioning is correct and the chest still does not rise, consider an airway obstruction with a foreign body (see page 21). After blowing the first two breaths into the victim, check for a pulse for 5 to 10 seconds (see page 26). If none is present, prepare to administer the chest compressions of CPR (see page 28).

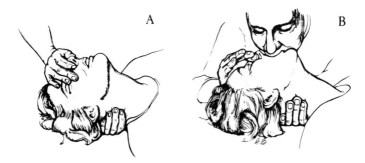

Figure 8. Mouth-to-mouth breathing. (A) While the neck is supported with one hand, the nose is pinched closed. (B) The rescuer covers the victim's mouth with his own and forces air into the victim until the chest rises.

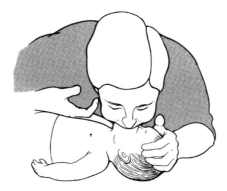

Figure 9. Mouth-to-mouth-and-nose breathing required to resuscitate a child.

5. Remove your mouth and allow the victim to exhale passively. Repeat the cycle every 5 seconds for adults, and every 3 seconds for children.

6. If you meet resistance trying to blow air into the victim's lungs, check the head positioning and reclear the mouth. You may need to lift the jaw in order to pull the base of the tongue up and out of the throat.

7. If it is impossible to blow any air into the victim's lungs, it might be that something is lodged in his airway. Turn the victim on his side and deliver four sharp blows between the shoulder blades, or perform the Heimlich maneuver (see page 22).

8. Mouth-to-mouth breathing usually forces air into the victim's stomach as well as into his lungs. If the stomach fills up with so much air that it

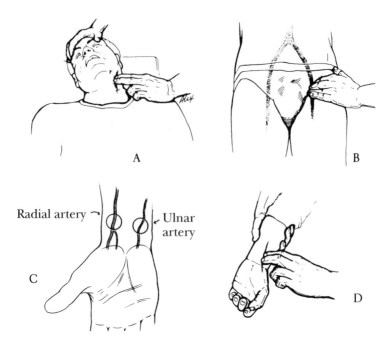

Figure 10. Location of the pulses. (A) Carotid artery in the neck. (B) Femoral artery in the groin. (C) Radial and ulnar arteries in the wrist. (D) Taking a radial artery pulse.

becomes tense and you cannot expand the lungs, turn the victim quickly on his side and press on the abdomen. This may make him vomit, so be prepared to clean out the mouth.

Check for Pulses (Circulation)

Assess the need for cardiopulmonary resuscitation (CPR). Check for pulses for 10 seconds at the neck (carotid artery: figure 10A) or groin (femoral artery: figure 10B). Use the tips of your index and middle fingers to feel for a pulse. Do not use your thumb, because this finger often has pulsations of its own, which you may confuse with the victim's pulse.

Do not rely upon the wrist (radial or ulnar artery: figures 10C and 10D) for the determination of heartbeat. The carotid artery is located (figure 10A) at the level of the Adam's apple, between this structure and the large muscle (sternocleidomastoid) that runs from the base of the ear to the collarbone. Pulsations from the femoral artery may be felt (figure

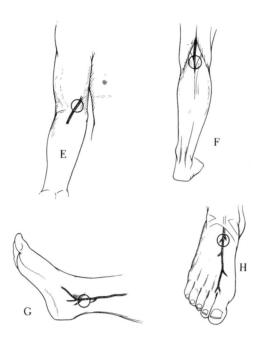

Figure 10. (CONT.) (E) Brachial artery in the arm. (F) Popliteal artery behind the knee. (G) Posterior tibial artery on the inner aspect of the ankle. (H) Dorsalis pedis artery on the top of the foot.

10B) below the abdomen in the groin crease where the front of the leg attaches to the trunk, two finger breadths medial (toward the center) to the midpoint in the line from the hipbone (anterior iliac spine) to the bony region directly under the pubic hair (the pubic symphysis). Other locations where the pulse may be felt (often with great difficulty) are on the inner aspect of the elbow (brachial artery: figure 10E); behind the knee (popliteal artery: figure 10F); directly behind the bony prominence (malleolus) on the inner side of the ankle (posterior tibial artery: figure 10G); and centrally on the top of the foot (dorsalis pedis artery: figure 10H).

A normal resting pulse rate is 55 to 90 per minute for adults, 80 to 110 per minute for small children, and 100 to 130 per minute for infants. A well-conditioned athlete will often have a resting pulse rate of 45 to 50 per minute, because the well-developed vagus nerve's impulses dominate. Failure to feel a pulse means that the heart is not beating (cardiac arrest), the pump (heart) is not squeezing with sufficient force (profound shock or hypothermia), the artery is constricted (hypothermia), there is an injury to

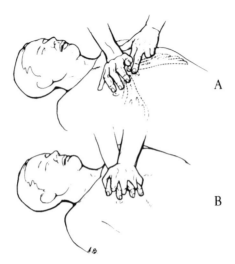

Figure 11. Positioning the hands for CPR (cardiopulmonary resuscitation). (A) The heel of the first hand is placed two finger breadths above the bottom edge of the breastbone. (B) The second hand is placed over the first and the fingers are interlocked.

the artery (from a fracture or severe cut), or you are feeling in the wrong place.

If no pulse is detected (and the victim is unconscious and not breathing), send someone for help, give two breaths to the victim (see page 24), and begin the chest compressions of cardiopulmonary resuscitation (CPR).

Chest compressions are performed as follows:

1. Place the victim on his back on a firm surface and position the heel of one of your hands over the center of his breastbone (figure 11A). The heel of your second hand is placed over the bottom hand. Interlock your fingers (figure 11B) and keep them held lightly off the victim's chest.

2. Your shoulders should line up directly over the victim's breastbone, with your arms straightened at the elbows (figure 12).

3. Using a stiff-arm technique, the breastbone is compressed 1½ to 2" (3.8 to 5 cm) and then released (figure 13). Keep your motions smooth. The compression phase should equal the relaxation phase, with a rate of 60 to 80 compressions per minute. Give an initial 15 compressions. With single-rescuer CPR, try to maintain a ratio of 15 compressions interrupted by two mouth-to-mouth breaths (see page 24). After the first four cycles of compressions and breaths, check for pulses and

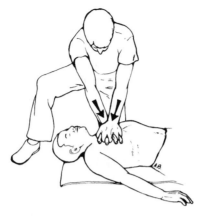

Figure 12. Proper arm and body position for CPR. The rescuer compresses the victim's chest by keeping the arms straight and dropping his upper-body weight directly over the victim.

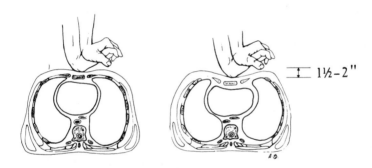

Figure 13. Compression of the chest during CPR. With proper technique, the adult breastbone should be compressed 1½ to 2", with 50 to 60 compressions per minute.

spontaneous breathing. If both are absent, resume your efforts, checking for signs of life every few minutes.

4. If two rescuers are working together, the second rescuer should give the victim mouth-to-mouth resuscitation, forcing a breath into him with every five chest compressions. The artificial breath does not have to be positioned precisely between compressions.

5. Continue CPR until you are relieved by someone, you become exhausted, the victim is revived, or a qualified person pronounces the victim dead. Situations in which CPR is unlikely to revive a victim include cardiac arrest associated with severe injuries, drowning in which the victim has been submerged for more than an hour (with the rare exception of cold-water immersion—see page 274), the victim having an incompressible chest (extreme cold or prolonged "downtime" with rigor mortis—see below), and after 30 minutes of resuscitation effort without any victim response (breathing or pulse).

Chest compressions in infants and small children can be performed by placing a stabilizing hand on the child's back and compressing hand (or fingers) on the chest (figure 14). With a small child, use one hand to perform the compressions. With an infant, use two fingers. Care should be taken to provide firm compressions without separating the ribs from the breastbone. The rate of chest compressions for a child is 80 to 100 per minute at a depth of 1 to 1½" (2.5 to 3.8 cm), with a breath after each five compressions. For an infant, the rate of compressions is 100 per minute at a depth of ½ to 1" (1.3 to 2.5 cm), with a breath after each five compressions.

Continue to administer rescue breathing and chest compressions until help arrives or you become too tired to continue. Miraculous survivals have been reported in victims of prolonged cardiac arrest from cold-water submersion or lightning strike. During a resuscitation, the rescuer(s) should check every few minutes for return of a pulse or spontaneous breathing.

The Condition of Death

CPR in a wilderness setting is rarely successful. Unfortunately, your best efforts at resuscitation may be to no avail and the victim will die. Signs of death include no movement or response to pain; no detectable pulse; absent breathing; dilated (and often irregularly shaped) pupils that do not contract when exposed to bright light; pale or blue-gray skin, fingernails, and lips; penile erection; uncontrolled urination or bowel movement; and cool body temperature. After a period of an hour or two, the muscles become stiff (rigor mortis), the skin mottles, and blood settles visibly in a dependent fashion due to gravity, causing large discolored blotches on the victim's back, buttocks, and legs (if he is kept supine). *However, it is essential to remember that hypothermic individuals, who are extremely cold, may appear to be dead* (see page 269). Therefore, if hypothermia is suspected, "no one is dead until he is warm and dead." In such a case, resuscitative efforts should be carried out until the victim is revived, the rescuers become exhausted or endangered, or a health care professional can pronounce

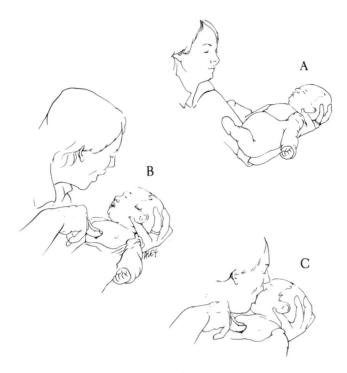

Figure 14. Infant CPR. (A) Positioning the infant on the forearm. (B) With the forearm for a back support, two fingers of the opposite hand are used to compress the breastbone. (C) The mouth and nose of the infant are covered by the rescuer's mouth for artificial breathing.

death. This is also true for a victim of lightning strike or cold-water drowning, and for children. If a victim is dead, the body should be decently covered and kept in a cool location until extrication is possible. If foul play is suspected, the body should not be moved.

Protect the Cervical Spine

If a victim has fallen, is unconscious, and/or has a face or head injury, he may have a fracture of the cervical spine (neck). *Never move the neck to reposition it.* You must immediately immobilize the head and neck. The neck can be immobilized by taping the head to a backboard or stretcher, by applying a rigid collar, or by placing sandbags or their equivalent on either side of the head (see figure 15). Do not use bags of snow to hold the head,

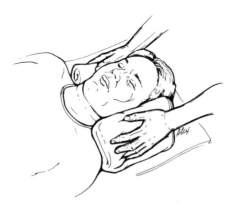

Figure 15. Immobilization of the neck using rolled towels. The rescuer's hands may be replaced with a strap or tape across the forehead to prevent movement.

because these may melt and allow too much motion; they can also contribute to hypothermia (see page 269).

In general, the most dangerous direction of motion for a neck- (spinal cord–) injured person is chin to chest (flexed). Circumferential neck collars that prevent flexion can be purchased preformed or be fashioned from cardboard, Ensolite sleeping pad material, foam-covered aluminum (the SAM Splint) (figure 16), a padded backpack hip belt, or other semirigid materials. Remember, for a neck collar to be effective, it must be rigid or semirigid, fit properly, not choke the victim, and allow the victim's mouth to open if he needs to vomit.

If no other equipment is available and if the victim is conscious and cooperative, a thick pad (rolled towel, jacket, or the like) may be placed at the base of his neck. This can be made more rigid by first wrapping (compressing) it with a wide elastic (Ace) bandage. Secure this by wrapping tape or cloth around the forehead, then crossing it over the pad and bringing it back out under the armpits to be tied across the chest (figure 17). Remember, this technique does not guarantee immobilization in a combative or confused victim.

In proportion to the torso, the head of a young child is larger than is the head of an adult. Therefore, when a child is flat on his back, his neck may be flexed instead of in a "neutral" position. To overcome this effect, tilt the head back slightly, or place a blanket or pad under the child's torso.

If the victim becomes uncooperative or agitated, you must hold his head until it can be firmly immobilized and the victim restrained from motion (see figures 15

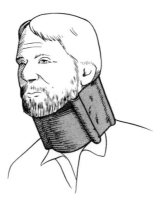

Figure 16. Cervical collar fashioned from a SAM Splint. The malleable foam-covered aluminum allows construction of rigid pillars.

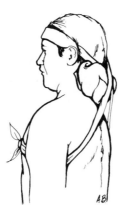

Figure 17. Immobilization of the neck. A rolled towel or shirt is secured behind the neck with a firmly wrapped cravat or cloth. This technique should be used solely for an alert and cooperative victim. It provides only enough support to remind the victim to not move his head and neck.

and 18). All of this is necessary to avoid injury to the spinal cord. If the victim must be moved or turned on his side (most commonly to allow vomiting or to place insulation beneath him), hold his head fixed between your forearms while you hold his shoulders with your hands. In this way the victim can be "logrolled," using as many rescuers as possible to avoid unnecessary motion.

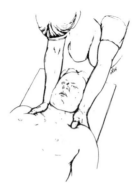

Figure 18. Immobilization of the neck. The rescuer grasps the victim's shoulders and controls the head between his forearms.

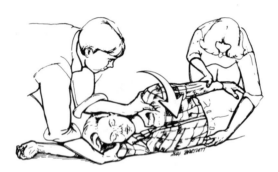

Figure 19. Logrolling the victim. The rescuer at the head immobilizes the neck with his forearms and the victim's extended arm, while an assistant helps turn the body.

Logrolling the Victim (Figure 19)

The best way to carry and immobilize a person who may have an injured spine is to use a scoop stretcher, or to slide a backboard underneath the victim. However, when these are not available and a spine-injured person must be turned, logrolling is the best alternative.

1. The first rescuer approaches the victim from the head, and keeps the head and shoulders in a fixed position (no neck movement).
2. The second rescuer extends the victim's arm (on the side over which

the victim is to be rolled) above the victim's head. The first rescuer takes this arm and uses it to help support the head in proper position.

3. All rescuers work together to roll the victim without moving his neck.

Lifting a Victim

See page 406.

CHEST INJURY

Broken Ribs

Direct force applied to the chest wall can break the ribs, causing extreme pain with breathing and/or collapse of a lung (pneumothorax). If the right lower ribs are broken, be alert to the possibility of a bruised or cracked liver, which lies directly below; if the left lower ribs are broken, the underlying spleen may be injured.

Flail Chest

If a number of ribs are broken or detached in series, so that the affected section of the chest wall cannot expand and contract in synchrony with the rest of the chest, then a flail chest (see figure 20) is present. Depending on the size of the flail segment, this can cause severe respiratory compromise. Occasionally, the flail segment moves with breathing in a direction opposite to the rest of the chest wall.

Pneumothorax

A pneumothorax is a collapsed lung created when there is an air leak (from the lung or from a penetrating wound of the chest wall) into the space between the lung and the inside of the chest wall (pleural space). In the normal situation, the pleural space is undetectable and filled with negative pressure, which allows the lung to expand and contract with chest wall movement (breathing). When air leaks into the pleural space, either from a lung injury or from a hole in the chest wall, the lung collapses. The lung may then be increasingly compressed if air accumulates in the pleural

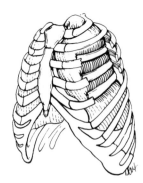

Figure 20. Flail chest. A section of detached (broken) ribs may seriously impede the mechanics of breathing.

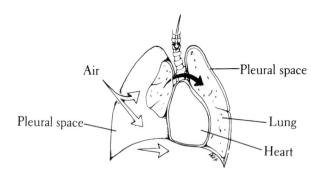

Figure 21. Pneumothorax. Air enters the pleural space lining the lung through the chest wall or from a lung leak, which causes the lung to collapse. A tension pneumothorax occurs when air in the pleural space accumulates under pressure, forcing the lung, heart, and trachea to the opposite side (dark arrow).

space under pressure (figure 21). A collapsed lung is recognized by diminished or absent breath sounds (heard through a stethoscope or an ear held against the chest wall) on the affected side, accompanied by chest pain, shortness of breath, and difficult breathing. If air accumulates under pressure in the affected pleural space, this becomes a "tension" pneumothorax. It is characterized by rapidly progressive difficulty in breathing associated with a pneumothorax, cyanosis (blue skin discoloration), distended neck (jugular) veins, and a shift of the windpipe away from the affected side.

Rarely, air that escapes from the lung to create a pneumothorax can become trapped under the skin, creating a "crackling" sensation when the skin is pressed, a sensation of fullness or visible swelling in the neck, a change in voice, and difficulty swallowing. While worrisome in appearance, this subcutaneous (under the skin) air absorbs over time and is not nearly as dangerous as a collapsed lung.

Bruised Lung

A bruised lung can result whenever sufficient force is applied to the chest wall. This injury typically causes increased difficulty with breathing after a delay of minutes to hours, as blood and tissue fluid accumulate in the injured lung. In a severe case, the victim will cough up clots of blood.

Treatment for Chest Injuries

1. Attend to any chest wounds. All open wounds (particularly those in which air is bubbling) should be rapidly covered, to avoid "sucking" chest wounds that could allow more air to enter the pleural space and thus continue to worsen a collapsed lung (see page 35). For a dressing, a Vaseline-impregnated gauze, heavy cloth, or adhesive tape (see figure 22) can be used. The dressing should be sealed to the chest on at least three sides. If the victim develops a tension pneumothorax following a penetrating wound to the chest and his condition deteriorates rapidly (difficulty breathing, cyanosis, distended neck veins, collapse followed by unconsciousness), force a finger through the wound into the chest to allow the air under pressure to escape. If your diagnosis is correct, you will hear a hissing noise as the air rushes out. This allows the lung to partially expand and may save the victim's life. After the release of air from a tension pneumothorax, cover the wound with a dressing and seal only three sides to create a flutter-valve effect (air can exit, but not enter) and prevent a recurrence—which might come with a complete seal.

2. Administer oxygen (see page 383). If an oxygen tank is available, oxygen should be administered at a rate of 5 liters per minute by face mask or nasal prongs. Elderly victims who have been heavy cigarette smokers (COPD: see page 42) should be watched carefully for signs of decreasing consciousness whenever oxygen is administered. If this occurs (in the absence of head trauma or shock), supplemental oxygen should be discontinued.

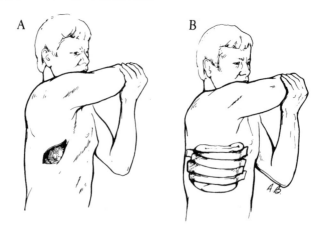

Figure 22. Chest wound dressing. (A) Open chest wound. (B) The dressing is held firmly in place with tape or a cloth wrap.

3. Assess the rate and adequacy of breathing. Watch for chest rise, feel and listen to the chest, place a hand near the nose and mouth to check for air movement, and observe skin color. If necessary, assist breathing. This may be done with mouth-to-mouth breathing (see page 24) or with a mask device. *If the victim is not breathing, check for pulses and assess the need for cardiopulmonary resuscitation* (CPR) (see page 28).

4. Anyone who has a significant flail chest will be unable to coordinate the muscular act of breathing and will need early assistance. The flail segment should be cushioned firmly with pillows, sandbags, or their equivalent (figure 23). This prevents movement (pain) and eases the act of breathing. If the victim is lying down, turn him onto the side with the flail segment. This stabilizes the injury and allows the good (upside) lung to more fully expand. Use padding underneath the victim to control pain.

5. Broken ribs are best managed with cushioning in a position of comfort and frequent reevaluation of the ability to breathe. Do not tape or tightly wrap the ribs, because this might prevent complete reexpansion of the chest (lung) with inspiration and therefore predispose the victim to shallow, inadequate breathing and subsequent pneumonia. Encourage the victim to take at least one deep breath or give one good cough each hour.

6. Evacuate the victim as soon as possible. If the chest is injured on one side, transport the victim on his side with the injured side down. This

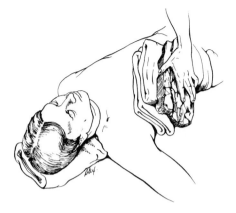

Figure 23. Method of cushioning a flail chest wall segment by applying firm pressure with a blanket and section of tree bark.

facilitates better expansion of the good (upside) lung and more complete oxygenation of the blood.

SERIOUS LUNG DISORDERS

Asthma

Asthma is a disease of the lungs that involves episodes of coughing, shortness of breath, wheezing, and increased secretions in the bronchi. Generally, most people will know that they are prone to asthma attacks; however, a first-time episode may occur during an allergic reaction, upon exertion or exposure to cold, or as a result of emotional stress. In most cases, the mechanism is the same: narrowing and spasm of the small airways, with increased mucus production.

The victim has difficulty breathing and wheezing on exhalation (most common) and/or with inspiration. Coughing is a major feature. The victim may become quite anxious ("air hunger"). Severe cases lead to rapid respiratory deterioration, cyanosis (blue discoloration of the skin), and the use of accessory muscles of respiration (the victim sits upright and attempts to expand the chest wall by contracting neck muscles and using body movements). When the attack is extreme, wheezing may diminish, because the lungs become so "tight" that there is not enough air movement to create the abnormal breath sounds.

Treatment for Severe Asthma

1. Administer oxygen (see page 383) by face mask at a rate of 10 liters per minute. If cold weather precipitated the attack, try to get the victim into a warmer climate.

2. Administer an inhaled (aerosol or "micronized") bronchodilator. Bronchodilators (airway openers) are drugs that carry the advantages of minimal side effects and direct delivery to the site of action. They are available in metered-dose handheld nebulizers ("mistometers") from which the victim inhales therapeutic puffs. An excellent drug for an acute attack is albuterol (Ventolin). The dose for an adult is two to four puffs initially, followed by two puffs every 3 to 6 hours. A mild to moderate asthma episode in an adult can frequently be controlled with an inhaled bronchodilator alone. Young children have difficulty using the inhaler, and therefore may require administration of the drug orally in pill or liquid form. The most effective technique for metered-dose inhalation appears to be discharging the aerosol through a spacer clamped between the lips. The drug should be released (canister pressed down or "triggered") at the beginning of a deep inspiration. After inhalation, the recipient should attempt to hold his breath for 10 seconds.

3. Administer epinephrine if the victim remains in severe distress after inhalation of a bronchodilator. Epinephrine is a powerful bronchodilator that is injected subcutaneously (see page 419) as an aqueous solution of 1:1,000 concentration in a dose of 0.3 to 0.5 ml for an adult and 0.01 ml per kg of body weight for a child (not to exceed 0.3 ml). For weight estimation, 1 kg equals 2.2 lb. The drug is not recommended for those known to have coronary artery heart disease (angina or recent heart attack) or older than 45 years. Epinephrine is the treatment of choice for a severe asthma attack in a child. When administering an injection, *never* share needles between people.

4. Administer a corticosteroid. A victim who has required steroids in the past in order to manage acute asthma attacks should be dosed with prednisone tablets at the earliest possible opportunity, because the onset of their action is delayed by 4 to 6 hours. The dose for an adult is 50 to 80 mg, tapered over 10 days (for example, give 80 mg on days 1 and 2; 60 mg on days 3 and 4; 40 mg on days 5 and 6;

20 mg on days 7 and 8; 10 mg on days 9 and 10). The initial dose for a child is 1 mg per kg (2.2 lb) of body weight, also tapered over 10 days. If a person with asthma improves greatly after using epinephrine and/or an inhaled bronchodilator, steroid administration is not necessary.

5. A person with asthma who is in more than minimal distress or who does not achieve great improvement with these basic pharmacological maneuvers should be transported rapidly to the nearest medical facility. Great care should be taken to keep him well supplied with oxygen and as exertion-free as possible.

Pulmonary Embolism

A pulmonary embolus is a blood clot that has traveled from a vein somewhere in the body to lodge in the circulation of a lung. Such a clot obstructs the flow of blood through a portion of the lung and prevents the normal transfer of oxygen to blood by the affected lung tissue.

The most common sources of the original blood clots are the veins of the pelvis or legs ("thrombophlebitis": inflammation of the veins with blood clots). Predisposing factors to thrombophlebitis include dehydration, underlying disease of the veins (such as varicose veins), injuries, cancer, medications (such as birth control pills), injury, and prolonged immobility (see page 257).

Symptoms of pulmonary embolism include sudden sharp chest pain (occasionally worse with deep breathing), cough (occasionally with blood), shortness of breath, increased rate of breathing, and increased heart rate. The victim may develop a fever. It is often difficult to distinguish pulmonary embolism from pneumonia (see page 43). If the clot is very large, the victim may collapse and die rapidly.

If a person develops symptoms that may represent pulmonary embolism, he should be rushed to medical attention. If oxygen (see page 383) is available, it should be administered by face mask at a flow rate of 10 liters per minute. If the victim can swallow purposefully, administer an aspirin tablet (325 mg) every 24 hours.

Heart Failure

Failure of the heart muscle to pump blood effectively may occur suddenly (usually with a large heart attack) or start gradually and worsen with time (after a heart attack; with infections of the heart muscle; from prolonged cocaine, anabolic steroid, or alcohol abuse; from chronic anemia; and so on). The symptoms include shortness of breath (particularly with exertion), swollen feet and ankles (fluid retention), bubbling noises in the lungs (fluid in the lungs), cough, wheezing, and blue skin discoloration (cyanosis) noted under the fingernails, around the lips, and at the earlobes. Frequently, a victim of heart failure cannot lie flat to sleep (because fluid collects in the lungs), so he wakes up at night suddenly short of breath.

If a victim with known heart failure suddenly worsens, or if a previously healthy individual develops signs of heart failure (which may represent a new heart attack), he should be kept sitting up, unless he is more comfortable lying on his back. Administer oxygen (see page 383) by face mask at a flow rate of 10 liters per minute, and immediately carry him to medical attention. If the victim must travel under his own power, all exertion should be kept to a minimum.

If traveling at high altitude, suspect high-altitude pulmonary edema (see page 294).

Chronic Obstructive Pulmonary Disease (COPD)

COPD refers to a number of diseases suffered by people who have exposed their lungs to long-term insults, particularly cigarette smoke. Chronic bronchitis (infection, inflammation, and/or bronchospasm—see page 181) or emphysema (scarring that leads to lack of elasticity, overinflation, and/or lung collapse) are the most common subsets of COPD. People with COPD have poor respiratory reserves, and cannot tolerate strenuous exercise or extremes of environment. A victim of COPD suffers attacks of shortness of breath and coughing similar to asthma, but can get into serious trouble much faster because of underlying debilitation. The earliest signs of respiratory fatigue should be heeded, and evacuation to a restful situation and physician evaluation are high priorities.

With the exception of epinephrine, you may treat a victim of COPD with the same drugs used for the management of asthma. However, administration of high-flow oxygen (greater than 1.5 to 2 liters per minute by nasal cannula, or tube) carries a risk, because correction of the low blood oxygen level (hypoxia) in some individuals with COPD will cause them to stop breathing. This is because they have lost sensitivity to high carbon dioxide levels in the blood as a stimulus for breathing (COPD victims always have a relatively high level of carbon dioxide in the blood), and administration of oxygen removes the remaining stimulus (hypoxia) for breathing. Therefore, any person with COPD who is given oxygen should be watched continuously. If his rate of breathing becomes dangerously slow, or he becomes confused or sleepy, the oxygen flow rate should be lessened. Severe COPD can be catastrophic. If necessary, the person may need to have his breathing assisted.

If a person with COPD shows signs of bronchitis (see page 181) or pneumonia (see below), the first-line antibiotic should be trimethoprim-sulfamethoxazole, amoxicillin, doxycycline, tetracycline, azithromycin, clarithromycin, levofloxacin, or sparfloxacin. Second-line antibiotics include ciprofloxacin, cefixime, cefprozil, ofloxacin, and amoxicillin-clavulanate.

Pneumonia

Pneumonia is an infection of the lung(s) characterized by combinations of fever, shaking chills (often with chattering teeth), cough, painful and difficult breathing, chest pain, weakness, and the expectoration of discolored (red, green, yellow, brown) phlegm. Pneumonia may evolve from bronchitis (see page 181) or arise independently.

Treatment for Pneumonia

1. If respiratory difficulty is extreme, administer oxygen (see page 383) at a flow rate of 5 to 10 liters per minute by face mask.
2. Administer an antibiotic. Although many different bacteria, viruses, mycoplasmas, fungi, and other agents can cause pneumonia, the organisms most commonly acquired outside the hospital ("community acquired") respond to the following drugs (for people under the age of 60 years): erythromycin (500 mg four times a day for 14 days), azithromycin (500 mg the first day, then 250 mg a day for four more days), or clarithromycin (500 mg twice a day for 14 days). If one of these is not available, use doxycycline or amoxicillin-clavulanate. A person over the age of 60 years or who is debilitated should be treated additionally with amoxicillin-clavulanate (875 mg twice a day), cefuroxime axetil (500 mg twice a day), or cefpodoxime (400 mg twice a day), or just with levofloxacin (500 mg once a day for 10 days). For a child 4 months to 6 years of age, use amoxicillin-clavulanate, azithromycin, erythromycin-sulfisoxazole, or cefuroxime axetil.
3. Evacuate the victim.

Serious lung problems related to specific environmental conditions are discussed in the sections on altitude illness (see page 292), drowning (see page 354), and smoke inhalation (see page 104).

CHEST PAIN

Chest pain may be a manifestation of a variety of disorders, ranging from a harmless chest cold or heartburn to a life-threatening heart attack. To try to attain a diagnosis, it is important to ask these questions:

1. Where is the pain?
2. What is the nature of the pain?
3. How severe is the pain?
4. How long have you had the pain?
5. Does the pain extend into the arm, neck, jaw, or abdomen?
6. What relieves the pain?

Angina

Angina is caused by narrowing or obstruction (spasm or actual occlusion) of the coronary arteries, which supply the heart muscle. The pain is most often described as heavy and pressurelike ("squeezing," like a weight on the chest); it is classically located beneath the breastbone, with radiation to the jaw, back (between the shoulder blades), and left arm. Rarely, it can radiate to the right arm. Associated symptoms include nausea, sweating, shortness of breath, anxiety, and weakness. It is commonly associated with exertion, and may be more frequent at high altitudes, where less oxygen is available. "Atypical" angina is pain that occurs at rest or that awakens a victim from sleep. A first-time angina episode, change in the pattern of existing angina episodes, or increased frequency of episodes may portend a heart attack. Angina may be relieved by rest.

The person who suffers from angina should be kept at absolute rest (sitting or supine) until the pain subsides. If he is carrying his medications, he should place a nitroglycerin tablet (0.4 mg) under his tongue (the tablet dissolves) or use sublingual nitroglycerin spray. If pain persists, this may be repeated after 3 to 4 minutes (not to exceed three tablets or spray applications in 10 minutes). Unless the victim is completely familiar with his angina and declares the episode typical and completely resolved, he should be transported with minimum exertion to an appropriate medical facility. If no relief is obtained, the victim may be suffering a heart attack. Expect a person with chest pain to trivialize his symptoms and deny the possibility of a heart attack.

Heart Attack (Acute Myocardial Infarction)

This is an emergency, because it may rapidly lead to complete cardiac arrest (standstill). A person suffering a heart attack will usually show some or all of the following symptoms: crushing substernal (under the breastbone) chest pain that may extend into the back, left arm or both arms, and/or neck; shortness of breath; profound weakness; nausea or vomiting; pale, moist, and cool skin; sweating; agitation; abnormal heart rate and rhythm—slow, fast, and/or irregular; and collapse. Typically, the chest pain does not subside with the administration of nitroglycerin. When cardiac arrest occurs, the victim stops breathing and has no heartbeat. Any elderly person with chest pain requires prompt physician evaluation.

A "silent" heart attack, in which there is a paucity of symptoms, more commonly occurs during sleep or in a diabetic victim.

Treatment for a Heart Attack

1. Send someone for help.
2. If the victim has a pulse and is breathing, he should be kept at absolute rest and arrangements made for immediate transport to a medical facility. If oxygen (see page 383) is available, it should be administered by face mask at a flow rate of 5 to 10 liters per minute.
3. If the victim collapses, *assess the need for cardiopulmonary resuscitation* (CPR) by feeling for a pulse (see page 26) and checking for breathing (see page 24). If these are absent, begin CPR (see page 28).

Rapid Heart Rate

Supraventricular tachycardia (SVT), sometimes called paroxysmal atrial tachycardia (PAT), is a disorder that causes a person's heart to beat very rapidly, sometimes up to 250 beats per minute. This can make the victim extremely uncomfortable, with a sensation of fluttering in the chest, palpitations, chest discomfort or tightness, anxiety, nausea, and weakness. If he is not carrying appropriate medications to treat this syndrome, you might try having the victim bear down and hold his breath as if straining to lift a heavy weight, or immerse his face in a pool of ice water. Another technique is to have him close his eyes, then have him press firmly on both eyeballs for 15 seconds to the point of moderate discomfort. Do not suggest this if the victim has glaucoma or recent eye surgery. Rubbing and pressing ("massaging") one of the carotid arteries (see page 26) in the victim's neck can sometimes send a reflex signal through the nervous system to the heart to cause it to slow to a normal rate ("break" the SVT). Carotid artery massage must be done in elders with extreme caution, because on rare occasion it has been noted to precipitate a stroke (see page 129). SVT is definitively treated by a physician with an intravenous injection of a specific medication, or in a dire emergency with a controlled (synchronized) electrical shock to the heart.

Noncardiac Causes of Chest Pain

Infection

Chest pain may be caused by a lung infection, such as pneumonia, bronchitis, or pleuritis. Typically, infection is characterized by pain that is sharp in nature and associated with fever, cough, weakness, and production of colored (nonwhite) sputum. Deep breathing usually makes the pain worse. The treatment of these disorders is discussed in other sections. Consult the index.

Heartburn

The pain of gastrointestinal upset (in particular, reflux of food and acid from the stomach into the esophagus) may closely mimic angina. Typically, heartburn occurs after a large meal, especially when the victim immediately lies down. Foods that are often troublesome include alcoholic and carbonated beverages, coffee, chocolate, and fats. The discomfort radiates sharply from the stomach through the breastbone and into the throat. Pain, belching, and a sour taste in the mouth may indicate a hiatal hernia, which allows reflux of stomach acid back up into the

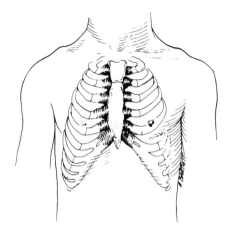

Figure 24. Costochondritis. The attachments of the ribs to the breastbone are inflamed and exquisitely tender to pressure.

esophagus. Treatment for heartburn is discussed on page 195. If there is any suggestion that angina (see page 44) is present, seek medical attention. Because the symptoms of a heart attack can be easily confused with those of heartburn, any elderly person with chest or abdominal pain requires prompt physician evaluation.

Muscle Injuries

Heavy physical exertion can lead to overuse syndromes. The pain is related to muscle motion and is accompanied by pain with motion and soreness to the touch. Treatment for these injuries is discussed on page 250.

Costochondritis

Costochondritis is an irritation of the cartilaginous ends of the ribs where they attach to the sternum (figure 24). The pain is sharp and well localized to the breastbone and adjacent rib ends. It is worsened considerably by pressing on the area or by deep breathing. Occasionally, slight painful swellings of the rib ends can be felt. The treatment is administration of aspirin or a nonsteroidal anti-inflammatory drug (such as ibuprofen).

BLEEDING

For a discussion of wound management (cleaning, closing, and dressing), see page 226.

Whenever you are going to be exposed to blood or other potentially infectious body fluids, wear sterile latex rubber gloves from your first-aid kit. If you are allergic to latex, use other nonpermeable gloves (such as nonlatex synthetic).

While it is occasionally visually distressing, bleeding can be one of the easiest problems to manage, because the treatment options are so straight-forward. The severity of the injury determines the rate of blood loss and what measures you must take to control the bleeding. Evaluate the follow-ing considerations:

1. Where is the bleeding? It is important to consider and identify internal bleeding as well as external bleeding. Considerable blood loss can be associated with blunt (nonpenetrating) abdominal injury (liver, spleen), as well as long bone or pelvic fracture (2 quarts, or liters, of blood can rapidly accumulate in the thigh following a broken femur). *Examine the entire victim!*

2. Is the bleeding from an artery or from a vein? Because arterial blood is under higher pressure, blood loss tends to be more rapid from a sev-ered artery than from a vein. Arterial bleeding can be recognized by its spurting nature and rapid outflow. All blood exposed to air, in the absence of unusual drug intoxications, turns red fairly quickly, so you cannot rely upon color to indicate origin.

Treatment for Bleeding

First, remove all clothing covering the wound so that you can see precisely where the bleeding is coming from. *Almost all external bleeding stops with firm, direct pressure.* This should be applied directly to the wound with the heel of your hand, using the cleanest available thick (four or five thick-nesses of a 4" by 4"—or 10 cm by 10 cm—sterile gauze pad, for instance) bandage or cloth compress (figure 25). Maintain pressure for a minimum of 10 minutes, to allow severed vessels to close by spasm (an artery con-tains small amounts of muscle tissue in its walls) and to allow early blood clot formation. Peeking at the wound under the compress interrupts the process and prolongs active bleeding. The application of cold packs or ice

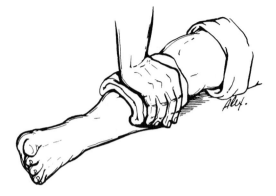

Figure 25. Firm pressure applied to a bleeding wound.

packs over the compress (*not* under it) may hasten the process by initiating spasm and closure of disrupted blood vessels. It is also useful to have the victim lie down, and to elevate the bleeding part above the level of his heart. A scalp wound tends to bleed freely, and may require prolonged pressure or wound closure for control (see page 57).

If direct pressure to the wound does not stop the bleeding, you must make certain that you are applying the pressure in the correct spot. Check quickly to see that you are pressing precisely over the bleeding point. If you are a fraction of an inch off, you can miss the best compression spot for a torn blood vessel; in this case, simply piling on more bandages may not solve the problem. Once you have repositioned your pressure, wait again for 5 to 10 minutes. If the pressure appears to be working, once the bleeding has substantially subsided you can apply a pressure dressing. Do this by covering the wound with a thick wad of sterile gauze pads or the cleanest dressing available, and wrapping the area firmly with a rolled gauze or elastic bandage. Do not apply the dressing so tightly that circulation beyond it is compromised (as indicated by blue fingertips or toes, or by numbness and tingling). Watch the dressing closely for blood soaking and dripping, which indicate continuous bleeding.

Some important things to be aware of with a serious wound are:

1. A victim who has lost 25 to 30% of his blood volume may suffer from shock. Treatment is discussed on page 54.
2. Prolonged uncontrollable bleeding is rare unless a major blood vessel or more than one vessel is disrupted, the victim is taking an

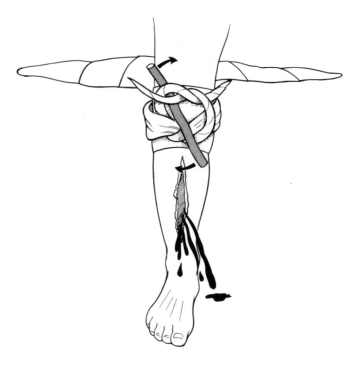

Figure 26. Application of a tourniquet. (A) Wrap the bandage around the limb, then tie a square knot. Tie a stick in place over the knot. Twist the stick to tighten the tourniquet just until the bleeding stops.

anticoagulant (blood thinner) medication, or the victim suffers from hemophilia. In such a case, heroic intervention may be lifesaving. The application of extreme compression to "pressure points," such as the radial, brachial, or femoral arteries, is both difficult and of considerable risk (since the purpose is to cut off all circulation).

A tourniquet is indicated only in a life-threatening situation and is best applied by an experienced person. Only in the case of torrential bleeding is a tourniquet more advantageous than continuous pressure. The decision to apply a tourniquet is one in which a limb is sacrificed to save a life.

A tourniquet should be applied to the limb between the bleeding site and the heart, as close to the injury as is effective, and tightened just to the point where the bleeding can be controlled with direct pressure over the wound.

To construct a tourniquet, use a 2 to 4" (5 to 10 cm) bandage—not something that will cut through the skin. Wrap the bandage around

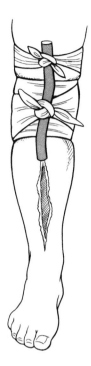

Figure 26. (CONT.) (B) Secure the stick.

the limb several times, then tie half or an entire square knot, leaving loose ends long enough to tie another knot (figure 26A). Place a stick or stiff rod over the knot, then tie it in place with the loose ends. Twist the stick until the bandage is tight enough to stop the bleeding, then secure it (figure 26B).

If possible, the tourniquet or a pressure-point occlusion should be released briefly every 10 to 15 minutes to see if it is still necessary. Always keep a tourniquet in plain view, so that it doesn't get left in place longer than necessary just because someone didn't know or forgot it was there.

3. If the victim has suffered a large wound through which internal organs (such as loops of bowel) (see figure 27A) or bones (see page 61) are protruding, *do not attempt to push these back inside the body or under the skin unless they slide back in without your assistance.* Cover extruded internal organs or bones with continually moistened bandages (pads of gauze or cloth) held in place without excess pressure (see figure 27B). Seek immediate medical attention.

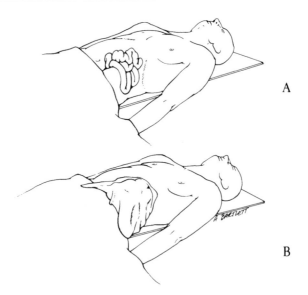

Figure 27. (A) Loops of bowel protrude from a laceration in the abdomen. (B) These should be covered gently with a moistened bandage or cloth. Do not try to push them back into the abdomen unless necessary for evacuation (for instance, if the victim must walk out under his own power and such activity is forcing more bowel to extrude from the wound).

4. If the victim has suffered a severe cut in his neck, take special care to not disturb the wound, because such disturbance might remove a blood clot that is controlling the bleeding from a large blood vessel. Apply a firm pressure dressing (don't choke the victim with the bandage) and seek immediate medical attention. Continually assess the airway (see page 17), because an expanding blood clot within the neck can compress the throat and windpipe. If the victim begins to have raspy breathing or a changed voice, evacuation is maximally urgent.

5. Bleeding can be quite brisk from a ruptured or torn varicose (dilated) vein in the leg. This can usually be managed with direct pressure, while elevating the leg. Follow this with a pressure dressing.

6. If a foreign object (such as a knife, tree limb, or arrow) becomes deeply embedded (impaled) in the body, do not attempt to remove it, because the internal portion may be occluding a blood vessel that will hemorrhage without this "plug." Any attempt at removal may create more damage than already exists, which includes increasing the bleeding. This is particularly true with a hunting (broadhead) arrow. Instead, pad and bandage the wound around the object, which should

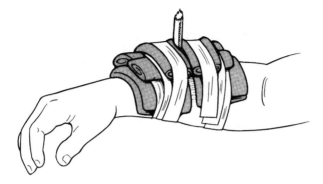

Figure 28. Padding and bandages to prevent motion of a penetrating object.

be fixed in place with tape if possible (figure 28). The external portion of the object may be cut to a shorter length (cut off the shaft of the arrow a few inches above the skin, for example), if necessary to facilitate splinting and transport of the victim.

7. A gunshot wound may cause severe internal damage that is not readily visible from the surface wound. Any victim who has suffered a gunshot wound should be brought to immediate medical attention, no matter how minor the external appearance.

Always disarm the victim. A head-injured or otherwise confused victim carrying a loaded weapon could accidentally create an additional victim. If you don't know how to handle a gun, move the weapon at least several feet away and point it in the direction where accidental discharge will do the least harm.

8. After the bleeding has stopped, immobilize the injury. Check all dressings regularly to be certain that swelling has not made them too tight.

Internal Bleeding

If bleeding is internal, such as from a bleeding ulcer, broken bone, injured spleen or liver, leaking abdominal aneurysm, or lung cancer, the victim may suffer from shock. Symptoms of internal (undetected) bleeding are the same as those of external bleeding, except that you don't see the blood. They include rapid heartbeat, shortness of breath, general weakness, thirst, dizziness or fainting when arising from a supine position, pale skin color (particularly in the fingernail beds and conjunctivae), and cool, clammy skin. Other signs include increasing pain and firmness of the abdomen after an injury, vomiting blood or "coffee grounds" (blood darkened by stomach acid), blood in the urine or feces, or large bruises over the flank or abdomen. Because it is difficult to predict the rate of internal blood loss and because the only effective treatment for many causes of severe internal bleeding is surgery, medical help should be sought immediately.

SHOCK

Shock is a condition in which the blood supply (which carries oxygen and nutrients) to various organs of the body is insufficient to meet metabolic demands. The signs and symptoms are restlessness, low blood pressure, weak and rapid (thready) pulse, altered mental status (restlessness, anxiety, confusion), moist and cool (clammy) skin, rapid shallow breathing, inability to control urination and bowel movements, nausea, and profound weakness. It is a life-threatening condition and may follow a large number of inciting events: Causes of shock include severe internal or external bleeding (25 to 30% acute loss of an adult's total blood volume, equivalent to 1.5 to 2 liters out of 6 liters), overwhelming infection, burns, dehydration, heart attack or disease, hormonal insufficiency, hypoglycemia, hypothermia, hyperthermia, allergic reaction, drug overdose, and spinal cord injury (loss of sympathetic nervous system support allows blood vessels to dilate as they lose tone).

Shock is a true emergency. Unfortunately, there is little that the rescuer can do in the field. The management of shock includes the following:

1. Position the victim on his back, with the legs elevated about 30 degrees (8 to 12", or 20 to 30 cm), in order to encourage blood in the leg veins to return to the central circulation (heart) and head (brain) (figure 29). Do not elevate the legs if the victim has a severe head injury (see page 55), difficulty breathing, a broken leg, neck or back injury, or if such a maneuver causes any pain. If the victim is short of breath because of heart failure (see page 41), he may be more comfortable in the sitting position.

2. Keep the victim covered and warm. Remove him from harsh weather conditions. Remember to insulate him from below. If insufficient bundling is available, lie next to the victim to share body heat. Take special care to keep his head, neck, and hands covered.

3. Administer oxygen (see page 383) at a flow rate of 10 liters per minute by mask.

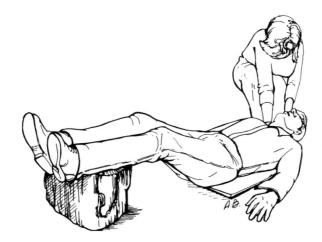

Figure 29. Positioning a victim who is in shock. Elevate the legs, cushion the back, protect the airway, and keep the victim warm.

4. Control any obvious sources of external bleeding (see page 48). Splint all broken bones.

5. If the victim is diabetic, consider a hypoglycemic reaction (see page 128). If the victim is conscious and can purposefully swallow, administer Glutose paste (see page 128) or a sugar-sweetened liquid by mouth in small sips. Otherwise, do not give the victim anything to eat or drink unless he is alert and thirsty or hungry. If the victim is in shock because of diarrhea and dehydration, attempt to initiate oral fluid intake (see page 184).

6. If the victim has been stung by an insect or appears to be suffering an allergic reaction (see page 58), treat the allergic reaction.

7. Transport the victim to a hospital as rapidly as possible.

HEAD INJURY

Victims of head injury can be divided into two groups, according to whether or not they have lost consciousness. Always remember that the dazed or unconscious victim cannot protect his airway; you must be vigilant in your observation. The most common complication of head injury is obstruction of the airway with the tongue, blood, or vomitus. The most common associated serious injury is a broken neck.

Loss of Consciousness

If a person struck in the head has lost consciousness, he has suffered at least a concussion.

1. *Protect the airway* (see page 17) and *cervical spine* (see page 31).
2. If the victim wakes up after no more than a minute or two and quickly regains his normal mental status and physical abilities, he has probably suffered a minor injury—so long as there is no relapse into unconsciousness or persistent lethargy, nausea or vomiting, or severe headache. If the victim is far from help, he should undertake no vigorous activity and be kept under close observation for at least 24 hours. Normal sleep should be interrupted every 2 to 3 hours to briefly ensure that his condition has not deteriorated. Confusion or amnesia for the event that caused the blackout is not uncommon and not necessarily serious, so long as the confusion does not persist for more than 30 to 45 minutes. Because a serious brain injury may not become apparent for hours, the wilderness traveler who has been knocked out should not venture farther from civilization for 24 hours. If headache and/or nausea persist beyond 2 to 3 hours, the victim should begin to make his way (assisted by rescuers) to medical care.
3. If the victim wakes up and is at first completely normal, only to become drowsy or disoriented, or to lapse back into unconsciousness (typically, after 30 to 60 minutes of normal behavior), he should be evacuated and rushed to a hospital. This may indicate bleeding from an artery inside the skull, causing an expanding blood clot (epidural hematoma) that compresses the brain. Frequently, the unconscious victim with an epidural hematoma will be noted to have one pupil significantly larger than the other (figure 30).
4. If the victim awakens but has a severe headache, bleeding from the ears or nose with no obvious external injury to those organs, clear fluid draining from the ear or nose, unequal-sized or poorly reactive (do not constrict promptly upon exposure to bright light) pupils, weakness, bruising behind the ears or under the eyes, vomiting, or persistent drowsiness, he might have a skull fracture. Such signs mandate immediate evacuation to a medical facility.
5. If the victim suffers a seizure (see page 59) after a head injury, no matter how brief, he should be transported to a medical facility.
6. If the victim does not wake up promptly after a head injury (unconscious for more than 10 minutes), has bleeding from an ear, has unequal or nonreactive (do not constrict to bright light) pupils, has clear fluid from the nose, has a profound headache, is weak in an arm or

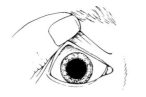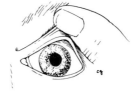

Figure 30. Unequal pupils.

leg, is disoriented, or has a fluctuating level of consciousness (normal one minute, drowsy the next), he may have suffered a significant brain injury and should be immediately rushed to a medical facility. Because there is a high incidence of associated neck injuries, any person with a serious head injury should have his cervical spine immobilized (see page 31). Remember, head injuries often cause vomiting. Therefore, be prepared to turn the victim on his side so that he doesn't choke (see page 21).

No Loss of Consciousness

If a person has been struck on the head but was never knocked out, he will rarely have incurred a serious injury to the brain. The scalp should be inspected for cuts, which generally bleed freely; it requires considerable pressure to stop the bleeding (see below). If the victim seems normal (answers questions appropriately; knows his name, the location, and the date; walks normally; appears coordinated; has normal muscle strength), there is probably no need to perform a hurried evacuation. If the victim is in any way abnormal, however, he should be rapidly transported to a medical facility. A small child who has been struck on the head and begins to vomit, refuses to eat, becomes drowsy, seems apathetic, or generally appears abnormal should be examined by a physician as soon as possible.

Lacerations of the Scalp

Cuts of the scalp tend to bleed freely, because the blood vessels are positioned in the thick skin in such a way that they cannot go into spasm and seal off after they are severed. For this reason, it is important to apply prolonged firm pressure to any head wound, and to seek care as soon as possible. If the wound is large and you do not have any bandages, you can bring the edges together by tying hair taken from opposite sides of the wound. If possible, this should be preceded by a quick, vigorous rinse of the wound to remove any large pieces of dirt, gravel, or other debris.

For information regarding wound repair and bandaging, see pages 226 and 241.

ALLERGIC REACTION

A severe allergic reaction (anaphylaxis) can be life threatening. It is caused by exposure to insect and animal venoms (such as wasp or jellyfish stings), plant products, medications, or any other agent to which the victim's immune system has been previously sensitized.

Symptoms include low blood pressure (shock); difficulty breathing (severe asthma) with wheezing; swelling of the lips, tongue, throat, and vocal cords (leading to airway obstruction); itching; hives (red, raised skin welts that may occur singly or in large patches); nausea and vomiting; diarrhea; abdominal pain; seizures; and abnormal heart rhythms. Any or all of these symptoms may be present in varying severity. The most common life-threatening problem is respiratory distress. Facial swelling indicates that the airway may soon become involved. *Be ready at all times to protect and support the airway.*

Treatment for an Allergic Reaction

1. Administer aqueous epinephrine (adrenaline) 1:1,000 in a subcutaneous injection (see page 419). The adult dose is 0.3 to 0.5 ml; the pediatric dose is 0.01 ml per kg of body weight, not to exceed a total dose of 0.3 ml. For weight estimation, 1 kg equals 2.2 lb. The drug is available in preloaded syringes in certain allergy kits, which include the Ana-Kit (Hollister-Stier) and the EpiPen and EpiPen Jr. (Dey). Instructions for use accompany the kits. The EpiPen products are generally easier for laypeople to use, because it requires less dexterity to accomplish injection with them. The Ana-Kit syringe is preloaded with enough epinephrine for a second (repeat) adult dose.

For dosing purposes, the EpiPen should be used for adults and children over 66 lb (30 kg) in weight. Children 66 lb and under should be injected with the EpiPen Jr.

Take particular care to handle preloaded syringes properly, to avoid inadvertent injection into a finger or toe. Do not intentionally inject epinephrine into the buttocks or a vein. Epinephrine should not be exposed to heat or sun, but does not need to be kept refrigerated. If clear (liquid) epinephrine turns brown, it should be discarded. When administering an injection, *never* share needles between people.

2. Administer diphenhydramine (Benadryl) by mouth. A milder reaction that does not require epinephrine or corticosteroids may be managed with diphenhydramine alone. The adult dose is 50 to 75 mg every 4 to 6 hours; the pediatric dose is 1 mg per kg (2.2 lb) of body weight, also every 4 to 6 hours. The major side effect of this medication is drowsiness.

3. In case of a severe reaction, administer corticosteroids. Prednisone tablets in a dose of 50 to 80 mg should be given to an adult; the pediatric dose is 1 mg per kg (2.2 lb) of body weight. The onset of action of steroids is delayed for 4 to 6 hours; therefore, this drug should be given early in the course of therapy.

4. Administer an inhaled (aerosol or "micronized") bronchodilator. Bronchodilators (airway openers) are drugs that have the advantages of minimal side effects and direct delivery to the site of action. They are available in metered-dose handheld nebulizers ("mistometers") from which the victim inhales therapeutic puffs. An excellent drug for an acute attack is albuterol (Ventolin). The dose for an adult is two to four puffs initially, followed by two puffs every 3 to 6 hours. A child over age 12 who can manage the device may use a handheld nebulizer; younger children often require oral (liquid) medication in the appropriate dose.

5. Transport the victim for medical evaluation.

Reactions to specific agents (such as bee stings, plant contact, hay fever) are discussed elsewhere. Consult the index.

SEIZURE

A seizure ("fit"; epilepsy) represents vigorous involuntary muscle activity and altered consciousness associated with abnormal electrical discharges within the brain. It may be caused by a number of underlying disorders, which include structural abnormalities of the brain (scars, birth defects), injury, tumor, infection, bleeding (stroke), uncontrolled hypertension, lack of oxygen, abnormal blood chemistries (calcium, sodium, glucose), and "recreational" drug abuse (including drug withdrawal).

Most seizures have been grouped into various classifications, which include the following types:

Partial. This seizure is initiated in a focal, or "restricted," part of the outermost layer (cortex) of the brain. Consciousness may (complex seizure) or may not (simple seizure) be impaired.

Generalized. This seizure involves the cortex of the brain in a symmetrical and synchronous manner, and may lead to "automatic," "absent," or profoundly agitated behavior patterns.

Grand mal (big illness). In this type of generalized seizure disorder, the victim classically becomes unconscious and has violent repetitive muscle activity with tongue biting, grunting, eye deviation to one side, difficulty breathing, and occasional loss of bladder and/or bowel control. Following the seizure, the victim will be confused or combative for a time (10 to 60 minutes) as he slowly returns to normal. He may sleep for a while after a seizure.

Status epilepticus. This is defined as prolongation of the seizure activity for a period that exceeds 1 to 2 minutes, or as multiple seizures without a return of normal consciousness between fits. Status epilepticus is a true medical emergency.

Petit mal (little illness). This is an "absence" attack generally seen in a child; in it, he seems to be daydreaming, distracted, or confused. It is not associated with violent, abnormal physical behavior.

Psychomotor (temporal lobe). This is an episode of patterned abnormal behavior, such as lip smacking, olfactory hallucinations, vulgar speech, or repetitive movements such as arm waving. The origin of the electrical activity is thought to reside in the temporal lobe of the brain.

Treatment for Seizure

1. Protect the airway (see page 17). If the victim vomits, do your best to clear the mouth and nose of debris. Turn the victim on his side. He may suddenly bite down and hold his teeth clenched, so take care not to get your fingers caught in the mouth. A padded object that cannot be bitten through (such as a leather wallet edge) may be used as a bite block to keep the teeth apart and prevent tongue biting, but take extreme care not to obstruct the airway. Do not place a hard object in the mouth that might break the teeth. Take care not to force the tongue backward into the throat. *Never try to pour liquids into the mouth of a seizing victim.*

2. Protect the cervical spine (see page 31).

3. Protect the victim from injuring himself during the seizure. This may be done with cushions, a sleeping bag, or constant repositioning of the victim. If he needs to be physically restrained, keep him on his side. Loosen all clothing around the neck.

4. In most cases, a grand mal seizure will only last 30 seconds to 2 minutes and will be self-limited. The victim will be confused for a few minutes to an hour after the seizure, and should be watched closely for recurrence or difficulty in breathing. If the victim continues to seize or does not wake up between seizures (status epilepticus), he must be transported to a medical facility as soon as possible for drug administration. Any victim who does not fully awaken, who awakens but has never previously had a seizure, or who appears weak or feverish after a seizure should be rapidly evacuated.

5. When the victim awakens, determine if he has ever had a seizure before and whether he is supposed to be taking anticonvulsants. The most common cause of a seizure is failure to take prescribed anti-seizure medication(s). If the victim has been delinquent, he should take his medicine as soon as possible. For an adult, common medications are phenytoin sodium (Dilantin) 300 to 400 mg per day, phenobarbital 30 to 60 mg three times a day, or diazepam (Valium) 5 to 10 mg three to four times a day. Never administer an oral medication to anyone unless he is awake and capable of purposeful swallowing.

6. A possible cause of unconsciousness or seizure in a person who suffers from diabetes is low blood sugar (hypoglycemia). If a diabetic suffers a seizure, he should be given sugar as soon as possible. This may be difficult to do away from the hospital, because intravenous injection will be required if the victim cannot swallow. If a diabetic feels weak, sweaty, dizzy, or nauseated, he should immediately ingest a sugar-containing beverage, food (see page 128), or concentrated liquid glucose (Glutose: one tube contains 25 g). If the victim is unconscious, sugar granules or small squirts of Glutose can be placed under the tongue, where they can be passively swallowed.

FRACTURES AND DISLOCATIONS

A bone fracture (break) may be simple (one clean break) or comminuted (multiple breaks or shattered) (see figure 31). Furthermore, it may be closed (skin intact) or open ("compound," with the skin broken, often with the bone visible in the wound). An open fracture is highly prone to infection. A fracture may be associated with injuries to adjacent nerves and blood vessels.

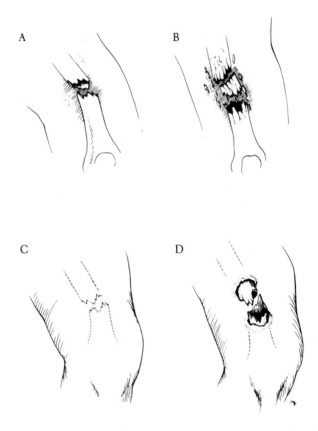

Figure 31. Fractured bones. (A) Simple fracture (one break). (B) Comminuted fracture (multiple breaks). (C) Closed fracture (skin unbroken). (D) Open, or compound, fracture (skin broken).

A broken bone or dislocation (displacement of a bone at the joint) should be suspected whenever there has been sufficient force to cause such an injury, if a snap or crack was heard, if the victim cannot move or bear weight upon the body part, or if an injured body part is painful, swollen, discolored, and/or deformed. A broken or dislocated bone should be compared with the normal opposite limb; asymmetry is a key sign of a significant injury. Pain with a broken bone tends to be instantaneous, constant, and worsened considerably with motion, which may also create a grating sensation and noise. A small child with a fracture or dislocation will not use the affected body part and will cry vigorously with the slightest manipulation. If you think that a bone may be broken, it is best to treat it as a break until an X ray can be obtained or the situation shows obvious marked improvement (which usually requires 4 to 6 days).

Because of the force necessary to break or displace a bone, any person with a fracture or dislocation should be examined carefully for other injuries. All fractures and some dislocations cause a certain amount of bleeding, which can be significant with the larger bones (femur, pelvis). Be prepared to treat the victim for shock (see page 54). Do not manipulate a broken limb unnecessarily if circulation to the limb seems normal; excess motion increases the risk of damage to the bones, nerves, and blood vessels. When examining an injury, always begin with an uninjured area and work toward the injury, so that the victim's response to pain doesn't interfere with your exam.

If the skin has been disrupted in the vicinity of the broken bone, the fracture is open. The bone end may or may not be visible through the wound, and bleeding may be minor or major. If a victim has sustained an open fracture, is alert enough to swallow liquids, and is more than 6 hours distant from a medical facility, administer penicillin, erythromycin, amoxicillin, or cephalexin 500 mg by mouth every 4 hours. Rinse the wound gently to remove any obvious dirt, then cover it with a sterile dressing. Do not vigorously scrub or irrigate the wound. Unless there are signs of loss of circulation (coldness, blue color or paleness, numbness) or it is necessary to realign the limb in order to allow splinting and evacuation, do not try to reposition the injury or to push the bone back under the skin. If you must manipulate the limb, rinse any visible bone with water or disinfectant (such as povidone iodine 10% solution), then allow the bone to slide under the skin without touching it. While holding traction (pulling on the end portion of a limb in a longitudinal axis in order to achieve correct anatomic alignment), immediately apply a splint (see page 65) to prevent further motion and damage.

In general, it is unwise to manipulate an injured limb. If the extremity is deformed, but the circulation is intact (normal pulses, sensation, temperature, and color), do not attempt to straighten it; instead, splint it in the position in which you found it ("splint 'em as they lie"). On the other hand, if the circulation to an extremity is obviously absent (the extremity is numb, cold, and blue or pale), if the victim is in extreme discomfort, or if gross deformity prevents moving the victim out of a dangerous situation or prevents the application of a splint, then an attempt to restore the part to a normal position is justified. Early realignment is easier than delayed, may alleviate a major amount of pain, and often allows easier splinting and transport. Be advised, however, that the relocation of a fracture or dislocation may be difficult and transiently very painful for the victim. If you are going to make an attempt to realign a limb, it should be done as soon as possible after the injury (preferably, within 3 hours), before swelling and increasing pain and muscle spasm make the maneuver impossible. If there

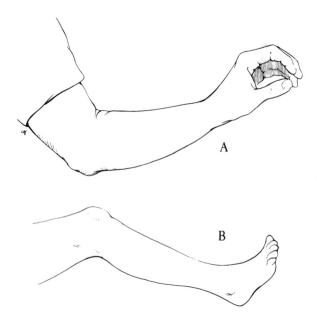

Figure 32. Position of function (normal anatomical resting position). Unless otherwise specified, the upper and lower limbs should be bandaged and/or splinted in these positions. (A) Upper extremity. (B) Lower extremity.

is no deformity, splint the injured body part in the "position of function" (the position it would assume if it were at rest) (figure 32).

To attempt to reposition a displaced body part, apply steadily increasing traction (pulling force) to the injury while applying countertraction above the injury. Do not forcefully lever or snap a bone back into position with a quick, forceful motion. To gain mobility in a deformed area, it is sometimes necessary to gently rock the body parts or slightly accentuate the deformity ("distract" the joint to create maneuvering space between the bones) while applying continuous traction away from the body. This allows the dislocated part to clear any obstruction and slip back into position. If the part is repositioned, it should be held in place while you splint it into position. After such maneuvers, check to see that circulation has been restored. *In no circumstance should you try to reposition a suspected cervical spine injury.*

Compartment Syndrome

Within the limbs (leg, arm, forearm, foot, hand, and fingers), there are "compartments" defined by inelastic boundaries of tough connective tissue, or fascia. These compartments contain bones, groups of muscles, blood vessels, and nerves. If swelling occurs within a compartment—typically caused by bleeding, continuous excessive external pressure, a crush injury, or envenomation (snakebite)—the pressure can exceed 30 mm of mercury, which is the pressure at which blood travels through microscopic blood vessels, such as capillaries. This effectively squeezes the tiniest blood vessels and occludes flow through them, cutting off circulation to the compartment and rapidly causing tissue death. The most common cause of a compartment syndrome in a wilderness enthusiast is swelling surrounding a broken bone or associated with a severe blunt injury, such as occurs after a fall. The lower leg and forearm are the most common sites.

Signs and symptoms include severe pain that seems out of proportion to the injury. The underlying tissue feels extremely tight, and pain is increased markedly with external pressure. Stretching the muscles that run through the compartment causes worsened pain. There may be decreased sensation in those skin areas supplied by the nerves that run through the compartment—for example, decreased sensation to pinprick or light touch on the top of the foot in the web space between the great and second toes because of pressure on the deep peroneal nerve, which runs through the anterior leg compartment.

Field treatment involves elevation of the affected limb, splinting, padding to protect against further injury, and rapid evacuation. A true compartment syndrome must be treated with surgery to open the compartment and allow the pressure to be reduced. Severe damage can occur within 12 hours of the onset of the syndrome. Do not administer aspirin to the victim. Cold packs are of limited, if any, benefit; never immerse in ice water.

Compartment syndrome is rare following snakebite (see page 300), because most of the swelling following a bite is confined to superficial soft tissues.

Splints and Slings

A splint should be applied to any broken bone, bad sprain, or severely lacerated body part after gross deformity is corrected, to maintain proper position and immobilize the injured part(s) so that it cannot be displaced. This prevents further nerve, blood vessel, and muscle damage, and keeps broken bone ends from grating against each other or from poking through the skin. A sling-and-swathe combination helps further immobilize a limb. Pain may be lessened or relieved by eliminating unnecessary motion, allowing more rapid transport.

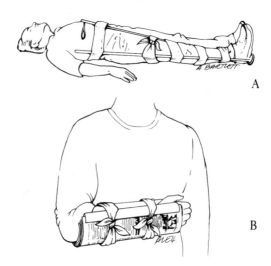

Figure 33. Splints may be fashioned from items such as (A) ski poles and (B) rolled newspaper.

General guidelines to follow in the application of splints are:

1. Examine every suspected fracture to see if it is open or closed (see page 61). Check the circulation below the fracture site by inspecting pulses, skin color, sensation, and movement of fingers and toes. In the arm, check the radial and brachial pulses; in the leg, check the popliteal, dorsalis pedis, and posterior tibial pulses (see figure 10).

2. Control bleeding (see page 48) and apply a dressing if necessary.

3. Splint the joint above and below the injury. For instance, to keep the knee from moving, you often need to prevent motion at the ankle, knee, and hip. There will be times when this is difficult, but do the best you can.

4. If possible, fashion the splint first on an uninjured body part, then transfer it to the injured area. This lessens manipulation of the injured part and minimizes pain associated with splinting.

5. Splints can be fashioned from sticks, cardboard, foam pads, rolled newspapers, pack frames, ski poles, or other similar objects (figure 33). The SAM Splint is made of padded (foam glued to each side) malleable aluminum (4¼" by 35½"; rolls easily to become a 3" by 4¼" cylinder) that can be shaped to splint a great number of body parts. Foldable or rollable wire splints can be constructed by cutting 6" by 30" (15 by 76 cm) and 18" by 36" (46 by 91 cm) pieces of ⅛" or ¼" (3 or 6 mm) wire mesh and covering the sharp edges with adhesive or duct tape.

An inflatable air splint is sometimes less desirable, in that it can only attain one shape and may create circulation problems by exerting too much pressure on injured tissues. If you use an air splint, be sure that it has a mechanism to adjust for volume expansion (heat and altitude). When stored at freezing temperatures, it should be kept partially inflated so that any frozen moisture (from inflating breaths) within the air bladder doesn't cause the walls to adhere.

Fasteners can include belts, triangular bandages, tape, elastic wraps, shirtsleeves, and blankets. Slings can be fashioned from triangular bandages, cravats, sheets, ropes, and vines.

6. When applying a splint, don't cut off the circulation. Pad all bony prominences, other pressure points, and injuries as best possible. This may be done with foam, a sleeping pad, pack material, or clothing.
7. If the injury is closed (skin unbroken) and there are no signs of decreased circulation, apply ice packs intermittently to the swollen area. Do not apply ice directly to the skin.
8. Remove all constrictive jewelry (watches, bracelets, rings, and so forth). Left in place, these can become inadvertent tourniquets on swollen limbs and fingers (see page 423).
9. Administer appropriate pain medication.
10. After a splint is applied, check the limb periodically to make certain that swelling inside the splint has not cut off the circulation. This is particularly important in cold weather, where numbness can be a confusing factor.
11. Elevate the injured part as much as possible, to minimize swelling.
12. Insist that all victims seek medical evaluation when they return home, to be certain that all bones are properly aligned and that no further intervention is needed.

To learn more about specific splints and slings, read about the specific injuries (below).

Specific Injuries

The major bones of the skeleton are illustrated in figure 34.

Neck

If a fracture of the cervical spine is suspected because of neck pain, weakness or loss of feeling in an arm or leg, tingling in an arm or leg, or mechanism

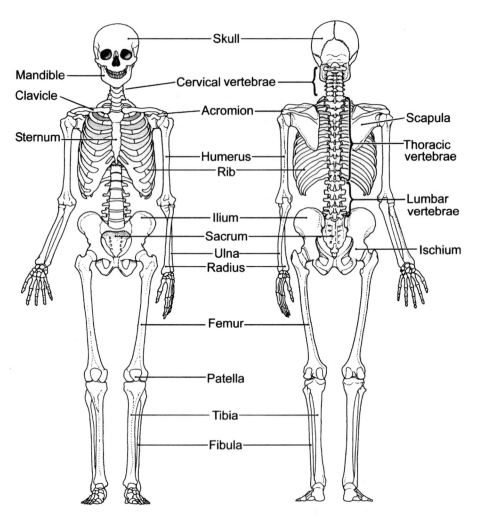

Figure 34. Major bones of the skeleton.

of injury (for instance, a victim who has fallen, is unconscious, and has a face or head injury), you must immediately immobilize the head and neck. This can be done by taping the head to a backboard or stretcher, by applying a rigid collar (which may be fashioned from a SAM Splint, as in figure 16), or by placing sandbags or their equivalent on either side of the head (see figure 15). *Never move the neck to reposition it.*

For the ambulatory, cooperative victim with minor neck discomfort, a thick pad (rolled towel, jacket) can be placed posteriorly at the base of the neck. Secure this by wrapping tape or cloth around the forehead, then crossing it over the pad and bringing it back out under the armpits to be tied across the chest (see figure 17). Alternately, use a thick removable waistband from a backpack or a rolled Ensolite pad in a horse-collar configuration. Soft-collar techniques should not be relied upon to hold the neck immobile; they merely offer gentle support.

If the victim is uncooperative or agitated, hold his head until you can firmly immobilize it and restrain the victim from motion (see figure 18). All of this is necessary to avoid injury to the spinal cord. If the victim must be moved or turned on his side (most commonly to allow vomiting or to place insulation beneath him), hold his head fixed between your forearms while you hold his shoulders with your hands. In this way the victim can be "logrolled," using as many rescuers as possible to avoid unnecessary head, neck, and spine motion.

Logrolling the Victim (Figure 19)

1. The first rescuer approaches the victim from the head, and keeps the head and shoulders in a fixed position so that the neck doesn't move.
2. The second rescuer extends the victim's arm (on the side over which the victim is to be rolled) above the victim's head. The first rescuer uses this arm to help hold the victim's head in proper position.
3. All rescuers work together to roll the victim without moving the neck.

In no circumstance should you try to reposition a suspected cervical spine injury. An alert victim with a broken neck or severely torn ligament will usually have enough discomfort from the injury and muscle spasm to force him to hold his neck still. However, someone with a head injury or who is under the influence of alcohol or drugs may feel no pain, and can have an undetected serious injury that will be worsened by motion.

Any victim with a suspected neck fracture should be transported on a firm board or in a scoop stretcher, if possible.

Skull

See page 55.

Nose

See page 170.

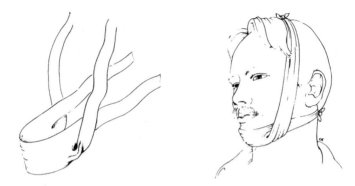

Figure 35. Bandage for a dislocated or fractured jaw. The bandage must be easy to remove, in case the victim needs to vomit.

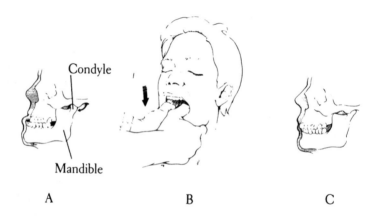

Figure 36. Dislocated jaw. (A) The condyle of the mandible slips forward out of the joint. The teeth do not fit together properly. (B) The rescuer applies firm downward pressure to relocate the jaw. (C) Normal position is restored, and the teeth fit properly.

Jaw

A fractured jaw is usually caused by a fall or a blow from a closed fist. The lower bone (mandible) may be broken in one or more places. The victim will complain of pain, swelling, inability to close his mouth, improper fit of the teeth, and difficulty talking. If the fracture extends into the oral cavity, there may be bleeding from the mouth. Treatment is to wrap a bandage over the top of the head and under the jaw for support (figure 35).

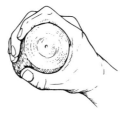

Figure 37. A rolled elastic bandage is gripped gently to maintain the hand in the "position of function."

It should be easily removable in case the victim needs to vomit. A liquid diet should be maintained until the victim can reach the hospital.

A dislocated jaw can occur from a blow, from a widemouthed yawn, or even during sleep. The mandible slips loose from its two bony sockets below the ears and slides forward (figure 36). To reposition the mandible, grasp the jaw by placing your thumbs (with cloth or gauze padding for traction) inside the mouth against the lower molars (rear teeth), holding the bone firmly with your remaining fingers. Exert steady pressure straight down until you feel the mandible "pop" back into place, and the victim says his teeth fit properly (figure 36B). After the jaw is repositioned, tie a bandage under the chin and over the top of the head to keep the jaw from easily dislocating again (see figure 35). *The bandage should be easily removable in case the victim needs to vomit.*

Wrist, Hand, and Finger

A fracture or dislocation of the hand, wrist, or finger should be positioned and splinted in the normal resting position (position of function; see figure 32A). For a wrist or hand injury, this may be accomplished by allowing the victim's fingers to rest around a padded object in his palm (such as a rolled pair of socks, rolled elastic bandage, or wadded cloth; figure 37), with a circumferential wrap to maintain position (see figure 38). Every attempt should be made to allow the fingertips to remain uncovered, in order to assess circulation. If the wrist is involved, place a rigid splint on the underside of the hand, wrist, and forearm to prevent motion (see figure 39). Fingers may be splinted independently or taped together (with padding in between) for support (see figures 40 and 41).

A sling can be applied to the forearm for support and pain relief. A swathe may be added for further immobilization. To make a classic arm

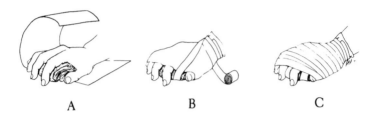

Figure 38. Hand dressing in the "position of function." (A) The fingers hold a pad of cloth in the palm. (B) A circumferential wrap is applied, taking care to pad between the fingers. (C) The completed wrap leaves the fingertips exposed, so that they can be checked for adequate circulation.

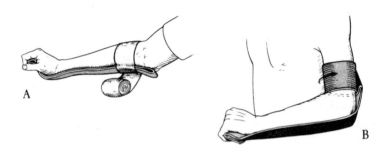

Figure 39. A SAM Splint fashioned to stabilize the wrist and forearm. (A) In this method, the elbow is free to bend. (B) The splint can be extended to immobilize the elbow.

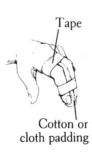

Figure 40. Buddy-taping method to immobilize a finger.

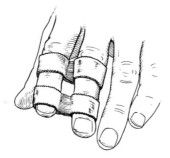

Figure 41. A variation of the buddy-taping method to immobilize a finger. If the fingers are taped together tightly, cotton or cloth should be placed between them for padding.

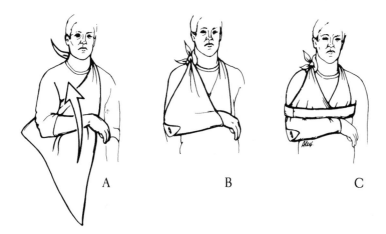

Figure 42. Sling and swathe. (A) A triangular bandage is draped under the arm and over the opposite shoulder. (B) Two corners are tied behind the neck, and the third is pinned at the elbow. (C) A cravat swathe holds the arm against the chest.

sling out of a triangular bandage, lay the bandage under the arm as shown in figure 42. Tie two corners together with a square knot at the opposite shoulder—which creates the arm cradle—then pin the remaining elbow corner up onto the body of the sling. A rolled or folded triangular bandage becomes a cravat (see page 244), which is wrapped around the sling-encased arm and chest (as a swathe) to hold the arm snug against the body wall (figure 42C). If materials to fashion a sling are not available, the victim's shirt can be pulled up and pinned to create a crude hammock for

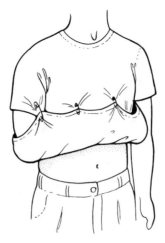

Figure 43. Pinning the shirt to make a hammock sling for the arm.

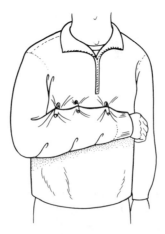

Figure 44. Pinning a shirt sleeve to the chest.

the arm (figure 43), or you can pin the shirt sleeve to the body of the shirt after the elbow is flexed to the proper position (figure 44).

If a finger is dislocated at the middle or distal joint, make a gentle attempt at relocation by applying steady, firm traction to the fingertip (figure 45). Do not try to reposition the joint with a sudden forceful snap. It may be easiest to relocate a finger if you hold the joint bent and push the distal (overriding) bone back into position with your thumb(s). It is nearly impossible to reduce a dislocation at the knuckle of the index finger

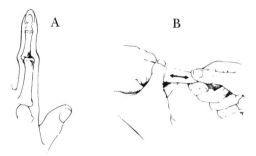

Figure 45. (A) Dislocation of a finger joint. (B) Relocation of the bones with firm steady traction.

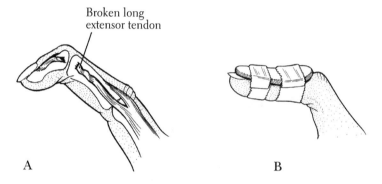

Figure 46. (A) Mallet finger. (B) Splinting a mallet finger.

without an operation. After a finger is realigned, it should be taped to one or two adjacent fingers for splinting (see figures 40 and 41).

A "mallet finger" (figure 46A) results from disruption of the extensor tendon, which pulls the tip of the finger into a straight position. The finger should be splinted with a slight amount of hyperextension (figure 46B).

If the thumb is dislocated or fractured, it can be taped to prevent further injury, by fixing it with an anchor to the index finger (figure 47A) or directly against the hand (figure 47B). You can use the anchor technique to hold any two fingers together.

Forearm

A fracture of the forearm should be splinted to immobilize the wrist and bent elbow (see figure 39B). Fashion sling and attach it to the trunk with a swathe (see figure 42).

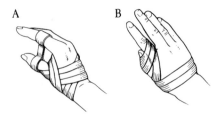

Figure 47. Taping the thumb for immobilization. (A) The buddy-taping method. (B) A thumb-lock. If possible, padding should be placed between the thumb and the forefinger.

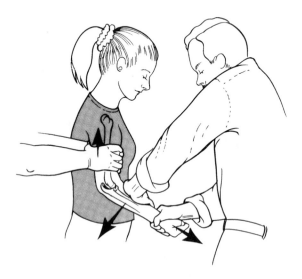

Figure 48. Repositioning a dislocated elbow.

Elbow

A fracture of the elbow should be splinted to include the wrist and shoulder, if possible, and at an angle of 60 to 90 degrees. However, if it is painful for the victim to move his elbow, splint it in the position in which you found it. A sling should be fashioned and attached to the trunk with a swathe. A dislocated elbow should be realigned if necessary to restore circulation to the hand. Hold the arm bent 45 to 90 degrees at the elbow and use a lever motion to pull the bones of the forearm back into position, while holding the upper arm fixed in countertraction (figure 48). This may require a fair amount of force to accomplish and is usually difficult if the victim cannot relax.

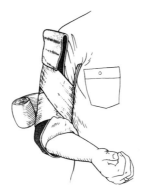

Figure 49. The SAM Splint can be conformed in a "sugar tong" to immobilize the upper arm.

Upper Arm

The entire length of the bone of the upper arm (humerus) can be palpated for tenderness or deformity from the arm's inner aspect. A fracture of the humerus can be differentiated from a dislocated shoulder by observing how the victim holds his arm. With a humeral fracture, the arm is often held close to the chest, while a dislocation of the head of the humerus from the shoulder socket (shoulder dislocation—see page 79) prevents the victim from pulling his arm into his body.

A fracture of the upper arm, particularly if it is close to the shoulder, is often quite difficult to splint. A "sugar tong" splint can be fashioned using a SAM Splint, by laying the splint along the inner and outer surfaces of the arm, with the U of the "tong" at the elbow (figure 49). If possible, the elbow should be kept bent at 90 degrees and the arm placed in a sling. Attach the sling to the body by using a circumferential (around the chest) swathe fashioned from a belt, rope, or long piece of cloth to prevent motion of the arm at the shoulder (see figure 42).

Two padded board splints can be used to stabilize an arm fracture above the elbow (see figure 50). The splints cross the upper part of the arm and the midforearm to create a triangle with the elbow. A sling is added for support.

Collarbone

A fracture of the collarbone is best managed with a sling and swathe (see figure 42) and/or a modified figure-of-eight bandage. The latter is created by draping a rope, cloth, or cravat behind the neck across the shoulders, then

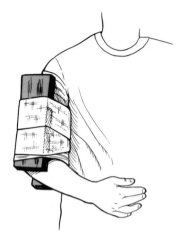

Figure 50. Padded boards to splint the upper arm.

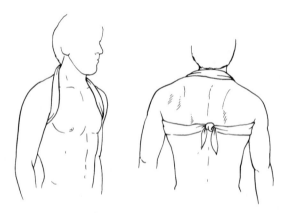

Figure 51. Modified figure-of-eight bandage for a broken collarbone.

forward over the shoulders and under the arms (pad the armpits, if possible), to be tied in the back (figure 51). This will pull the shoulders back into the military position. To provide a tighter fit, tie the cross-shoulder section to the lower knot (giving a figure-of-eight appearance). After the figure-of-eight bandage is pulled snug, the affected arm may be fixed to the chest using a sling and swathe. Another technique is to weave a figure-of-eight bandage with a long, rolled elastic bandage (figure 52). If any figure-of-eight bandage increases the victim's discomfort, you can use a sling and swathe alone. A collarbone fracture appears to heal equally well with either technique, so the major issue is immobilization for comfort.

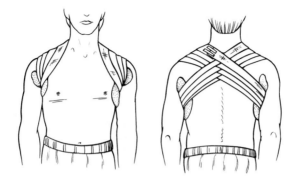

Figure 52. Woven figure-of-eight bandage for a broken collarbone.

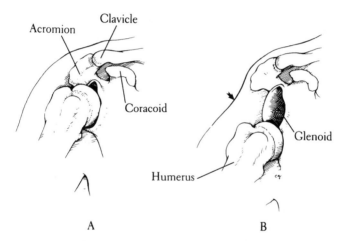

Figure 53. Dislocated shoulder. (A) Normal anatomy. (B) With dislocation, the head of the humerus slips out of the glenoid (socket), and a depression (arrow) is noted in the external appearance of the shoulder.

Another alternative is to have the victim wear a properly fitted backpack with shoulder straps and carry approximately 15 pounds of weight in the pack.

Shoulder Dislocation

The long bone (humerus) of the upper arm fits into the shoulder joint with a ball-and-socket mechanism, held in place by muscles and tendons (figure 53A). When a person falls onto his shoulder or an outstretched

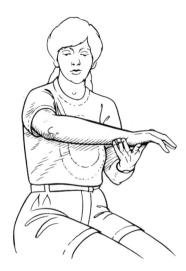

Figure 54. The victim with a dislocated shoulder carries the arm up and away from the body.

arm, or has his arm twisted or pulled forcefully, the head of the humerus can dislocate out of the shoulder joint (see figure 53B). This is usually quite painful and may be associated with a fracture of the humerus or the lip of the shoulder socket. The diagnosis of shoulder dislocation is made by observing and feeling a depression in the shoulder where the upper arm bone should be (see figure 53B), noting that the victim holds the arm up and away from the body (figure 54), and feeling the head of the humerus as a firm ball 2 to 3" (5 to 7.5 cm) below its normal location. Those who have previously suffered shoulder dislocations are often prone to recurrent episodes with lesser forces applied to the joint.

If the injured victim can be transported to a medical facility within 3 hours, there is no need to attempt relocation of the arm unless he is in extreme pain. Place the arm in a sling, position some padding underneath the arm and against the chest, and secure the sling to the victim's chest with a swathe to minimize motion and discomfort (see figure 42).

If more than 3 hours will elapse before medical help is obtained, if the dislocation is recurrent (has happened to the same shoulder before), or if the victim is suffering intolerable pain, you can make an attempt to reposition the arm bone in its socket. Do not attempt relocation if the upper arm or elbow is deformed (indicating a broken bone). The safest and simplest technique for relocation is to pull with steady, forceful traction on the injured arm, directed at a 45- to 90-degree angle away from the body.

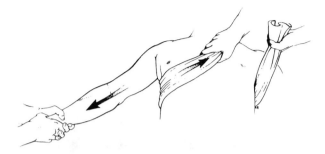

Figure 55. Technique for relocating a shoulder dislocation. One rescuer applies traction at the forearm while another applies countertraction at the chest.

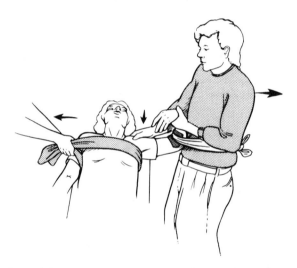

Figure 56. Repositioning a dislocated shoulder. Attached to the victim's forearm with a strap, rope, or sheet, the rescuer uses his body weight to apply traction, leaving his hands free to manipulate the victim's arm. A second rescuer applies countertraction, or the victim can be held motionless by fixing the chest sheet to a tree or ground stake.

At the same time, someone should provide countertraction by holding a sheet or blanket that is wrapped across the victim's chest and under the affected armpit (figure 55). The easiest technique is to tie a sheet, belt, webbed strapping, or avalanche cord around the rescuer's waist and the victim's bent forearm, so that the rescuer (standing or kneeling) can lean back to apply traction, keeping his hands free to guide the head of the humerus back into position (figure 56). In all cases, place padding in the

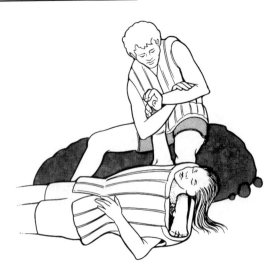

Figure 57. Life jacket brace to assist in the relocation of a dislocated humerus.

armpit and bend of the elbow to prevent a pressure injury to sensitive nerves beneath the skin. A single rescuer can provide countertraction by placing his foot against the victim's chest just below the armpit, or fixing the countertraction sheet or rope to a tree or ice ax buried in the ground; he can also use a life jacket as a foot brace (figure 57). *Do not jerk the arm, attempt to twist or lever it into position, or pull with a tugging motion.*

Another technique is to have the victim lie prone so that his injured arm can dangle free. Place a thick pad under the injured shoulder. Attach a 10 to 20 lb (4.5 to 9 kg) weight to the wrist or forearm (do not have the victim attempt to hold the weight) and allow it to exert steady traction on the arm, using gravity to relocate the humeral head (figure 58). Alternately, have the standing victim bend forward at the waist as you pull steadily downward on his arm to simulate the gravity effect, with gentle side-to-side (at the wrist) rotation (figure 59).

In the scapular manipulation technique, the victim is placed in a prone position so that his injured arm can dangle free. Apply traction for 5 to 10 minutes. Then, while maintaining traction, push the tip (lower edge) of the scapula ("wingbone") in toward the spine while pulling the upper portion (toward the shoulder) of the scapula away from the midline. This can also be done with the victim in a standing position (see figure 60A). If the victim is standing, it may help to pull the arm forward as well as down (see figure 60B).

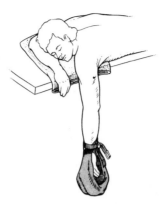

Figure 58. A fanny pack filled with rocks can be used for a weight in the "dangle" method of shoulder relocation.

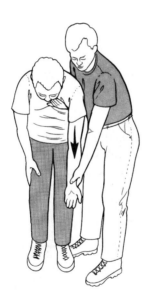

Figure 59. Pulling on the hanging arm to relocate a dislocated humerus.

If pain medicine is available, the victim should be medicated before relocation is attempted, to allow the greatest possible shoulder and chest muscle relaxation. As the arm bone moves back into proper position (this may require 15 minutes of steady traction), it will sometimes "give" in little movements, with a final "pop" back into the socket. Once the

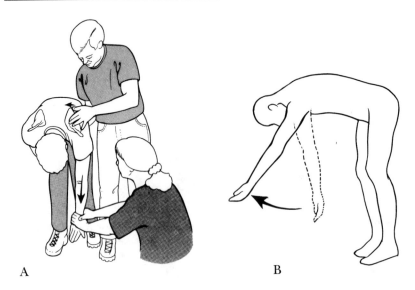

A   B

Figure 60. (A) Pushing the lower edge of the scapula toward the spine while an assistant pulls downward on the hanging arm to assist in the relocation of a dislocated humerus. (B) The downward pull on the arm may be slightly forward to help put the arm bone back in the shoulder socket.

bone is back in place, the victim will be able to bring his arm across the chest. If the victim cannot relax his muscles sufficiently to allow relocation, if your attempts cause excruciating pain, or if you are otherwise unsuccessful after 30 minutes, leave well enough alone (no one ever died of a dislocated shoulder). Place padding in the armpit and fix the arm near the body in as comfortable a position as possible with swathe bandages, then head for help. A shoulder harness (figure 61) may be useful. The victim who cannot walk should be transported in a sitting (for comfort) position, if possible. If the shoulder relocates, it should be placed in a sling and swathe, to prevent a repeat dislocation (see figure 42). A first-time shoulder dislocation that is relocated should be immobilized for 3 weeks. A recurrent dislocation that is relocated can be exercised gently after 3 to 5 days.

Shoulder Separation

A shoulder separation, as contrasted with a dislocation, occurs when the collarbone's ligamentous attachments to the acromion and coracoid structures of the triangular scapula ("wingbone") are weakened or disrupted

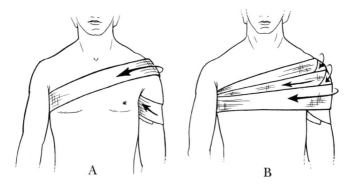

Figure 61. Shoulder harness.

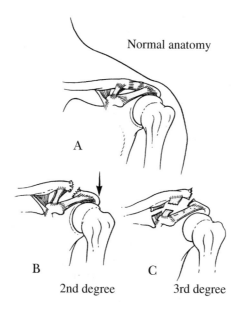

Figure 62. (A) Ligamentous attachments of the collarbone at the shoulder. (B) Second-degree shoulder separation. (C) Third-degree shoulder separation.

(figure 62). This can range from small tears in the ligaments, which do not result in a visible deformity, to full disruption of the ligaments, leading to a "free-floating" collarbone. The injury usually follows a direct blow to the shoulder, such as occurs when you fall onto your side and cannot break the fall with an outstretched arm.

If tenderness is elicited when pressing directly over the acromio-clavicular joint (AC joint), particularly with swelling and a spongy sensation over the end of the collarbone, suspect a shoulder separation. Treat as for a broken collarbone (see page 77).

Rib

A broken rib can be very painful, but there is little that the rescuer can do to improve the situation. Pad the chest wall with blankets or clothing (if the victim needs to be carried out on a stretcher) to restrict unnecessary motion and contact. Never bind the chest tightly; this inhibits deep breathing and prevents full expansion of the lungs, which predisposes the victim to partial lung collapse and pneumonia. Encourage the victim to breathe deeply (sigh) or cough a few times an hour. If there is a segment of detached (flail) ribs (see page 35), attempt to stabilize its position with padding (see figures 20 and 23). Because of the force necessary to break a rib, anticipate internal bleeding (lungs, liver, and spleen) (see page 53). A rib will sometimes break during forceful coughing. In this case, internal injury is not a concern.

Spine (Chest and Lower Back)

A victim who falls a great distance and lands on his feet frequently fractures his heel(s), ankle(s), and lumbar vertebrae (lower bones of the spine—see figure 34). Symptoms of spinal cord injury include back pain, weakness, numbness or tingling below the injury, loss of bladder or bowel control, and low blood pressure ("spinal shock"). If a fractured spine is suspected, the victim must be completely immobilized to avoid damage to the spinal cord. Position him on a firm litter or backboard, and secure him so that no motion of the back is possible (see page 31). If a scoop stretcher or backboard is not available and the victim must be moved, he should be logrolled (see page 34).

Pelvis

If pressing inward on the victim's hips or downward on the pubic bone causes pain, suspect a fracture of the pelvis, and immobilize the victim from his waist on down. A pelvic fracture is frequently associated with severe internal injuries and bleeding, so rapid evacuation is a high priority. Be prepared to treat the victim for shock (see page 54). Do not allow a victim with a suspected pelvic fracture to walk.

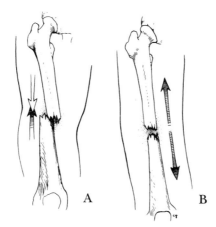

Figure 63. Fracture of the femur. (A) Without traction, strong muscles of the thigh pull the broken bone ends together, causing pain and deformity. (B) Traction straightens the leg and helps control bleeding and pain.

Femur

A fracture of the femur (the large bone of the upper leg) can be diagnosed by severe pain, inability to bear weight, deformity, and rapid swelling (from bleeding). Often, the affected leg is shortened and the foot is rotated away from the other leg. This injury requires splinting from the hip to the ankle. Because the muscles of the thigh are quite powerful and will tend to force the broken bone ends to overlap, traction is often necessary to control bleeding, maintain position, decrease pain, and prevent further internal muscle and blood vessel damage (figure 63). If sufficient rescuers are available, one person should maintain firm traction on the leg at the ankle to oppose the strong muscle contractions of the thigh (see figure 64). A broken femur can bleed 2 quarts (liters) of blood into the thigh rapidly, so evacuation is a high priority. Be prepared to treat the victim for shock (see page 54).

The standard Thomas ("half ring") splint allows traction to be applied to the femur. A Hare splint has a ratchet mechanism at the end to provide mechanical traction. A Sager splint allows traction by facilitating lengthening of its long, rigid axis rod. The Kendrick Traction Device (Medix Choice, El Cajon, California) is a lightweight, portable field traction apparatus that operates on the same principle and can easily be carried and applied in a wilderness setting.

You can also prepare an improvised traction splint that replicates the features of a Thomas splint: a half ring to anchor up against the pelvic

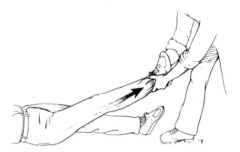

Figure 64. Technique for applying traction to the lower leg.

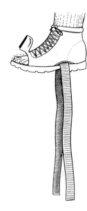

Figure 65. The toe section of a boot can be cut away to allow inspection for adequate circulation. A cravat or piece of webbing can be passed through a boot as the first step in creating a traction harness.

bone (ischial tuberosity) underneath the lower crease of the buttock, two longitudinal rigid rods to run the length of the leg, a fixed spacer at the lower (foot) end between the two rods, and a traction mechanism to pull on the leg in order to align the fracture.

The ankle should be padded with foam or cloth pads, or a boot should be worn. If the latter is done, you can cut away the toe section to assess the circulation (skin color, sensation) (figure 65).

A traction harness must be created to pull the leg straight down away from the head. One method is to cut two slits through the victim's sturdy boot, above the sole just in front of the heel and directly below the leg bones. Pass a cravat or nylon webbing (such as a pack strap) through the opening (figure 65); the ends of the strap will be secured to the rigid object that will form the spacer at the foot end of the leg splint. The paired-loop method of creating an ankle hitch uses paired lengths of

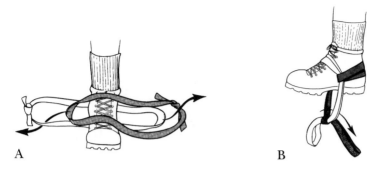

Figure 66. Paired-looped webbing to create an ankle hitch. (A) Position the webbing around the ankle. (B) Pull the harness tight with the ends pointed down for fixation to the splint.

cravat, nylon webbing, or rope (figure 66). Fold each in half, creating a single turn at one end. Lay one cravat over the top of the ankle and one behind the ankle (behind the Achilles tendon), with the curved ends pointed in opposite directions. Pass the free ends of each cravat through the loop in the other cravat, and tighten the cravats so that they fit snugly and flat against the ankle. The free ends should now hang down (figure 66B) and will be secured to the spacer, directly or with an interposed pulley system, that connects the long, rigid rods of the splint.

The traction splint rods can be fashioned from two ski poles, rigid tree limbs or saplings, tent poles, or anything else that is approximately a foot (30 cm) longer than the distance from the top of the thigh to the bottom of the foot. To measure the proper length, lay the rods next to the victim on either side of the thigh, with the top of the inner rod tucked up against the groin crease and the top of the outer at the top of the thigh. Cut the lengths to be even at a distance of approximately 8 to 12" (20 to 30 cm) below the foot (see figure 67).

Construct the splint away from the victim. Using a cravat, ski pole straps, webbing, or rope, attach the tops of the two poles with a length that approximates half the circumference of the thigh at this point, to create the "half ring" that will be snugged up underneath the victim into the lower buttock crease (see figure 68). At the lower (foot) ends of the rods, attach a perpendicular rigid spacer about 8" (20 cm) in length (see figure 69). This could be a piece of ski pole, a wrench, a piece of tree limb, or the like. Then lay four cravats (two for above the knee, two for below) or straps (that can be fastened) over the rods and wind them to be configured as cradle hitches (see figure 70). These will fix the rods to the leg after traction has been applied. Velcro straps are nice, if you have them.

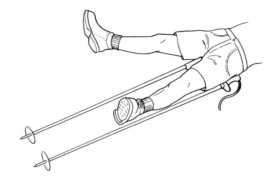

Figure 67. Proper length of traction splint rods.

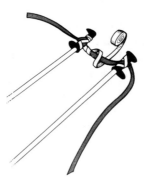

Figure 68. Creation of the half ring, which snugs up into the buttock crease.

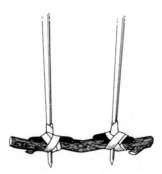

Figure 69. Attachment of the spacer at the foot end between the splint rods.

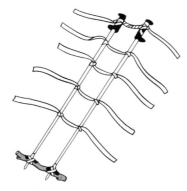

Figure 70. Configuration of cravats for cradle hitches.

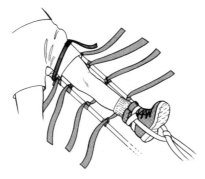

Figure 71. Attaching the splint to the leg above the suspected point of the fracture.

Holding traction on the leg, lift it enough to slide the splint underneath. Snug the half ring up into the buttock crease, remembering to keep the shorter rod on the inside of the leg. Attach the splint firmly to the leg with tape or a cravat around the front of the thigh (over thick padding, if available) at the top of the splint above the suspected point of the fracture (figure 71).

Tie the free ends from the traction harness (which you created through the boot or around the ankle) to the spacer at the end of the long splint. Create a "Spanish windlass" by inserting a short, rigid stick or rod between the tied-down free ends and twisting to produce the desired amount of traction (see figure 72). Fix the twister rod in place by tying it to the adjacent long splint rods (see figure 73).

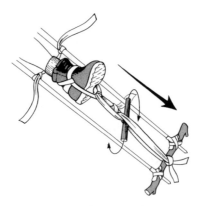

Figure 72. Tie the free ends of the foot harness to the spacer. Then twist the Spanish windlass to create downward traction on the leg.

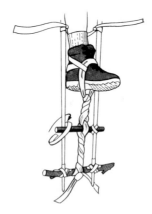

Figure 73. After the windlass is twisted to achieve the desired traction, tie the windlass rod to the long struts of the splint to maintain the traction.

Finally, secure the splint to the leg with the cradle hitches, two above the knee and two below (figure 74). Pad everything. The victim may be more comfortable if you apply traction while his knee is slightly bent.

Hip

If a person (usually elderly) falls with great force directly onto his knee, the large leg bone may be forced backward out of his hip socket and create a posterior hip dislocation. In such a case, the affected leg appears

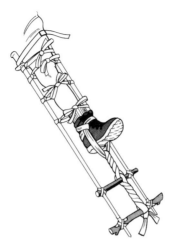

Figure 74. Secure the splint in place by tying off the cradle hitches.

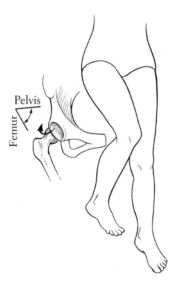

Figure 75. Position of the leg with posterior hip dislocation.

shorter and is bent at the knee; the foot and knee are also turned inward (toward the other leg) (figure 75). With an anterior hip dislocation, the ball of the femur slips forward out of the hip socket, and the leg is shorter and externally rotated (knee and foot face outward) (see figure 76). Either dislocation is a serious condition, because the blood supply to the head of the femur (the "ball" of this ball-and-socket joint) is disrupted. If

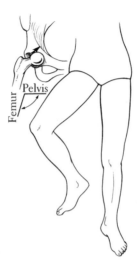

Figure 76. Position of the leg with anterior hip dislocation.

medical attention cannot be reached within 1 hour, make an attempt at relocation—*unless there is a deformity of the upper leg or knee (indicating a fracture).* Hold the leg and knee of the victim firmly, and exert forceful traction pulling on the thigh directly down toward the victim's feet, in an attempt to slide the head of the femur back into the hip socket. If this is successful, you will feel a "give," and the leg, knee, and foot will regain proper alignment.

Because of the force required to perform this maneuver, it is generally necessary to have a second rescuer provide countertraction to the victim's upper body. The two-rescuer method involves the first rescuer straddling the supine victim directly over his hips, facing toward the victim's head and holding the victim's bent leg between his knees. The second rescuer holds the victim's pelvis to the ground while the first lifts upward on the dislocated femur (figure 77). If relocation is successful, firmly splint the hip by securing the victim's legs together, slightly bent at the hips and knees with padding in between; he should be promptly evacuated, and should not attempt to walk.

Knee and Kneecap

A suspected fracture of the knee or kneecap should be splinted from hip to ankle. If there is such great deformity that the foot becomes numb and

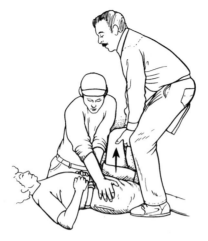

Figure 77. Two-rescuer method for repositioning a dislocated hip.

turns blue or pale and cold (usually with severe dislocation of the knee joint), and pulses cannot be felt, use traction to attempt to realign the leg in a position of function (with the knee bent at a 15- to 30-degree angle; see figure 32B) in order to reestablish circulation. If pulses do not return after the knee is repositioned, the major artery that traverses the knee joint may have been torn or crushed and occluded. This is a surgical emergency.

If the kneecap becomes dislocated, gently straighten the leg while pushing the kneecap from the lateral side back into place. Occasionally, the kneecap will not pop back into position. If the maneuver is painful or not easily accomplished, do not apply force. After the kneecap is repositioned, splint the leg straight or at a 15-degree bend (knee) using an Ensolite or foam pad and elastic bandage(s).

If the knee has been dislocated or fractured, the victim must be carried. If a kneecap dislocation is the only injury, however, successful treatment will allow the victim to walk, using an ice ax, ski pole, or other object as a crutch.

The knee can be sprained (or strained) when it twists or withstands impact. The supporting ligaments that bind the joint on the outside and inside (lateral and medial collateral ligaments) and those that cross front to back through the interior of the knee joint (cruciate ligaments) can be stretched, slightly torn, or completely disrupted. This causes immediate pain with weight bearing (walking), motion (trying to bend the knee or extend the leg), or touch (pressing against the injured side of the knee). Often, there is swelling and a spongy feel to the knee. As swelling increases, the knee becomes less flexible and more difficult to bend. If you suspect

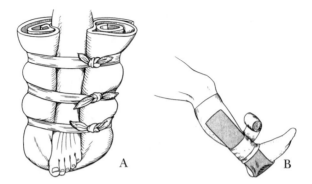

Figure 78. Methods of foot and ankle immobilization. (A) A piece of rolled foam can be used as a "stirrup" to hold the foot and ankle motionless. (B) The SAM Splint is easily configured in a similar fashion.

more than a minor sprain, immobilize the knee as if for a fracture; the victim should avoid weight bearing.

Lower Leg

A fracture of the lower leg should be splinted from knee to ankle. If necessary, the legs can be attached side by side with padding in between. If the knee is not involved, keep it bent at 15 to 30 degrees.

Ankle

A fracture of the ankle can be stirrup-splinted or wrapped to prevent movement. This can be accomplished using a SAM Splint, parka, or piece of rolled foam taped or wrapped into place (figures 78 and 79). Remove or loosen the boot or shoe to avoid entrapment due to swelling, which could impair circulation. However, if the victim must walk out under his own power, replace footwear as soon as possible, before swelling makes this impossible.

Toe

A fractured toe may be splinted by buddy-taping. This is performed by placing some padding (cloth or cotton) between the toes and taping the injured toe to a healthy adjacent toe for support.

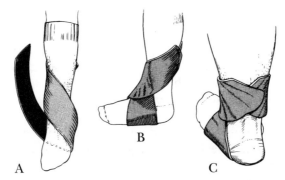

Figure 79. Ankle fixation with the SAM Splint. (A) The splint is wrapped in a figure-of-eight over the top of the ankle. (B) The aluminum is molded to fit snugly against the foot and lower leg. (C) Rear view of completed splint.

AMPUTATION

Amputation is detachment of a body part, such as an ear, finger, or foot. It is usually associated with a serious force or crushing injury, such as an animal bite. The immediate threats to life are bleeding and shock (see page 54).

If a body part is detached, apply firm pressure to the site of the bleeding where the tissue loss has occurred. Manage any serious bleeding (see page 48). Cover the wound with the cleanest available bandage, then wrap firmly. *Do not attempt to reattach the detached body part.* If a digit is hanging on by a small "bridge" of skin or muscle, attempt to bandage it without completing the separation.

If the body part can be easily recovered and the victim can be brought to a hospital within 6 hours of the injury, do the following:

1. Gently rinse the body part if the cut end is contaminated with dirt.
2. Wrap the body part in clean cloth or gauze and keep the covering moist. The ideal solution is saline (*not* ocean water, because of infection risk), if that is available; if not, fresh water will do. Do not immerse the part in a bag of water; merely keep the covering moist. Keep the body part cool by placing it on ice after wrapping it securely in a bandage, cloth, or towel. To avoid a frostbite injury, *do not apply ice directly to the body part or immerse it in ice water.*
3. Bring the body part with the victim to the hospital.

The application of a tourniquet to stop bleeding is essentially a decision to sacrifice the limb in order to preserve life. If any salvageable part of the limb is still attached, do not apply a tourniquet to stop bleeding until you have exhausted all pressure techniques (see page 48). If the limb is completely severed and the bleeding is torrential, a tourniquet may be applied until the muscular walls of the arteries constrict and bleeding can be controlled by direct pressure. Tie a cloth or rope circumferentially an inch or two above the wound and tighten it just enough to allow direct pressure to stop the bleeding (see page 50). After 5 to 10 minutes, loosen the tourniquet briefly to see if the bleeding can be controlled with pressure techniques alone.

BURNS

Definitions (Figure 80)

First-degree burn. This is a burn that involves the outermost layer of skin, the epidermis. It is often quite painful. The skin is reddened, but there is no blister formation. When a large surface area is involved, as with a severe sunburn, the victim may become quite ill, with fever, weakness, chills, and vomiting.

Second-degree burn. This is a burn that involves the epidermis and portions of the next-deeper layer of the skin, called the dermis, which contains the sweat glands, hair follicles, and small blood vessels. It is usually more painful than a first-degree burn, and blisters are present. Large areas of second-degree injury impair the body's ability to control temperature and retain moisture. Thus, a severely burned victim loses large amounts of fluid and can rapidly become hypothermic in a cold environment.

Third-degree burn. This is a burn that has penetrated the entire thickness of the skin, and may involve muscle, bone, and so on. It is typically painless because of nerve destruction. The appearance is dry, hard, leathery, and charred. Occasionally, the skin will appear waxy and white with small clotted blood vessels visible as purple or maroon lines below the surface. Because a third-degree burn is usually surrounded by an area of second-degree injury, the edges of the wound may be quite painful. Third-degree burns nearly always require a skin graft for coverage.

Partial-thickness burn. First-degree or second-degree burn.

Full-thickness burn. Third-degree burn.

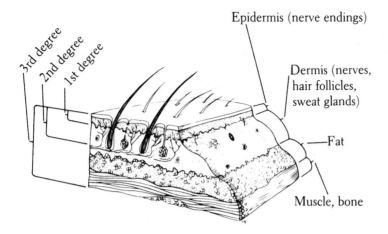

Figure 80. Burn wound. Note that third-degree (full-thickness) burns completely destroy nerves and are painless.

Inhalation injury. This is a burn that involves any portion of the airway. Inhalation injury occurs when a victim is trapped in a fire and/or inhales smoke, steam, or superheated air (see page 103).

Treatment for Burns

1. Remove the victim from the source of the burn. If his clothing is on fire, roll him on the ground or smother him in a blanket to extinguish the flames. If the victim has been burned with chemicals, *gallons* of water should be used to wash off the harmful agents. If the eyes are involved, they should be irrigated copiously. Phosphorus ignites upon contact with air, so any phosphorus in contact with the skin must be kept covered with water. Do not attempt to neutralize acid burns with alkaline solutions or vice versa; the resultant chemical reaction may liberate heat and worsen the injury. Stick to irrigation with water. If clothing remains stuck to the skin and does not fall away with irrigation, do not tear the clothing away. Cut around it.

2. Evaluate the airway. Look for evidence of an inhalation injury: burns of the face and mouth, singed nasal hairs, soot in the mouth, swollen tongue, drooling and difficulty in swallowing saliva, muffled voice, coarse or difficult breathing, coughing, and wheezing. If it appears that an inhalation injury has occurred, administer oxygen (see page 383) by face mask at a flow rate of 5 to 10 liters per minute, and transport the victim to a hospital as quickly as possible.

3. Examine the victim for other injuries. Unless the airway is involved or the victim is horribly burned, the burn injury will not be immediately life threatening. In your eagerness to treat the burn, don't overlook a serious injury such as a broken neck. Control all bleeding and attend to broken bones before applying burn dressings.

4. Treat the burn:

First-degree: A first degree burn, such as a mild to moderate sunburn, may be treated with cool, wet compresses. If the burn is acquired suddenly (as when a child grabs a hot rock), immediate application of very cold water (not solid ice) may help limit the extent of the tissue damage. Oral administration of an anti-inflammatory drug, such as aspirin or ibuprofen, may provide considerable relief. For severe sunburn ("lobster body"), the administration of oral prednisone in a rapid taper (80 mg the first day, 60 mg the second, 40 mg the third, 20 mg the fourth, 10 mg the fifth) may be extremely helpful. Corticosteroids should always be taken with the understanding that a rare side effect is serious deterioration of the head ("ball" of the ball-and-socket joint) of the femur, the long bone of the thigh.

Topical corticosteroid creams or ointments are of no benefit in treating a burn wound. Anesthetic sprays that contain benzocaine work for a few hours, but may induce allergic reactions. They should be used sparingly. If no blisters are present, a moisturizing cream (such as Vaseline Intensive Care) will help soothe the skin. Aloe vera gel or lotion seems to promote resolution of extensive first-degree burns. Burnaid first-aid burn gel (Rye Pharmaceuticals, Marina del Rey, California), which also comes in an impregnated dressing, contains 2 to 4% melaleuca oil and is advertised to provide relief from the pain of minor burns and scalds.

Second-degree: A second-degree burn should be irrigated gently to remove all loose dirt and skin. This should be done with the cleanest cool water available. *Never apply ice directly to a burn;* this may cause more extensive tissue damage. Cool compresses may be used for pain relief.

After the wound is clean and dry, cover it with a soft, bulky dressing made of gauze or cloth bandages, taking care to keep the dressing snug but not tight. If antiseptic cream such as silver sulfadiazine (Silvadene) is available, it should be applied under the dressing. An alternative is mupirocin ointment or cream, or bacitracin ointment. A nonadherent dressing layer directly over the antiseptic is easier to change than coarse gauze. Another excellent covering is Spenco 2nd Skin underneath an absorbent sterile dressing. Spenco 2nd Skin is an inert hydrogel composed of water and polyethylene oxide. It absorbs fluids (so long as it doesn't dry out), which "wicks" serum and secretions away from the wound and promotes wound healing. Other occlusive hydrogel-type dressings are NU-GEL (preserved polyvinyl pyrrolidone in water) and Hydrogel, which can absorb up to 2½ times its weight in exuded (from the wound) fluids. Yet another covering for a burn is a layer of petrolatum-impregnated Aquaphor gauze under a dry (absorbent) gauze dressing.

Do not apply butter, lanolin, vitamin E cream, or any steroid preparation to a burn. These can all inhibit wound healing, and may facilitate infections with increased scarring.

Dressings should be changed each day to readjust for swelling and to check for signs of infection. Be certain to keep burned arms and legs elevated as best possible, to minimize swelling and pain.

Blisters should not be opened, unless they are obviously infected and contain pus (this will generally not occur until 24 to 48 hours after the burn injury). If a blister remains filled with clear fluid, it is an excellent covering for the wound and will minimize fluid loss and infection. There is no rush to remove charred skin from a burn wound. As the wound matures and dressings are changed, gentle scrubbing will lift off dead tissue.

A victim with large areas of second-degree burns may need to be treated for shock (see page 54).

Third-degree: A third-degree burn should be irrigated gently and covered with antiseptic cream or ointment or Spenco 2nd Skin, and a dry sterile dressing.

If a first-degree burn involves more than 20% of the body surface area and the victim suffers from fever, chills, or vomiting, a physician evaluation is required. If a second-degree burn involves a significant portion of the face, eyes, hands, feet, genitals, or an area greater than 5% of the total body surface area, a physician evaluation is required. Body surface area can be estimated using the "palm of hand" rule: The surface area of the victim's palm without the fingers represents approximately 1 to 1.5% of his total body surface area. All third-degree burns are serious and should be seen by a physician.

Wet versus Dry Dressings

If the burn surface area is small (less than 10% of total body surface area), then cool, moist dressings *(not ice)* may be used to initially cover the burn wound. These often provide greater pain relief than do dry dressings. If the surface area involved is large, however, dry, nonadherent dressings should be used, in order to avoid overcooling the victim and introducing hypothermia (see page 269). Because the skin is the major thermoregulatory organ of the body, it is difficult for an extensively burned victim to control his body temperature, so great care must be taken when wetting down such a person. If the victim begins to shiver, the cooling is too extreme.

Fluid Replacement

A person who has suffered an extensive burn will rapidly become dehydrated. Because water quickly shifts from the blood volume into the tissues of the body, the injured skin cannot retain moisture, and associated immune suppression leads to overwhelming infection and shock. Oral rehydration with balanced salt solutions is little help, but in the wilderness, it is usually the only option. Try to get the victim to drink—in sips, if necessary—enough liquid to keep the urine copious and clear (see page 286). If a burned victim cannot drink because his airway is injured, consciousness is altered, weakness prevails, or vomiting is persistent, immediately call for an evacuation.

Antibiotics

Antibiotics are not necessary for burns unless they become infected. This is indicated by the presence of pus, foul odor, cloudy blisters, increased redness and swelling in the normal skin that surrounds the burn, and fever greater than 101°F (38.3°C). If a burn becomes infected, administer dicloxacillin, cephalexin, or erythromycin, and be certain to change all dressings daily. If a person sustains a serious burn that becomes infected after exposure to ocean water, administer ciprofloxacin or trimethoprim-sulfamethoxazole in addition to the other antibiotic chosen (above). Blisters that appear infected should be "unroofed" and drained, then covered with a proper dressing.

Tar Burn

If a victim is splashed with hot roofing tar or paving asphalt, immediately immerse the affected area in cool water to solidify the tar and limit the burn. If a small area is covered with tar and you cannot reach a physician, you can remove the tar by gently massaging it with repeated coatings of bacitracin or mupirocin ointment, or mayonnaise, which will turn brown as the tar dissolves into it. Do not injure the skin by attempting to roughly peel off the tar. After the tar is removed, treat the burn as described above. If you cannot dissolve the tar, cover the wound with bacitracin ointment or mupirocin ointment or cream, and a clean dressing.

INHALATION INJURIES

Inhalation injuries include thermal (heat) and chemical (smoke, noxious gas) inhalations. A third type of inhalation injury is aspiration (inhalation) of stomach contents; blood; and/or ocean, river, lake, or pool water into the lungs. The severity of the injury is determined by the chemical nature of the substance, temperature, volume of inhaled material, and underlying health of the victim. In a likely scenario, such as a boating accident or a seizure that occurred in the water, you must have a high index of suspicion for an inhalation injury. Drowning is discussed on page 360.

Thermal Injury

In thermal inhalation, the airway is injured by the introduction of super-heated air or steam. Such injuries almost always occur in an enclosed environment, although occasional mishaps occur in association with wildland fires (see page 288). Because water conducts heat approximately 30 times as efficiently as air, the risk of injury is far greater with steam than with dry superheated air.

The heat injures the inside of the mouth and nose, throat, vocal cords, trachea, bronchi, and occasionally lungs. External signs of an inhalation injury include burns of the face and mouth, singed nasal hairs, and soot in the mouth and nose. Symptoms include shortness of breath; wheezing; coughing (particularly of carbonaceous black sputum); raspy coarse breathing (stridor) noted most often during inspiration, with a barking quality that seems to originate in the neck; muffled voice; drooling; difficulty swallowing; swollen tongue; and agitation.

Once the burn injury has occurred, there is no effective way to limit its progress, so *the victim should be transported as rapidly as possible to an emergency facility*. If oxygen (see page 383) is available, it should be administered at a flow rate of 5 to 10 liters per minute by face mask. If the victim's condition deteriorates rapidly because the airway becomes swollen and obstructed, the only hope for survival is the placement of a tube directly through the vocal cords and into the trachea, or the creation of an air passage through the neck (tracheotomy).

Smoke (Chemical) Injury

Most smoke is composed of soot and various chemicals. Although each specific substance causes its own variation on the basic lung injury, the immediate first-aid approach is the same: Remove the victim from the offending agent, and *immediately administer oxygen* at a flow rate of 5 to 10 liters per minute (see page 383) by face mask. If the victim is having difficulty breathing or is without respirations, he should be supported with mouth-to-mouth breathing (see page 24). Difficulty in breathing may be delayed for a few hours after smoke inhalation, so a victim should seek immediate medical attention even if he feels fine initially.

The utmost caution must be exercised when removing a victim from the source of suspected toxic gases, so as not to create additional victims. Rescuers should wear gas masks if they are available. Carbon monoxide intoxication is discussed on page 291.

Aspiration Injury

Vomiting and inhalation of stomach contents is a common complication of severe hypothermia or drug overdose, and often follows head injury. The key factor is altered mental status, because a person who has a depressed level of consciousness does not protect his airway. In any situation in which a victim is unconscious and prone to vomit, *and the neck is known to be uninjured,* place the victim on his side so that vomitus and blood will drain from his mouth rather than into his lungs. If you suspect a neck injury, and the victim must be kept on his back with the neck immobilized, keep constant watch for vomiting. If the victim vomits, he must be quickly turned on a stretcher or backboard or logrolled (see page 34), and his mouth manually cleared of debris.

POISONING

See page 368.

ABDOMINAL PAIN

The causes of abdominal pain are myriad, but may be categorized by classical symptom complexes. As with most disorders, there are serious causes and minor disturbances. The purpose of taking a history and performing a physical examination is to determine the urgency of the situation, in order to plan for evacuation if necessary. Because differentiation between various causes is often difficult, the recommendations that follow are ultraconservative. Any person with severe abdominal pain should be seen by a physician as soon as possible.

General Evaluation

Obtain the following history:

1. *Nature of the pain.* Is the pain sharp (knifelike), aching (constant), colicky (intermittent and severe), or cramplike (squeezing)? Has the victim ever suffered a similar episode? Been given a specific diagnosis?
2. *Location of the pain.* Is the pain well localized to one particular area, or does it radiate to another region (from the back to the groin, for example)? Did the pain begin in one region and move to another?
3. *Mode of onset of the pain.* Did the pain occur suddenly or has it gradually increased in intensity? How long has the victim been in pain?
4. *Associated symptoms.* Is the victim short of breath, nauseated, vomiting, suffering from diarrhea or constipation, or dizzy? Is the victim vomiting blood, bile (green liquid produced by the gallbladder), or "coffee grounds" (blood darkened by stomach acid)? Does the vomit smell like feces?
5. *Relief of pain.* Is there a position that the victim can assume that will lessen the pain? Does the victim feel better in a quiet position, or is he agitated and constantly moving around?
6. *Menstrual history.* In the female victim, it is important to determine if there is any chance that the abdominal pain is related to a disorder of pregnancy.

Physical Examination

Perform the following physical examination:

1. Observe the victim. Note whether he is active or avoids movement. If possible, note the severity of distress when the victim has his

attention diverted (and so is not focusing all of his attention on your examination).

2. Note the victim's skin color, pulse rate and strength, rate of respirations, effort of breathing, mental status, and temperature. Abnormalities of any of these heighten the possibility of a serious problem.

3. Examine the abdomen. This is best done by having the victim lie quietly on his back, with his knees drawn up. Gently press on the abdomen, *proceeding from the area of least discomfort to the area of greatest discomfort.* For the purposes of examination, the abdomen can be divided by perpendicular lines through the navel into four quadrants: right upper, left upper, right lower, and left lower (figure 81). The epigastrium is the area of the abdomen directly below (not underneath) the breastbone in the midline. Note where the victim complains of pain and whether the pain is affected by your examination. If the victim has increased sharp pain when you suddenly release your hands from his abdomen after a pressing maneuver, this may indicate "rebound" pain associated with general inflammation of the lining of the abdominal cavity (peritonitis). Rebound pain may be caused by severe infection or leakage of blood or stomach/bowel contents into the abdominal (peritoneal) cavity, or other problems that are generally quite severe.

When a specific area of the abdomen is tender, there are certain disorders to consider:

Epigastrium. Heart attack, ulcer, gastroenteritis, heartburn, pancreatitis.
Right upper quadrant. Injured liver, hepatitis, gallstones, pneumonia.
Left upper quadrant. Injured spleen, gastroenteritis, pancreatitis, pneumonia.
Right lower quadrant. Appendicitis, kidney stone, ovarian infection, ectopic fallopian tube (tubal) pregnancy, colitis, bowel obstruction, hernia.
Left lower quadrant. Diverticulitis, colitis, kidney stone, ovarian infection, ectopic fallopian tube (tubal) pregnancy, bowel obstruction, hernia.
Lower abdomen (central). Abdominal aortic aneurysm, ovarian infection, ovulation disorder, ectopic fallopian tube (tubal) pregnancy, bladder infection, colitis, bowel obstruction.
Flank. Abdominal aortic aneurysm, kidney stone, kidney infection, pneumonia.

By quadrant, brief descriptions of and treatments for these disorders follow.

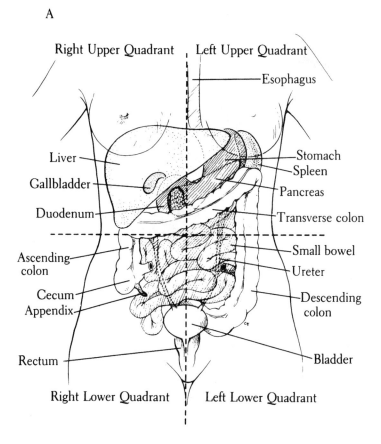

A

Right Upper Quadrant   Left Upper Quadrant

Esophagus

Liver
Gallbladder
Duodenum

Stomach
Spleen
Pancreas
Transverse colon

Ascending colon
Cecum
Appendix

Small bowel
Ureter

Descending colon

Rectum

Bladder

Right Lower Quadrant   Left Lower Quadrant

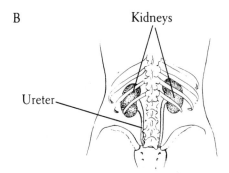

B   Kidneys

Ureter

Figure 81. Location of the abdominal organs. (A) View from the front, with the abdomen divided into four quadrants. (B) The kidneys are located posteriorly, and may be the cause of flank or back pain.

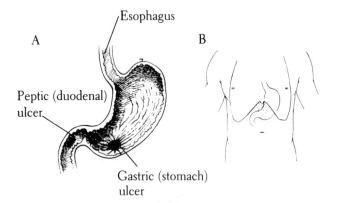

A

B

Esophagus

Peptic (duodenal) ulcer

Gastric (stomach) ulcer

Figure 82. Ulcers. (A) Location of ulcer craters in the duodenum and stomach. (B) Epigastric region of the abdomen, where ulcer pain is often noted.

Epigastrium

Heart Attack (See Page 45)

The symptoms of a heart attack can include pain that is located in the epigastrium, rather than in the chest. If the victim has a history of heart disease and complains of dull epigastric pain, nausea, shortness of breath, and weakness, consider the possibility of a heart attack. If you suspect a heart attack, even minimally, plan for immediate rescue or evacuation.

Ulcer (See Also Page 196)

An ulcer is an erosion in the lining of the stomach (gastric ulcer) or duodenum (peptic ulcer) that penetrates the protective mucous layer and allows acid and digestive juices to erode deeper into the tissues (figure 82). This causes extreme pain and can lead to bleeding from leaking blood vessels in the ulcer crater. Symptoms include constant burning pain in the epigastrium that is made worse by pressing and is often associated with nausea and/or belching. In a minor case, the pain may be relieved by a meal. In a severe case, when the ulcer has eroded into a blood vessel or has perforated the wall of the stomach or bowel, the victim will vomit red blood or dark brown clotted blood ("coffee grounds") and complain of pain that may radiate to his back. Rebound tenderness and peritonitis may be present. Dark black tarry bowel movements (melena) are caused by blood that has made its transit through the bowel. Bright red blood or blood clots with a bowel movement can be caused by brisk bleeding from an ulcer, but more commonly originate from bleeding that is occurring within the large intestine (colon) or from hemorrhoids (see page 193). Mild bleeding from an ulcer may actually transiently decrease the pain, because blood acts as an antacid. Some ulcers are caused by bacterial infection. To eradicate the bacteria and allow the ulcer to heal, a physician must prescribe specific, intense antibiotic therapy.

Gastroenteritis

Gastroenteritis is the "stomach flu" (see the discussion of diarrhea on page 183). Symptoms include waves of crampy upper and/or lower abdominal pain, followed by loose bowel movements. Nausea and vomiting may be present. Occasionally, the victim has symptoms of an upper-respiratory infection, with cough, runny nose, sore throat, headache, and fever. The treatment for viral gastroenteritis consists of a clear liquid diet (adequate hydration is the key to recovery—see page 286) and medicine for intractable vomiting (see page 195). When a victim vomits green bile, this should be taken as a sign that the problem is more serious than straightforward gastroenteritis, although bilious vomiting can occur with repetitive retching, when the stomach has been emptied and duodenal contents are all that is left for regurgitation.

Heartburn

See page 195.

Pancreatitis

The pancreas is an organ situated in the posterior upper abdomen that secretes a number of enzymes used to digest food. The pancreas also secretes insulin, the hormone that allows us to use and store glucose. The digestive enzymes travel from the pancreas through a duct, from which they are released through a small opening into the duodenum (the first portion of the bowel after the stomach). If the pancreas becomes inflamed, either by alcohol abuse (heavy drinking is far and away the most common cause), viral infection, or blockage of the main secretory duct by a gallstone, severe epigastric pain is the rule. This is accompanied by nausea and vomiting (which may contain bile). A person with pancreatitis needs to be hospitalized, because the most effective treatment is to eliminate oral intake for a time (to decrease stimulation of the pancreas). Out of the hospital, allow the victim clear liquids and antacids only, and pain medicine if pills can be kept down. Seek immediate physician care.

Right Upper Quadrant

Injured Liver

If a fall or blow to the abdomen, right flank, or right lower chest is followed by abdominal pain that is worsened by pressing on the right upper quadrant, a torn or bruised liver should be considered. The victim is at risk for severe internal bleeding and should be observed for signs of shock (see page 54). Evacuate him as soon as possible.

Hepatitis

See page 198.

Gallstones (Cholelithiasis)

Gallstones are formed in the gallbladder, which lies under the liver in the right upper quadrant of the abdomen. The gallbladder stores bile (manufactured in the liver), which is released into the duodenum to aid in digestion following each meal (figure 83). An attack of gallbladder inflammation (cholecystitis) occurs when the outlet from the gallbladder or the main bile duct into the duodenum becomes obstructed (usually by a gallstone) and the gallbladder cannot empty. This causes stretching of the gallbladder, inflammation, and painful contraction against an impenetrable passage. There is often an element of infection.

A typical attack occurs immediately after a meal and is sudden in onset. The pain is colicky and located in the right upper quadrant or epigastrium. It may be associated with nausea, vomiting, and fever. Occasionally, it radiates to the back or right shoulder. Examination of the abdomen demonstrates tenderness in the right upper quadrant. Occasionally, you can feel a tennis-ball-sized tender mass—the swollen gallbladder.

The definitive treatment for cholecystitis is removal of the gallbladder, although many surgeons prefer to "quiet down" the situation first with

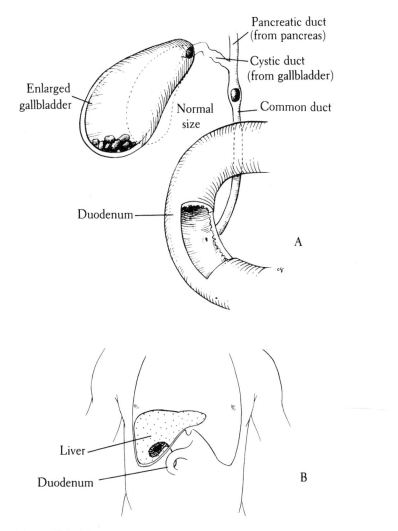

Figure 83. Gallbladder with gallstones. (A) The stones are formed in the gallbladder and travel through a narrow passageway (cystic and common ducts), which is easily blocked. (B) Location of the gallbladder adjacent to the liver in the right upper quadrant of the abdomen.

antibiotics, pain medicine, and intravenous fluids. The victim of a gallbladder attack should be transported to a hospital for evaluation. Pain medicines can be given safely, although certain narcotics may increase spasm of the bile passage and, paradoxically, briefly worsen pain. Solid foods (particularly fats) are prohibited during an attack. Maintain the victim on clear liquids and begin combination antibiotic therapy with ampicillin, amoxicillin, or amoxicillin-clavulanate combined with metronidazole, if pills can be kept down.

Pneumonia

See page 43.

Left Upper Quadrant

Injured Spleen

If a fall or blow to the abdomen, left flank, or left lower chest is followed by abdominal pain that is worsened by pressing on the left upper quadrant, consider a torn or bruised spleen. The victim is at risk for severe internal bleeding and should be observed for signs of shock (see page 54). Evacuate the victim as soon as possible.

Gastroenteritis

See page 109.

Pancreatitis

See page 109.

Pneumonia

See page 43.

Right Lower Quadrant

Appendicitis

The appendix is a small sausage-shaped bowel appendage, with no modern physiological function, that is located near the transition point

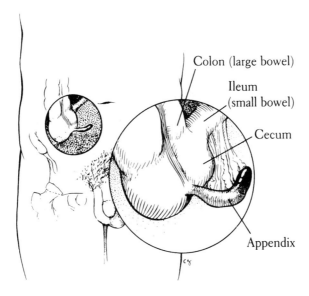

Figure 84. Appendicitis. Pain is felt in the right lower quadrant of the abdomen.

where the small bowel becomes the large bowel (colon) (figure 84). When it becomes obstructed or infected/inflamed (acute appendicitis), the victim typically has a history of crampy pain that begins in the central abdomen, then moves, over the course of a few hours, to become constant in the right lower quadrant. He may also suffer constipation or diarrhea, vomiting, fever, and weakness. There may be burning on urination if the appendix rests against a ureter carrying urine from the kidney to the bladder.

Examination of the abdomen demonstrates tenderness in the right lower quadrant. Frequently, the victim will resist any movement of the body or legs, because such movement causes abdominal pain. Rebound tenderness is associated with a swollen appendix that is ready to burst or has already ruptured. After the appendix ruptures, the pain may diminish considerably for a few days while an abscess forms. If you suspect appendicitis, transport the victim to a hospital for surgical evaluation. If transport will take more than 24 hours and the victim can tolerate oral fluids (is not actively vomiting), allow clear liquid intake to prevent dehydration. An antibiotic (cephalexin, amoxicillin-clavulanate, cefixime, or cefpodoxime) should be administered if more than 24 hours will elapse prior to arrival at a hospital.

Kidney Stone

See page 121.

Ovarian Infection (and Other Disorders of the Female Reproductive System)

See page 117.

Colitis

See page 192.

Bowel Obstruction

If the intestine becomes obstructed, by either scar tissue, cancer, injury, or feces, the victim rapidly becomes quite ill. Symptoms include nausea and vomiting, frequently of green bile or feculent (feceslike) material. The victim has waves of cramping pain associated with waves of bowel motion (contractions) that may be visible through the abdominal wall, which is often distended by the dilated loops of bowel. Occasionally, the victim will have small, squirting bowel movements, as a little liquid slips past the obstruction. If a bowel obstruction is suspected, the victim should be immediately evacuated to a hospital.

An ileus is functional inactivity (no food or fluid absorption, lack of normal peristalsis) of the bowel that leads to intestinal dilatation, vomiting, and abdominal pain. It commonly follows an intra-abdominal injury or physiological catastrophe (such as extensive burns, disseminated infection, or shock).

Hernia

If the intestine slips through the muscles of the abdominal wall, usually in the groin or around the umbilicus (navel), a hernia is formed (figure 85). Symptoms include a visible bulge, abdominal pain, and pain at the site of the hernia. The victim should be made to lie quietly on his back with his knees drawn up; place cold packs directly upon the bulge. Give pain medicine to control the discomfort. If sufficient relaxation is obtained, the hernia may slip back through the wall, and the bulge will disappear. Afterward, the victim should wear a support (truss or belt) to prevent recurrence until the problem can be corrected surgically. Straining and heavy lifting should be avoided.

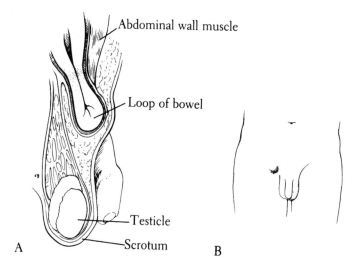

Figure 85. Inguinal (groin) hernia. (A) A loop of bowel bulges through a defect in the lower abdominal wall. (B) Location of external bulge. In some cases, the swelling extends into the scrotum.

If a victim has a painless hernia (bulge) that cannot be corrected, he should avoid straining, particularly when holding his breath, and seek the advice of a physician.

If the intestine will not slip back through, the hernia is trapped (incarcerated). This is an emergency, because if the blood supply to the bowel is pinched off, the tissue can be severely damaged or die, and/or a bowel obstruction (see page 114) can be created. An incarcerated hernia is extremely painful, and if the bowel is injured, the overlying skin frequently becomes reddened or dusky in appearance. Because the aforementioned maneuvers for reduction of a hernia will not be successful and pain will increase, the victim should be rapidly evacuated to a hospital.

Left Lower Quadrant

Diverticulitis

Diverticula are small outpouchings that develop at weak points along the wall of the colon (large bowel), probably because of high pressures associated with muscle contractions during the passage of stool. When these sacs become obstructed and/or inflamed (most frequently in middle-aged or elderly individuals), they enlarge and create pain and fever. Usually, the left lower quadrant is involved, because diverticula tend to form in the left-side portion of the colon (descending colon) more frequently than in the right-side portion (ascending colon) or horizontal connecting section (transverse colon). A ruptured diverticulum can cause a clinical picture much like that of a ruptured appendix (see page 112), with pain in the left side of the abdomen instead of the right side. The victim should seek medical attention, and his diet be limited to clear fluids. An antibiotic (amoxicillin-clavulanate alone or metronidazole with cefixime or cefpodoxime) should be administered if help is more than 24 hours away.

Colitis

See page 192.

Kidney Stone

See page 121.

Ovarian Infection (and Other Disorders of the Female Reproductive System)

See page 117.

Bowel Obstruction

See page 114.

Hernia

See page 114.

Lower Abdomen (Central)

Abdominal Aortic Aneurysm

An aneurysm is a dilated blood vessel that has been weakened by the ravages of age, high blood pressure, and atherosclerosis (figure 86). At a certain point, the wear and tear become too much and the blood vessel rips, causing either a slow leak or rapid massive bleeding that leads to sudden

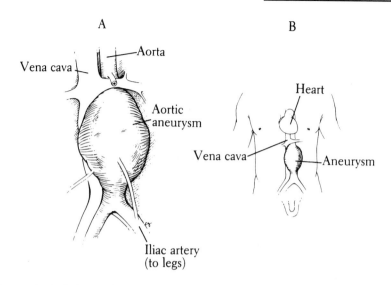

Figure 86. Abdominal aortic aneurysm. (A) Age, high blood pressure, and disease ravage the dilated aorta. (B) Location of the aorta in the abdomen. Leaking or rupture causes pain in the abdomen, back, and flank.

collapse and death. This generally occurs spontaneously only in the elderly, unless there is a congenital defect; traumatic tears of the aorta occur in all age groups.

The aorta is the large artery that carries blood from the left ventricle of the heart to the body. The symptoms of a ruptured abdominal aortic aneurysm are intense, unrelenting, ripping pain in the abdomen that may radiate to the back or chest; weakness; discoloration of the legs with mottling; and rapid collapse. Gentle examination of the abdomen may demonstrate a pulsating, expanding mass. Abdominal rigidity is due to the rapid accumulation of blood.

Any elderly person who suddenly develops abdominal pain or back pain associated with weakness, a fainting spell, decreased sensation and/or abnormal color in the legs or feet (even if transient), or shortness of breath should be immediately rushed to a hospital. In the best of circumstances, this is a highly critical situation. Be prepared to treat the victim for shock (see page 54).

Ovarian Infection

The ovaries and fallopian tubes (see figures 87 and 88), which carry eggs from the ovaries to the uterus, may become infected, commonly with the

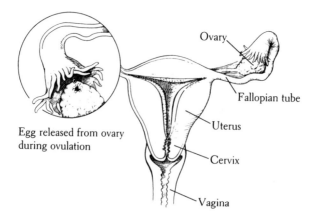

Figure 87. Female reproductive tract.

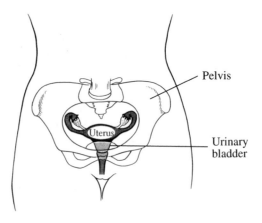

Figure 88. Location of female reproductive tract within the pelvis.

bacteria that cause gonorrhea (a form of venereal disease) or by other infectious agents, such as *Chlamydia trachomatis*. Symptoms include abdominal pain in the lower quadrants (greatest on the side of the affected ovary), fever, shaking, chills, nausea, vomiting, and weakness. Occasionally, the victim will complain of a yellow-greenish vaginal discharge. If you suspect an infection, take the victim to a hospital immediately. If more than 24 hours will pass before a doctor can be reached, the victim should be started on tetracycline 500 mg four times a day, or doxycycline 100 mg two times a day, for 10 days (to treat *Chlamydia*). Azithromycin 1 g in a single dose is also effective against chlamydial infection. If you suspect gonorrhea, administer cefixime 400 mg orally as a single dose (for other single-dose therapies for gonorrhea, see page 262). To treat gonorrhea and chlamydial infection at the same time (the two germs often "travel" together), administer azithromycin in a 2 g single dose (again, see page 262).

Ovulation, Ovarian Cyst, and Torsed (Twisted) Ovary

Some women suffer intense sudden abdominal pain at the time of ovulation (when the egg is released from the ovary) (figure 87). This is caused by a small amount of blood and ovarian fluid, which irritates the lining of the abdomen. Symptoms include pain that suddenly develops in the right or left lower quadrant, and is worsened by movement or deep palpation of the area. Treatment is pain medicine and rest. A ruptured ovarian cyst (which releases tissue fluid or blood) or torsed (twisted) ovary causes similar but much more severe symptoms, which may include excruciating pain, nausea and vomiting, and a rigid (to the pressing hand) abdomen. Any of these conditions may be difficult to distinguish from appendicitis (see page 112) if the right ovary is involved. Treatment for a torsed ovary may require surgery. *Any sudden abdominal discomfort in a woman of childbearing age should be promptly evaluated by a physician.*

Bleeding from the Vagina

If bleeding from the vagina accompanied by abdominal pain is not clearly part of a normal menstrual period, a woman should seek prompt medical attention. If the bleeding is clearly part of a normal menstrual period, and the pain is unquestionably due to menstrual cramps, the victim may benefit from the administration of a nonsteroidal anti-inflammatory drug.

If abnormal (in amount or character) pain and/or bleeding occurs during or between menstrual periods, the cause should be determined by a physician. Until the evaluation is performed, exertion should be kept to a minimum. If periods have been missed (or if the victim is known to be pregnant) and copious vaginal bleeding develops, place the victim at rest and transport her rapidly—by litter, if possible—to a physician. If the bleeding is spotty, the victim may walk with assistance. A ruptured tubal (ectopic) pregnancy can rapidly become life threatening. In this situation, a pregnancy situated in a fallopian tube (rather than in the uterus) causes the tube to rupture. The symptoms include vaginal bleeding, lower abdominal pain (which can become severe), and signs of shock (see page 54). This is a true medical emergency.

Vaginitis

Vaginitis is a condition of irritation and inflammation of the vagina, commonly noted as a secondary condition that follows administration of an antibiotic, such as ampicillin, to a woman. The antibiotic alters the normal bacterial population of the vagina and allows overgrowth of the causative (for vaginitis) agent, which is often yeast. With a *Candida albicans* yeast (candidiasis or moniliasis) infection, the victim notes a white and creamy or curdy ("cottage cheese") discharge, vulvar and vaginal itching and redness, and burning pain on urination. She should use clotrimazole (Gyne-Lotrimin). Administer vaginal 100 mg tablets once a day for 7 days, or twice a day for 3 days; a vaginal 500 mg tablet for 1 day (single dose); or 1% cream in a 5 g dose for 7 to 14 days. An alternative drug is miconazole nitrate (Monistat); administer 100 mg vaginal suppositories once a day for 7 days, 200 mg vaginal suppositories once a day for 3 days, 1,200 mg vaginal suppository one dose, or 2% cream in a 5 g dose for 7 days. Other acceptable treatments are a single fluconazole (Diflucan) 150 mg tablet by mouth; tioconazole 6.5% (Vagistat-1) ointment in a single 5 g application; butoconazole nitrate 2% (Femstat) cream in a 5 g dose for 3 days; and terconazole (Terazol) vaginal cream 0.8% in a 5 g dose once a day for 3 days, vaginal cream 0.4% in a 5 g dose once a day for 7 days, or vaginal suppositories 80 mg once a day for 3 days.

If the infection is due to trichomoniasis (caused by *Trichomonas vaginalis*), the victim will suffer a frothy white-gray discharge and may also have abdominal pain and fever. In such a case, the antibiotic of choice is metronidazole 250 mg three times a day, or 375 mg two times a day, for 7 days. If metronidazole is in short supply, administer 2 g in a single dose. Do not drink alcohol while taking metronidazole or for 3 days thereafter. The male sex partner should be treated with metronidazole 2 g in a single dose.

If a woman has a thin whitish discharge without the curdy appearance typical of a yeast infection, and with more vulvovaginal irritation than abdominal pain, the cause may be an infection with *Gardnerella* species (bacterial "vaginosis"). Treatment should be started with 0.5 or 0.75% metronidazole vaginal gel (such as MetroGel-Vaginal) twice a day for 5 days, or oral metronidazole 500 mg twice a day for 7 days. An alternative is clindamycin phosphate (Cleocin) 2% vaginal cream 5 g at bedtime for 7 days.

Upon return to civilization, an appropriate gynecological exam should be sought to exclude other causes of vaginal infection, which include herpes simplex virus, *Neisseria gonorrhoeae* (the causative agent of gonorrhea), and *Chlamydia trachomatis.*

Bladder Infection

See page 258.

Colitis

See page 192.

Bowel Obstruction

See page 114.

Flank

Abdominal Aortic Aneurysm

See page 116.

Kidney Stone

A kidney stone originates in the urine-collecting system of the kidney, and most commonly causes pain when it travels down the ureter to the bladder (see figure 89). After traversing the bladder, it may enter the urethra and continue to wreak havoc.

The pain of a kidney stone is usually sudden in onset and often becomes intolerable. The location of the pain is related to the location of the stone. If the stone is high in the ureter, the pain localizes to the victim's back (on the affected side), with some radiation to the abdomen. Lightly tapping over the flank and lower ribs on the back of a victim with a kidney stone will often cause extreme pain. If the stone is passing through the lower ureter, the victim will have extreme pain in the back, abdomen, and genitals. When the stone is not moving, the pain (renal "colic") may disappear as quickly as it began.

A victim who is passing a kidney stone finds no relief from remaining motionless, and will appear quite agitated, constantly changing positions.

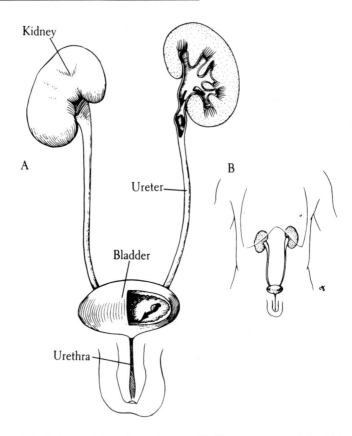

Figure 89. Kidney with kidney stones. (A) The stones are formed in the kidney and travel through the ureter, bladder, and urethra before they are passed in the urine. (B) Location of the genitourinary (urogenital) system.

Associated symptoms include nausea, vomiting, bloody urine, pain on urination, and sweating.

If the diagnosis of a kidney stone appears relatively certain, give the victim the strongest pain medicine that is available and encourage him to drink copious amounts of fluid. Seek physician evaluation as soon as possible. *If the victim is elderly, consider the diagnosis of ruptured aortic aneurysm* (see page 116). If you have any suspicion that the victim might have an aneurysm, evacuate him immediately.

Kidney Infection

See page 259.

Pneumonia

See page 43.

EMERGENCY CHILDBIRTH

When a woman is ready to give birth, the contractions of labor are usually intense and uninterrupted, or separated by intervals of less than 3 to 5 minutes. If the child to be born is not the woman's first, labor can progress very quickly, so don't wait until the last minute to set up. On the other hand, don't deliver a baby in the woods if it isn't necessary. If the child is the mother's first, if the contractions are more than 5 minutes apart, if the waters have not "broken" (a gush of fluid from the ruptured amniotic sac) and there has been no passage of bloody mucus, and if no bulging is present in the vaginal area, consider whether you have time to make it to the hospital. If the waters have broken and labor has not begun, it is best to evacuate the mother, because delivery must occur or be induced within 24 hours to avoid the onset of an infection that could jeopardize the infant and mother. *If the umbilical cord or any other part of the infant other than the head is showing at the vagina, the delivery will be difficult and should be performed if at all possible by a skilled obstetrician.*

If delivery is imminent (the mother wishes to push) and you are outdoors, spread a towel or blanket. The birthing process is fairly messy, so don't expect to salvage the ground cloth. Wear sterile latex rubber gloves from your first-aid kit. If you are allergic to latex, use other nonpermeable gloves (such as nonlatex synthetic). If you don't have gloves, wash your hands with soap and water. Have the following supplies ready: four towels for drapes; two sturdy strings to tie the umbilical cord; a sharp scissors, scalpel, or knife to cut the umbilical cord; a towel to dry the baby; a blanket to wrap the baby; a rubber suction bulb for the baby's mouth and nose; and a large plastic bag to carry the placenta.

Have the mother undress below the waist and cover her with a blanket or sheet. She should lie on her side between contractions until she feels she is ready to push. When she wants to push, have her lie on her back with her legs spread as far apart as possible. Place a towel (drape) over each thigh, across the abdomen, and under the buttocks to "frame" the vagina.

It is extremely helpful to elevate the buttocks with a folded blanket or pile of towels. This is because the most difficult part of a normal birth is

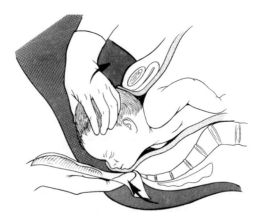

Figure 90. Appearance of the head and face during childbirth.

delivery of the upper shoulder, which is facilitated by pushing the infant downward at the proper time.

When the mother is undergoing a contraction, and you see some wrinkled skin and a wisp of hair from the infant's head showing in her vagina, have the mother grab behind her legs and pull them up toward her head, or plant her feet firmly, while she bears down (like having a bowel movement) and pushes. This may go on while the vaginal entrance stretches to accommodate the infant's head. If the fluid-filled, transparent amniotic sac is bulging out in front of the infant's head, it can be nicked with a sharp blade or scissors to allow the fluid to be released and the delivery to proceed. Do not do this unless you are absolutely certain that the childbirth will occur away from a hospital. A mother may prefer to squat during delivery, but this makes assisting her more awkward.

During a push, put one hand gently on the infant's head and another underneath his head, providing countertraction against the woman's perineum (the area between the anus and the vaginal opening) to allow gradual stretching of the opening and to then assist delivery of the head and control the speed of delivery. You do not want the head to "pop out," to avoid a large tear in the vagina.

A baby is delivered in (ideally) two stages. First, the head and face appear, usually with the face down (figure 90). Once the infant has appeared to the level of his eyebrows, instruct the mother to stop pushing. The baby will be extremely slippery. When his face appears, run your fingers around the infant's neck to see if the umbilical cord is wrapped around it. If it is, see if you can slip it over the head. If not, tie (clamp) it off tightly twice, with about 1½" (3.8 cm) between ties, and cut carefully

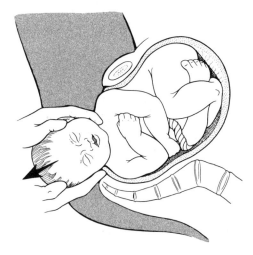

Figure 91. Gentle downward pressure to deliver upper shoulder.

between the ties. The ties must be tight and not slip off, or the baby could suffer severe bleeding.

In the moment between the delivery of the head and the beginning of shoulders' emergence, support the head with one hand and gently wipe the face with a clean cloth. Gently suction the nose, using the bulb syringe, by squeezing the air out, placing the tip in each nostril, and letting the bulb inflate. Squirt out any extracted material before each insertion of the tip. Suction each nostril at least twice, then suction out the mouth. If a device for suction isn't available, wipe out as much amniotic fluid as you can with a finger, tissue, or cloth.

The baby's head and body will spontaneously rotate 90 degrees (don't twist them) to one side as the body starts to emerge. Have the mother resume pushing. While supporting the head, grasp the uppermost (with respect to the ground) shoulder and apply gentle downward pressure until the upper shoulder is delivered from the vagina (figure 91). Don't tug on the head or pull from underneath the infant's armpits. After the upper shoulder is out, exert gentle upward pressure to free the lower shoulder (see figure 92). At this point, be prepared to hang on tight, because the rest of the baby will shoot out, usually with a big gush of amniotic fluid and some blood.

Hold the baby in a towel or blanket and dry him. Hold him firmly by the ankles, but don't dangle him upside down. If you have not already done so, tie (clamp) the umbilical cord with two ties (preferably sterile— dipped in boiling water, for example), one at 6" (15 cm) and one at 8"

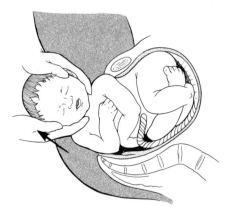

Figure 92. Gentle upward pressure to deliver lower shoulder.

(20 cm) from the child. Use cord that won't slip a knot, shoelace material, or cotton tape. Cut carefully between the ties. Suction the baby's mouth and nose (newborns are nose breathers) again, and stimulate him by rubbing with a towel until he begins to cry. Wrap the child in a blanket and hand him to the mother to hold. The mother may begin to breast-feed at this point.

The long end of the umbilical cord, which is still attached to the placenta that is attached to the inside wall of the uterus, will be hanging from the mother's vagina. The placenta will deliver spontaneously, so do not pull on the umbilical cord. Do not massage the mother's abdomen (uterus) until after the placenta is delivered. Place the placenta in a plastic bag and bring it to civilization for inspection. After the placenta is delivered, gently massage the mother's abdomen for 30 minutes. This stimulates the uterus to contract and helps control bleeding. It will feel like a firm, rounded, grapefruit-sized mass in the middle of the lower abdomen just above the pubic bone. If bleeding starts again, massage more vigorously. You may have to repeat this a few times during the hours immediately following childbirth. It may be uncomfortable for the mother.

If bleeding seems profuse after the placenta is delivered, or if the placenta does not spontaneously deliver after 60 minutes, be prepared to treat for shock (see page 54).

If the vagina is torn, apply pressure with a sterile compress. After the bleeding slows, the vaginal area can be gently washed, with the mother on her back, so that rinse water flows away from the vagina toward the anus. Take care to keep any contaminating material or solutions out of the vagina. Lay a sterile compress or clean sanitary napkin over the vagina.

After a wilderness birth, administer an antibiotic (cephalexin, amoxicillin–clavulanate, or erythromycin) to the mother for 48 hours.

Complicated Deliveries

Breech Delivery

In a breech delivery, the infant's buttocks and legs come out first. Let him deliver spontaneously (do not pull) until the level of his umbilicus (where the umbilical cord attaches) appears. At this point, take a firm hold on the baby's pelvis and apply gentle traction. Do not pull on his legs or back.

Determine which shoulder is lower, and try to swing the baby's body to the other side to allow that shoulder to exit the vagina. Gently move him to the opposite side to deliver the other shoulder. Don't let go of the baby. If the first shoulder won't deliver, you may need to reach inside the vagina with two fingers to locate one of the infant's arms and swing it down across his anterior chest, so that the hand and forearm are delivered. Repeat this procedure for the second arm.

Position the baby so that his face is down. With one hand tightly holding the baby by his ankles, slide your other hand underneath him and slip your middle finger into the vagina, then into the baby's mouth for a grip. During a contraction, when the mother is pushing, extract the baby. If the extraction takes a few minutes, let the baby rest on your forearm with your finger in his mouth and his arms and legs dangling on either side, and use your other hand to push the vaginal tissues away from his face.

Prolapsed Umbilical Cord; Single Arm or Foot

A prolapsed umbilical cord occurs when the cord falls out of the vagina and becomes trapped between the baby and the opening. This can be a catastrophe, because if the cord is pinched and obstructed, the blood supply to the baby will be interrupted.

Turn the mother on her side or have her kneel in the knee-to-chest position and try to interrupt labor. Do not encourage pushing. Place a moistened (with disinfected saline, preferably) towel over the cord and vagina and expedite an emergency evacuation of the mother from the wilderness. If the delivery continues, try to have it occur without undue delay. Do your best to keep the head from compressing the cord.

If a single arm or foot hangs out of the vagina, have the mother kneel in the knee-to-chest position and try to get her to a hospital as quickly as possible.

DIABETES

Diabetes mellitus is a disorder in which the pancreas cannot create sufficient insulin (Type I or insulin dependent) and/or in which insulin is not effective (Type II or non–insulin dependent). Insulin allows the body to use and store sugar; in the diabetic state, the victim suffers from high blood sugar and an array of physiological derangements (kidney failure, skin ulcers, bleeding into the vitreous of the eye) associated with deterioration of small blood vessels. Many diabetics need to take insulin by injection to manage the disease; others can control their blood sugar by diet and/or oral medications (hypoglycemic agents).

The most common dangerous acute situation incurred by a diabetic is a hypoglycemic reaction (low blood sugar) induced by an inadvertent overdose of insulin, or after a normal dose of insulin or glucose-lowering agent accompanied by extraordinary exercise or insufficient food intake. The manifestations of an insulin reaction are weakness, sweating, hunger, abdominal pain, and altered mental status (which may include confusion, belligerent behavior, fainting, seizures, or coma). The solution is to administer sugar as rapidly as possible. If the victim is unconscious, it is generally prohibited to administer anything by mouth, because of the danger of choking and aspiration of food or fluid into the lungs. However, sugar granules or concentrated liquid glucose (Glutose: one tube contains 25 g) can be inserted under the tongue, to dissolve and be passively swallowed. Otherwise, sterile glucose solution must be injected intravenously, which obviously requires a trained individual. If the victim is awake and capable of swallowing, a naturally sweetened solution (apple or orange juice, sugar-containing soft drink), banana, or candy bar (chocolate, sugar cube) should be eaten. As soon as the victim feels better, he should eat a meal, in order to avoid a recurrence.

It is important that anyone who suffers from diabetes wear appropriate identification, in case he requires assistance. No one who is insulin dependent should attempt physical exertion in a dangerous environment without adequate glucose intake. Even a person taking an oral hypoglycemic drug, such as micronized glyburide or glipizide, should be similarly cautious.

If the blood sugar gets dangerously high, the diabetic may become very ill, because the blood becomes acidotic with the by-products of metabolism (known as ketones), dehydration increases, and body chemistries become unbalanced. Such a patient is confused, combative, or comatose. His breathing rate increases, breathing becomes shallow, and exhaled breaths have a fruity or acetone (like fingernail polish remover) odor. Because of dehydration, the skin is very dry and there is little sweating (dry armpits). Such a clinical picture calls for immediate transport of the victim to the hospital. If he can drink, he should be encouraged to force unsweetened fluids. The definitive treatment for ketoacidosis is intravenous fluids and insulin injections, which must be carefully dosed according to the measured blood sugar level.

If you cannot differentiate between an insulin reaction (low blood sugar) and altered mental status due to excessively high blood sugar, you should err on the side of predicting a hypoglycemic episode and give the victim something sweet to eat or drink. If you have guessed correctly, the improvement will be dramatic; if your diagnosis was wrong, the extra sugar will not cause any significant harm. If a diabetic person is carrying a blood glucose monitor (such as FastTake, Accu-Chek, or SureStep), be sure you are instructed in its proper use before you need to use it.

If a person with diabetes develops a skin infection, particularly if it is on the foot, an appropriate antibiotic choice is dicloxacillin, amoxicillin-clavulanate, or ciprofloxacin.

STROKE

A stroke is caused by a blood clot that blocks an artery supplying part of the brain, or by bleeding from a leaking vessel into the brain. It occurs suddenly and can be minor or major, depending on the area and amount of the brain involved. If a stroke involves the brain stem, it may affect the breathing center and cause rapid death.

Symptoms include sudden headache, nausea, vomiting, blurred or double vision, weakness or paralysis of the arms and/or legs, difficulty speaking or understanding speech, difficulty walking, dizziness, confusion, loss of consciousness, coma, seizure, and collapse. If someone has stroke symptoms that last for a few minutes to an hour and then gradually resolve, he has suffered a transient ischemic attack (TIA), which is a warning that he may soon suffer a full-blown stroke. Even if stroke symptoms are fleeting, the victim should see a physician as soon as possible.

A rapid simple neurological examination may reveal subtle changes indicative of a stroke. This exam consists of the following:

Mental status. Ask the victim his name, age, and location, as well as time, day, and year.

Vision. Have the victim count fingers that you display. Check each eye by itself and then both eyes together. Check that the pupils are equal. Ask the victim to follow a moving object with his eyes.

Facial muscles. Ask the victim to pucker his lips, and then to whistle. Check the cheeks and mouth for symmetry. Have the victim clench his jaw while you feel the jaw muscles on each side. Have the victim tightly close his eyes. Have him relax with his eyes closed; lightly touch his face to locate any numb spots.

Hearing. Make a soft noise (yet loud enough that you can hear it) in each of the victim's ears.

Swallowing and speech. Ask the victim to swallow. Ask him to stick his tongue out and move it from side to side voluntarily. Listen carefully to note if his speech is clear or slurred.

Muscle strength. Have the victim squeeze one of your fingers with each hand, straighten each leg against resistance, bend each leg against resistance, bend and straighten each elbow and wrist against resistance, extend and flex each ankle against resistance, and shrug both shoulders against resistance.

Sensation. Using a light touch, move your fingers over the entire body and try to identify any areas of decreased sensation.

Coordination. Ask the victim to stand perfectly still in an upright position with his eyes closed and his arms at his sides. Be prepared to catch him if he begins to fall. Ask him to clap one hand into the palm of the other as fast as possible. Ask him to move an index finger back and forth between the tip of his nose and your finger, held 18" (46 cm) away. Have him walk heel to toe and on tiptoes.

If someone displays the symptoms of a stroke, he should be placed at absolute rest with his upper body and head elevated by an angle of at least 30 degrees. If his level of consciousness declines, pay attention to his airway (see page 17) so that he does not vomit and choke. Seek immediate medical attention. Remember that low blood sugar may cause symptoms that mimic a stroke. If the victim can swallow purposefully without choking, sugar granules or concentrated liquid glucose (Glutose: one tube contains 25 g) can be inserted under the tongue, to dissolve and be passively swallowed (see page 128).

If stroke symptoms are associated with scuba diving, they might indicate an air embolism (see page 355). In this case, the victim needs to be transported in a head-up and/or left-side-down position and delivered to a recompression chamber as soon as possible.

INFECTIOUS DISEASES

Foreign travel is increasingly a component of the wilderness experience, and thus American travelers are exposed to numerous diseases that are not indigenous to the United States. In addition, domestic outdoor activities expose us to the vectors (carriers, such as mosquitoes or ticks) and microorganisms that generate diseases such as malaria, Rocky Mountain spotted fever, and Lyme disease. People who handle wild animals or ingest animal products are at increased risk. This section addresses some of the more common and worrisome infectious diseases associated with outdoor activities. Immunizations are discussed on page 397.

Recommendations for drugs to treat these diseases are based on current literature. These recommendations may change—and some undoubtedly will, because new and better treatments are being discovered, organisms can acquire resistance to certain chemical agents, and toxic side effects to certain drugs will be revealed. It is important for physicians and laypeople who will assume responsibility for treating others to remain informed about current therapies.

Malaria

Malaria is caused by infection with one of four microscopic parasites: *Plasmodium falciparum, P. vivax, P. malariae,* or *P. ovale.* These are transmitted in the wild by the bite of an infected *Anopheles* mosquito. Most cases of malaria acquired by U.S. citizens are contracted in sub-Saharan Africa; most of the remainder are linked to travel in Southeast Asia, Central and South America, the Indian subcontinent, the Middle East, and Oceania.

When an infected mosquito bites a human, it releases malaria sporozoites (an immature form of the parasite), which mature in the liver to become merozoites, and then invade red blood cells. From these locations, the organisms can penetrate the vital organs, such as the brain, lungs, liver, and kidneys. The incubation period between acquisition of the parasites and the onset of symptoms is 8 to 40 days, depending on the species. Typical symptoms include a flulike illness, with headache, chills, sweats, fatigue, loss of appetite, muscle aches, nausea, and vomiting. These are soon followed by episodes of headache, intense chills, high fever, and sweating. Jaundice and anemia may occur. The episodes last 1 to 8 hours and are separated by 2 to 3 days.

Those infected with falciparum malaria may be significantly more ill, with episodes of fever and chills at closer intervals and lasting for more than 30 hours. Severe malaria can be fatal or lead to anemia, heart and kidney failure, and/or coma; untreated infections can cause recurrent illness for years.

Identification of the specific plasmodium is accomplished by observing the parasites under the microscope in blood smears. People infected with *P. falciparum* are treated with quinine sulfate in combination with pyrimethamine-sulfadoxine (Fansidar) or tetracycline. In recent studies, artemether (an artemisinin, or *quinghaosu*, derivative) has been shown to be as effective as quinine in the treatment of severe *P. falciparum* malaria. A person infected with *P. vivax, P. malariae,* or *P. ovale* is treated with chloroquine and primaquine phosphate.

Unfortunately, there is not yet a useful vaccine against malaria. Avoidance of mosquito bites is key to prevention. Because the *Anopheles* mosquito tends to feed during the evening and nighttime, it is particularly important to sleep under nets or screens; spray living quarters (with, for instance, a pyrethrin-containing product) and clothing (with, for example, permethrin 0.5%, Duranon, or Permanone; or concentrated Perma-Kill 4 Week Tick Killer, diluted and applied to clothing); and wear adequate clothing and insect repellent (N,N-diethyl-3-methylbenzamide, called DEET) at these times (see page 453).

If you travel to a region where *P. falciparum* is resistant to chloroquine and pyrimethamine-sulfadoxine, then prophylaxis (prevention) can be accomplished with mefloquine. The adult dose is 250 mg (salt) weekly. The pediatric dose varies according to the weight of the child: weight 15 to 19 kg, 63 mg; weight 20 to 30 kg, 125 mg; weight 31 to 45 kg, 188 mg; and over 45 kg, 250 mg. (For estimating purposes, 1 kg equals 2.2 lb.) Mefloquine should be started 1 to 2 weeks before travel, then administered once a week during travel in malarious areas and for 4 weeks after you leave such areas. Mefloquine should not be taken during pregnancy.

An alternative drug for travelers who cannot take mefloquine is doxycycline (the adult dose is 100 mg a day beginning 1 to 2 days prior to travel and continuing for 5 to 6 weeks after; the pediatric dose for those aged more than 8 years is 2 mg per kg of body weight a day, up to the adult dose). Doxycycline is not advised for pregnant women or children under the age of 8 years, and may cause increased skin sensitivity to sunlight.

A final alternative drug prophylaxis against malaria is chloroquine phosphate (the adult dose is 300 mg of the base once a week; the pediatric dose, 5 mg per kg of the base, up to the adult dose, once a week), which should be taken 1 to 2 weeks before you enter a malarious region and continued until 1 month after your journey. Chloroquine is recommended for travelers, particularly pregnant women and children who weigh less than 33 lb (15 kg), who cannot take mefloquine or doxycycline. If you use chloroquine for prophylaxis, you should also carry three tablets of Fansidar to be taken in the event of a flulike illness or other unexplained fever, assuming the absence of an allergy to sulfonamide antibiotics.

Proguanil (Paludrine) is a drug that may be used for antimalarial prophylaxis in areas where *P. falciparum* is resistant to chloroquine. The drug is available without prescription in parts of Europe, Scandinavia, and Africa, but is as yet unavailable in the United States. It is administered in an adult dose of 200 mg daily (pediatric dose: under 2 years, 50 mg; age 2 to 6 years, 100 mg; age 7 to 10 years, 150 mg; over 10 years, 200 mg), along with weekly chloroquine (the latter to protect against other forms of malaria). It can be used by those who will spend more than 3 weeks in rural areas of East Africa (particularly Kenya and Tanzania), but does not appear to be useful in Papua New Guinea, West Africa, or Thailand.

Pyrimethamine plus dapsone (drug combination: Maloprim) is prescribed in many malaria-endemic regions outside the United States. This drug cannot be used by pregnant women; it can also cause bone marrow suppression.

If you are stricken with malaria in an area where the malaria organism(s) is felt to be sensitive to chloroquine, but you have not been taking prophylaxis, begin treatment with chloroquine (adult dose, 600 mg of the base immediately, followed with 300 mg at 6 hours and once a day on days 2 and 3; pediatric dose, 10 mg per kg of body weight [up to 600 mg] of the base immediately, followed by 5 mg per kg at 6 hours and once a day on days 2 and 3). In a region where *P. falciparum* is resistant to chloroquine, administer quinine sulfate (adult dose, 650 mg every 8 hours for 3 days; pediatric dose, 8 mg per kg [up to 650 mg] every 8 hours for 3 days) *plus* tetracycline (adult dose, 250 mg four times a day for 7 days; pediatric dose, 5 mg per kg [up to 250 mg] four times a day for 7 days) or Fansidar (adult dose, 3 tablets; pediatric dose: weight 5 to 10 kg, ½ tablet; weight 11 to 20 kg, 1 tablet; weight 21 to 30 kg, 1½ tablets; weight 31 to 45 kg, 2 tablets; weight over 45 kg, 3 tablets. For purposes of estimation, 1 kg equals 2.2 lb.). *In any case of suspected malaria, seek the advice of a physician as soon as possible.*

Halofantrine (Halfan) is used to treat chloroquine-resistant *P. falciparum* infections in a dose of 500 mg every 6 hours for three doses, with repeat therapy in 7 days.

To determine the malaria risk within a specific country and to learn of the most recent recommendations for prophylaxis and drug therapy, you can call the Malaria Hotline sponsored by the Centers for Disease Control in Atlanta at (404) 332–4555.

Yellow Fever

Yellow fever is a viral disease transmitted in the jungle by mosquitoes of the genus *Haemogogus* and in urban areas by the *Aedes aegypti* mosquito. "Jungle" yellow fever is seen in forest-savanna zones of tropical Africa, parts of Central America, forested areas of South America, and Trinidad. The "urban" variety is seen in South America and West Africa. The disease has not yet been noted in Asia.

The illness begins 3 to 6 days after the culprit mosquito bite(s). Symptoms include sudden onset of fever, headache, red eyes, muscle aching, nausea, and vomiting. These symptoms last for 3 to 4 days, after which there may be 12 to 24 hours of remission. Soon thereafter comes an "intoxication phase," in which the seriously stricken victim develops fever, skin rashes, altered mental status, low blood pressure, and liver and kidney failure. In such cases, the victim becomes jaundiced (hence, "yellow" fever) and bleeds easily. The disease can be fatal. Treatment is supportive and based upon symptoms. Because of the bleeding problems, do not use aspirin to control fever.

Since yellow fever is so difficult to treat, it is essential to use yellow fever vaccine and mosquito control measures (see page 132). A live-virus vaccine is available. A single injection induces immunity after 10 days that is adequate for 10 years (see page 400).

Dengue Fever

Dengue fever is a viral disease transmitted by *Aedes albopictus* and female *A. aegypti* mosquitoes. The most active feeding times for these mosquitoes is for a few hours after daybreak and in the afternoon for a few hours just after dark. As opposed to the night-feeding mosquitoes that transmit malaria, these species tend to be "urban," may also feed during daylight hours (also indoors, in the shade, and during an overcast), and are known to bite below the waist. Dengue fever is seen chiefly in the Caribbean and South America, as well as other tropical and semitropical areas, such as Southeast Asia, Africa, and Mexico. In the United States, cases have been noted in Texas. The larvae flourish in artificial water containers, often in a domestic environment.

The incubation period following a mosquito bite is 2 to 8 days. The disease is self-limited (5 to 7 days) and characterized by a sudden onset of severe headache, fever, chills, muscle aches, sore throat, reddened eyes, bone and joint pain ("breakbone fever"), and a fine, red, itchy skin rash that typically appears simultaneously with the fever on the proximal arms, legs, and trunk (it spares the face, palms, and soles). It may then spread to the face, and farther out on the arms and legs. Although the fever usually remits spontaneously, an occasional victim will relapse. Children under 1 year of age appear to be particularly vulnerable to especially severe forms of dengue virus infection, associated with severe bleeding problems that can lead to extremely low blood pressure (shock—see page 54).

Treatment is supportive and based upon symptoms. There is no vaccine available against dengue fever. Insect repellents (particularly those containing DEET; see page 347) are critical for prevention.

Relapsing Fever

The sporadic (in occurrence) form of relapsing fever is caused by various borrelial organisms transmitted by argasid (soft) ticks of multiple *Ornithodoros* species. For instance, tick-borne relapsing fever in the western United States and Canada is caused by *Borrelia hermsii*, transmitted by the *Ornithodoros hermsi* tick. The epidemic form of relapsing fever is transmitted by the human body louse. In the U.S., relapsing fever is largely confined to the western portion of the country, where the ticks inhabit the coniferous forests in the remains of dead trees and burrows occupied by mice, rats, and chipmunks.

The disease is more common in men, who may occupy the poorly maintained cabins and huts that rodents like to visit. The classic case involves a tick bite and a 7-day incubation period, followed by the abrupt onset of high fever, shaking chills, severe headache, muscle and joint aches, abdominal pain, nausea, and vomiting. This lasts for about 3 (but may be 1 to 17) days, until there is a crisis wherein the fever drops while the victim undergoes drenching sweats and intense thirst. For a subsequent period that averages 7 days, there is no fever and minimal symptoms, then a relapse into illness. This cycle recurs an average of three times, with each episode of illness generally less severe. The sporadic (tickborne) variation tends to be less severe; mortality of up to 40% has occurred in louse-borne epidemics.

A physician can make the diagnosis by examining a smear of the victim's blood under the lens of a microscope and observing the causative organisms. Treatment is tetracycline or erythromycin 500 mg by mouth four times a day for 10 days. When the victim ingests the antibiotics, he may suffer a high fever and low blood pressure (shock—see page 54) as a reaction to the death of the organisms within his bloodstream. Therefore, if you suspect relapsing fever, unless the victim is extremely ill, it is best to have him treated in a hospital, where this reaction can be anticipated and managed. If you are forced to treat in the field, be certain that the victim is well hydrated (see page 286), and administer a lower dose (250 mg) of antibiotic for the first four doses.

Typhoid Fever

Typhoid fever is caused by the bacteria *Salmonella typhi,* which are transmitted among humans through ingestion of contaminated food or water. Most cases are acquired abroad under conditions of poor hygiene.

After an incubation period of 10 to 14 days, victims suffer fever with or without diarrhea and abdominal pain. Most victims also complain of headache, fatigue, and loss of appetite. "Rose spots," which are 2 to 4 mm red spots on the trunk that blanch (lose their color) when pressed, are seen in some cases. The liver may become inflamed.

Most cases resolve in 3 to 4 weeks. The seriously stricken individual may suffer a severely inflamed bowel, bleeding from the gastrointestinal tract, pneumonia, heart failure, severe fever, and death.

A physician who diagnoses typhoid fever will treat the victim with an intravenous antibiotic. The layperson can use trimethoprim-sulfamethoxazole; administer one double-strength tablet twice a day for 2 to 3 weeks. You can also use ampicillin 100 mg per kg (2.2 lb) of body weight in four divided doses for 2 to 3 weeks. It is important to keep the victim from becoming dehydrated (see page 286).

Injectable and oral vaccines (see page 402) to prevent typhoid fever are available to people traveling to areas of high risk.

Lassa Fever

Lassa fever is a viral disease transmitted to humans principally through the body secretions of the *Mastomys natalensis* rat. It occurs primarily in sub-Saharan West Africa.

The infected victim suffers a gradual onset of headache, fever, and fatigue. There is often a severe sore throat, and there may be diarrhea and/or reddened eyes. Victims often complain of chest pain behind the breastbone, which may be caused by inflammation of the throat and esophagus. Roughly a quarter of victims develop bleeding complications. If the case is nonfatal, resolution begins in 8 to 10 days. In a fatal case, the victim progresses to develop altered mental status, shock, and severe breathing disorders.

The viral hemorrhagic (bleeding) fevers (Lassa, Marburg, Ebola, and Crimean-Congo) can all be spread among humans by transfer of secretions (blood and body fluids). Therefore, it is important to isolate suspected victims as best possible from other humans during their care. Transfer to a medical facility for specific drug therapy may be critical to survival. Field care is supportive and similar to that for yellow fever (see page 134).

Schistosomiasis

Schistosomiasis is a term that describes a variety of diseases caused by different species of parasitic flatworms. The intermediate hosts are freshwater snails, which release the immature infective stages into the water; thus, the infections are acquired by people who bathe or swim in contaminated water. The early symptoms caused by all of the species of worms are similar. When the fork-tailed cercariae (early stages of the immature worm) penetrate the skin, they cause itching and a rash at the site of entry that lasts for 1 to 2 days. Four to 6 weeks later, the victim shows loss of appetite, fatigue, night sweating, hives, and late-afternoon fever lasting 5 to 10 days ("snail," "safari," "Katayama," or "Yangtze River" fever). After a few months, the different species cause specific organ damage.

Schistosoma haematobium is prevalent in Africa, the Middle East, the islands of Madagascar and Mauritius, and India. The worms take residence in the blood vessels of the bladder and genitalia, and induce bloody, painful, and frequent urination. *S. mansoni* is prevalent in Africa, the Arabian peninsula, Madagascar, Brazil, Suriname, Venezuela, and some Caribbean islands. The worms take residence in the blood vessels surrounding the large bowel and induce bloody and mucus-laden diarrhea. In late stages of the disease, the liver can be severely damaged. *S. japonicum* is prevalent in China, the Philippines, Japan, and the island of Sulawesi. The worms take residence in the blood vessels supplying the small bowel and induce severe, bloody, and mucus-laden diarrhea. Other schistosomal species are less virulent.

Treatment for schistosomiasis includes the prescription antihelminthic (antiparasitic) drug praziquantel.

To prevent schistosomiasis, it is necessary to prevent the entry of cercariae into the body. In a region of high risk, it is unwise to bathe or swim in an untreated pond or stream. Shallow, stagnant water is more contaminated than that in swift-moving currents. Always wear hip boots or waders when passing through streams or swamps. If contact with water occurs, apply rubbing alcohol to your skin and briskly towel off. Boil or disinfect all bathing water, or store it for 3 days (the life span of the cercariae) before using it; also be certain that it is free of snails. There is not yet an effective repellent or vaccine against schistosomiasis.

Rocky Mountain Spotted Fever

Rocky Mountain spotted fever is caused by *Rickettsia rickettii,* a tick-borne parasite. The disease is most commonly noted in late spring and early summer, when people are more likely to be outside and become hosts for the dog tick (*Dermacentor variabilis*) or western wood tick (*D. andersoni*). Other ticks can also carry the parasite. Most infections are reported in the southeastern states: North Carolina, South Carolina, Texas, Tennessee, Virginia, Maryland, and Georgia.

The incubation period is 2 to 14 (average 7) days after the tick bite, at which time a high fever begins abruptly. Two to 6 days after the onset of fever, the red-spotted rash typically begins on the hands (including the palms), wrists, feet (including the soles), and ankles, then spreads toward the trunk. The face is less often involved. At first, the rash is composed of pink spots that blanch with pressure; they later become darker red or purplish. As the disease advances, the spots coalesce to form purple blotches. However, some victims never develop a rash (Rocky Mountain "spotless" fever).

Other symptoms include headache (common), chills, joint and muscle aching, cough, puffy eyelids and face, swollen hands and feet, reddened eyes, abdominal pain, nausea, and vomiting. Severe cases can affect multiple organ systems and cause death.

If you suspect that someone is suffering from Rocky Mountain spotted fever, seek a physician's help immediately. Tetracycline (adult dose, 500 mg four times a day; pediatric dose, 10 mg/kg four times a day) or doxycycline (adult dose only, 100 mg twice a day) should be given for 6 days, or continued until the victim is without fever for 3 days. Although it is generally not recommended that you administer tetracycline to a pregnant woman or to a child less than 6 years of age, because of the risk of tooth discoloration or abnormal bone development (the latter in a fetus during pregnancy), in a case of suspected Rocky Mountain spotted fever when a physician is not available to administer an alternative antibiotic, tetracycline should be given.

Colorado Tick Fever

Colorado tick fever is caused by a virus transmitted to humans by the wood tick *Dermacentor andersoni,* and perhaps by other species. It is a seasonal illness that occurs from late March to early October, with peak incidence in May and June, usually in people who recreate outdoors.

The usual incubation period—from tick bite to symptoms—is 3 to 6 days. The victim complains of sudden onset of fever, severe headache, muscle aches, and fatigue. Other symptoms may include aversion to light, eye pain, loss of appetite, abdominal pain, and nausea and vomiting. Only 5 to 10% of victims develop a skin rash. The hallmark feature, which is only observed in half of victims, is a distinctive fever pattern: There is a fever for 2 to 3 days, a 1- to 2-day remission, and then an additional 2 to 3 days of fever. Permanent effects and serious complications are rare, but do occur, more commonly in children under the age of 10 years.

A victim of Colorado tick fever may require 3 weeks or longer to recover fully; the most common persistent symptoms are fatigue and weakness. However, infection appears to confer lifelong immunity to subsequent exposures to the virus.

Lyme Disease

Lyme disease, caused by infection with the spirochete *Borrelia burgdorferi,* is the most common tick-borne illness in the United States. Occurrence is most frequent in summer and early autumn, during peak outdoor activities. The two hard ticks implicated in transmission of the spirochete from mammal to mammal (for example, from white-footed mouse *Peromyscus leucopus* to the white-tailed deer *Odocoileus virginianus* in the South; from the dusky-footed wood rat *Neotoma fuscipes* and the California kangaroo rat *Dipodomys californicus* to larger mammals in northern California) are the *Ixodes scapularis* (formerly *dammini*) (deer tick) in the Northeast, South, and Midwest, and the *I. pacificus* (western black-legged tick) in the West.

The adult ticks of the these species are extremely small—about the size of a sesame seed. Worse yet, the disease can be transmitted by the nymphal forms, which may appear only as minuscule black spots on the skin. Other potential carriers of *Borrelia burgdorferi* in the United States include the dog tick, wood tick, rabbit tick, and Lone Star tick (*Amblyomma americanum*); however, these ticks may not transmit the disease. Lyme disease has been reported in Canada, the Soviet Union, Australia, Europe (linked to the sheep tick *Ixodes ricinus*), Scandinavia, Japan, and China.

The distinctive skin lesion of Lyme disease, erythema (chronicum) migrans, appears 3 to 32 days (usually, about a week) after the tick bite. It is attributed to *B. burgdorferi* that are spreading locally in the skin, and is usually found on the trunk, upper arm (or armpit), or thigh as a small red spot that expands into a large (average 7" or 18 cm, but up to 30" or 76 cm, in diameter) and irregular circle or oval with a red, raised, or flat outer border surrounding paler ("fading," but slightly red) skin in the center. The rash may itch or burn, and is warm to the touch. The initial central spot may turn into a blister or small ulcer, or it may turn blue in color. In some cases, multiple similar red areas appear simultaneously, occasionally within the larger primary lesion, but never on the palms or soles. These areas clear spontaneously over 1 to 14 (average 4) weeks. Variations of the rash include diffuse hives or a more measleslike eruption. An untreated victim may develop recurrent rashes 1 to 14 months after the initial rash disappears.

Within days to weeks of infecting a human, the *B. burgdorferi* organisms spread from the skin through the bloodstream and lymphatic system to affect other organs. Therefore, appearing just prior to, or coincident with, the skin rash(es) are flulike symptoms that include muscle aching (particularly of the calves, thighs, and back), stiff neck, fatigue, low-grade fever, chills, painful joints, loss of appetite, nausea, cough, sore throat, swollen lymph glands, enlarged spleen, headache, abdominal pain (particularly in the right upper quadrant), irritated eyes (conjunctivitis), swelling around the eyes, and aversion to light. Most of the symptoms disappear in 2 to 3 weeks (along with the rash), but fatigue and muscle aching may last for months.

More serious symptoms include severe headaches and a stiff neck suggestive of meningitis (see page 156), confusion, profound sleepiness or insomnia, memory disturbances, emotional changes, and poor balance. Pain in the joints and symptoms of hepatitis may also occur.

Pets can also contract this disease, suffering lameness, swollen joints, lethargy, and loss of appetite.

If Lyme disease is not treated with an antibiotic, the disease can progress to facial paralysis and severe heart and nervous system disorders weeks to months after the initial rash disappears. Months or years later, up to 60% of untreated victims will suffer arthritis.

The current recommendation for antibiotic therapy for an adult with Lyme disease at the time of the initial rash or symptoms is tetracycline 500 mg four times a day for 3 days, then 250 mg four times a day for 3 weeks; or doxycycline 200 mg twice a day for 3 days, then 100 mg four times a day for 3 weeks. An alternative is amoxicillin 1 g orally three times a day for 4 weeks. A child should be treated with amoxicillin 7 mg per kg (2.2 lb) of body weight (up to 250 mg) three times a day; or phenoxymethyl penicillin in a dose of 13 mg per kg (up to 500 mg) four times a day for 3 weeks. The drugs of second choice are: adult—phenoxymethyl penicillin 500 mg, or erythromycin 250 mg, four times a day for 4 weeks; child—erythromycin 8 mg per kg (up to 250 mg) four times a day for 4 weeks.

A physician may elect to treat certain Lyme disease victims with a daily injection of ceftriaxone for 2 weeks. There are occasional treatment failures; these people may require hospitalization for another intravenous antibiotic. Other antibiotics currently being tested against Lyme disease include cefuroxime axetil, cefixime, and azithromycin.

Prevention is key. Avoid tick bites by wearing proper clothing (light colored for spotting ticks, tightly woven collared shirts, closed boots, long sleeves and pant legs, hats) impregnated with 0.5% permethrin (Permanone) insecticide or N, N-diethyl-3-methylbenzamide (DEET) repellent in the critical locations (see page 347). When traveling in tick country, keep shirts and pant cuffs tucked in. All hair-covered areas and warm, moist locations on the skin should be inspected carefully. Any tick found on the skin should be removed promptly and properly (see page 342). Following a tick bite, watch for the characteristic rash and symptoms. Some authorities believe that a tick must be attached to a human for at least 24 hours to transmit Lyme disease, but this has not yet been proven.

It has also not yet been proven that administration of an antibiotic to every person bitten by an *Ixodes* tick is a cost-effective method to prevent this disease. However, in an area where carrier ticks and the disease are frequent, it is not unreasonable to administer an appropriate antibiotic (phenoxymethyl penicillin or tetracycline 250 mg four times a day) for 10 days following removal of an embedded or blood-engorged tick. In the absence of an allergic reaction to the antibiotic, this therapy is generally safe.

LYMErix (SmithKline Beecham PLC) is a vaccine in development. At this time, it appears that humans may require 6 months to one year to develop immunity to Lyme disease when injected with this vaccine, which is administered in three doses. The vaccine creates antibodies that recognize a protein in the Lyme bacterium present in the tick's saliva.

Ehrlichiosis

Human ehrlichiosis (there is also a canine form) is present in two forms, one caused by a rickettsial organism known as *Ehrlichia chaffeensis*, which is spread by *Amblyomma americanum* tick bites, and the other caused by the rickettsial organisms *E. phagocytophila* and *E. equi*, spread by *Ixodes* tick bites. Infection is usually acquired by a person who inhabits a rural environment. The average incubation period after a bite is approximately 7 to 10 days. The victims, who are more commonly middle-aged adults than children and young adults, complain of a flulike syndrome with high fever, chills, fatigue, headache, muscle aches, vomiting, and a variety of skin rashes, which can be punctate, bumpy, like tiny bruises, or broad and reddened. A victim often has decreased counts of various types of blood cells, as well as liver dysfunction. The treatment is tetracycline 500 mg four times a day, or doxycycline 100 mg twice a day, for 10 days. The few children who have been diagnosed with ehrichiosis have been treated with doxycycline 3 mg per kg body weight in two divided doses per day. Untreated or treated after a delay in diagnosis, up to 15% of victims can develop severe infections, kidney failure, bleeding disorders, seizures, and/or coma.

Babesiosis

Babesiosis is caused by protozoan parasites that invade human red blood cells. They are transmitted from mammals and rodents to humans by the bite of certain hard ticks. For instance, *Babesia microti* in New England is transmitted by the northern deer tick *Ixodes scapularis*, which can also transmit the spirochete agent of Lyme disease.

An infection manifests itself in a human with symptoms of fatigue, loss of appetite, and weakness, followed within a few days to a week by fever, sweats, and muscle aches. Less common symptoms include headache, nausea, vomiting, and chills. There is rarely a rash. The victim may suffer anemia and an enlarged spleen. A person who no longer has a spleen may suffer a more serious or prolonged illness.

A physician can make the diagnosis by observing the parasites in a smear of human blood under the lens of a microscope. Most victims recover without treatment. In severe cases, a physician may administer drugs, such as quinine and clindamycin.

Trichinellosis (Trichinosis)

Trichinellosis (trichinosis) is a disease that occurs in humans who consume the larvae of *Trichinella* species (such as *spiralis* and *nativa*) that have encysted in animal muscle tissue (meat). Most of us are familiar with the risk associated with eating undercooked pork, but be aware that cases have resulted from consumption of horse meat, wild boar, bear, walrus, and cougar, the latter in jerky form (which was brined and smoked, but never heated during preparation). Squirrels, woodchucks, capybaras, mice, and rats are infected in nature.

Victims of trichinellosis first develop gastrointestinal distress (nausea, vomiting, diarrhea, and abdominal pain) during the week following ingestion of infested meat. This may continue for 4 to 6 weeks. During the second week, when the larvae are invading human muscle tissue, high fever, muscle aches, swelling (edema, puffiness) of the soft tissues around the eyes, weakness, skin rash, and joint aches develop. There may be tiny red hemorrhages under the fingernails or visible within the skin. In addition, analysis of human blood shows an unusually high count of eosinophils, which are a cell type associated with allergies and certain parasite infestations.

The migrating larvae can cause damage to the lungs (cough, bloody sputum, shortness of breath, pain with breathing), heart, and brain.

The larvae encyst in the muscle tissues, beginning the second or third week of infection, which causes muscle aches and stiffness. Then the larvae die; they become calcified 6 to 18 months after the infection first occurred.

The definitive diagnosis is made in humans by a blood test or muscle biopsy (examining a small piece of muscle harvested from the patient for *Trichinella* cysts and muscle inflammation with a concentration of eosinophils). Treatment for a person with trichinellosis is not yet totally satisfactory; it involves administration of the drug thiabendazole or mebendazole.

Although most species of *Trichinella* are killed by freezing, there are freeze-resistant strains, so all meat that is at a high risk for carrying the parasite should be cooked thoroughly to a temperature of at least 150 to 170° F (65.6 to 77° C), which generally occurs when the meat turns from pink or red to gray. Certain brining solutions may kill *Trichinella;* however, the curing temperature must be sufficiently high.

Leptospirosis

Leptospirosis is caused by the spirochetes of *Leptospira* species. The organisms are shed in the urine of wild and domestic animals, including cows, dogs, and pigs. Humans acquire the disease by contacting contaminated soil or water, which includes freshwater ponds and streams. The spirochetes can enter through nicked or abraded skin, through the mucous membranes of the eye and mouth, or by being ingested.

After an incubation period of 7 to 12 days, many victims display a fever, chills, fatigue, muscle aches, headache, swollen lymph glands, and red eyes without a discharge. Nausea, vomiting, abdominal pain, and cough are common symptoms as well. This presentation lasts for about a week, then is followed by a few days of improvement, after which a second stage of the disease begins. This is characterized by more muscle aches, nausea and vomiting, and a diffuse skin rash (red or purplish patches of skin). A sore throat, enlarged spleen, abnormal heart rhythms, and enlarged liver with jaundice may develop.

The treatment is doxycycline 100 mg by mouth twice a day, or tetracycline 500 mg four times a day, for 7 days. Other antibiotics that can be used are amoxicillin, cefuroxime axetil, and erythromycin.

To avoid infection, it is best not to swim in freshwater ponds and streams likely to be heavily contaminated by urine from livestock or wildlife.

Tularemia

Tularemia is caused by the bacterium *Francisella tularensis,* which can be transmitted to humans by tick bites, or by handling, skinning, or eating improperly cooked infected rabbit meat. Rarely, it can be transmitted from a cat, bear, deer, beaver, or muskrat.

There are multiple clinical presentations of the disease, with combinations of the following signs and symptoms: painful and tender ulcers on the hand (from handling an infected animal) with associated swollen lymph glands behind the elbow and in the armpit; swollen lymph glands in the groin, associated with insect bites of the legs; sore throat; conjunctivitis in one eye with a swollen lymph gland in front of the ear on the same side; fever; chills; weakness; pneumonia; weakness; and weight loss.

A physician will use blood tests to confirm the diagnosis. Treatment is best rendered with intramuscular injections of streptomycin. If the victim cannot be brought to medical attention promptly, therapy may be initiated with tetracycline 500 mg four times a day, or ciprofloxacin 750 mg twice a day.

Meningococcal Disease

One of the most feared infectious diseases is meningitis caused by the bacterium *Neisseria meningitidis* (*meningococcus*). The infection can appear in outbreaks, most commonly abroad, particularly in sub-Saharan Africa and China. The infection is spread in the respiratory secretions of humans.

The disease appears in many forms, the most common of which are meningitis, pneumonia, and disseminated bacterial infection. The typical presentation of meningitis is fever, headache, and a stiff neck (see page 156). If the cause is meningococcus, the victim may develop a skin rash, which consists of red dots or bumps, or a flat, more patchy dark red discoloration. If the dark red dots begin to enlarge and coalesce into large purplish bruiselike discolorations, this is a bad sign. In the worst cases, the victim develops shock, diffuse bleeding, and death. Approximately 1 in 10 victims of meningococcal meningitis dies.

This is a true emergency. The victim needs large doses of intravenous antibiotics. If these are not available, administer a high oral dose of penicillin, cephalexin, cefixime, cefpodoxime, or amoxicillin–clavulanate acid for 10 days. If the victim is allergic to penicillin, use trimethoprim-sulfamethoxazole. This should also be administered to all close ("household") contact people for 3 days. In an ideal situation, these people would also be given the drug rifampin for 2 days.

An effective meningococcal vaccine is available (see page 401).

PART THREE

Minor Medical Problems

Although the afflictions discussed in this section are rarely life threatening, they account for the majority of health care problems encountered in a recreational or wilderness setting. For the sake of simplicity, this section is organized by body organ system. Specific disorders can be rapidly located by using the index.

Whenever a person becomes ill, it is wise to consider how the disorder can become worse. For instance, bronchitis can progress to pneumonia in situations of stress and suboptimal environmental conditions. Therefore, if someone develops severe bronchitis, he should not continue to travel farther from civilization until it is clear that medical management is going to halt progression of the illness.

I have not included all of the problems that originate from substance abuse or indiscriminate sexual encounters. However, it is critical to observe that drinking alcohol or using mind-altering drugs impairs judgment and is a major contributor to injuries. It is inexcusable to dull your senses when such activity places you and others at risk.

GENERAL SYMPTOMS

Unconscious (or Semiconscious) Victim

As discussed in detail in the section "Major Medical Problems" (see page 15), a proper approach to the unconscious (comatose) victim may make the difference between life and death. You must evaluate the semiconscious (stuporous, dazed, confused, or combative) individual with the same degree of concern. To discover the cause of an altered mental status, you must be a bit of a detective, while also performing the tasks that prevent the victim from hurting himself. Always assume that an unconscious person may be seriously injured.

1. Open and maintain the airway (see page 17). Check for adequacy of the pulse (see page 26).
2. Protect the cervical spine (see page 31). *Every injured person has a broken neck until proven otherwise.*
3. Carefully examine the victim for evidence of an obvious injury and treat accordingly.
4. Consider low blood sugar, and treat the victim with glucose if he is alert enough to cooperate (see page 128).

Don't:

1. Don't shake a victim vigorously to awaken him without first protecting the neck. *Never* shake a victim to awaken him if you suspect that hypothermia (see page 269) is present. If you think that the victim is merely intoxicated, you may snap an ammonia inhalant or hold "smelling salts" under his nose, and allow him a few whiffs to stimulate awakening. If there is any chance of a neck injury, do not perform this maneuver without maintaining the head and neck in a stable position.
2. Don't attempt to carry an unconscious victim or manage a belligerent person if this might exhaust you. Send someone for help and stay with the victim until help arrives.
3. Unless there is no other way to get lifesaving help, never leave an unconscious or dazed person unattended.

Fainting

Fainting is defined as sudden brief loss of consciousness not associated with a head injury. There are innumerable causes of fainting, but most episodes are associated with decreased blood flow (oxygen and/or glucose) to the brain. This may be caused by low blood sugar (hypoglycemia—see page 128), slow heart rate (vagal reaction, in which the vagus nerve, which slows the heart rate, is overstimulated: fright, anxiety, stomach irritation, bowel dilatation, drugs, fatigue, prolonged standing in one position), rhythm disturbances of the heart, dehydration, heat exhaustion, anemia, or bleeding.

If you witness a fainting episode, or are with someone who is becoming lightheaded (sweating, weak, ashen colored, dizzy), quickly help the person lie down and elevate his legs 8 to 12" (20 to 30 cm). This position increases venous blood flow back to the heart, which in turn pumps more blood to the brain. If the victim begins to vomit, turn him on his side. If he has fallen, examine him for injuries. A cool, moistened cloth wiped on his forehead, on his face, and behind his neck may make the victim feel better. Do not splash or pour water on his face or routinely use smelling salts or ammonia inhalants. Do not slap the victim's face.

After a victim suffers a fainting episode, he should be examined for any sign of serious illness or injury. If you don't suspect anything serious, have him lie still for a few minutes, then sit for a few minutes. If the victim is alert and capable of purposeful swallowing, offer him cool sweetened liquids to drink—preferably one that contains electrolytes (see page 286)—to correct dehydration. When the victim feels normal, he may slowly regain an upright posture. If the victim is elderly, and particularly if his pulse is irregular or he has chest discomfort, seek immediate medical assistance. Anticipate a heart attack (see page 45).

Fatigue

Fatigue (lethargy, tiredness, exhaustion, generalized weakness, decreasing exercise tolerance) can be a sign of any disorder or dysfunction that diminishes a person's energy level. Accompanied by fever, it can be indicative of an infection; accompanied by certain associated symptoms, it may indicate a hypoactive thyroid. In the outdoors, anyone who began the trip in good condition but is now fatigued should be examined carefully for signs and symptoms of hypothermia (see page 269), hyperthermia (see page 281), high-altitude illness (see page 292), infection, mental depression (see page 264), anemia (pale membranes inside the eyelid, pale fingernail beds, sallow skin complexion), dehydration (see page 286), or starvation. A diabetic who becomes fatigued may suffer from high or low blood sugar (see page 128). If fatigue is accompanied by shortness of breath, do not travel any farther from civilization until you determine a treatable cause, or the victim clearly improves. Sudden onset of fatigue can be indicative of a heart attack (see page 45).

If a person is suffering physical exhaustion, allow him at least 12 hours of rest, encourage adequate food intake, and take particular care to correct dehydration.

In a situation of extreme exercise upon a particular muscle group—the legs during forced or military-style marching, or long-distance or marathon running; the arms during repetitive, relentless exertion such as weight lifting—muscle tissue can be broken down. This is more common under conditions of environmental heat (see page 281). Substances (particularly myoglobin, a pigment that carries oxygen) are released into the bloodstream, which in large concentrations can cause the kidneys to fail. The victim has very darkened (brown) urine (myoglobinuria), sore muscles, and extreme fatigue. In this situation, remove the victim from environmental heat, place him at as near complete rest as possible, and encourage him to drink as much liquid as he can to correct dehydration (see page 286).

Fever and Chills

Fever is an elevation in body temperature caused by infection. The causative organism (most commonly a bacterium or virus) releases substances into the bloodstream; these quickly reach the part of the brain that acts as the body thermostat. Thus, body temperature is "reset" at a higher level. This probably helps fight infection, but the temperature may need to be lowered if the elevation is extreme or prolonged.

Normal body temperature is 98.6° F (37° C) measured orally, and 99.6°F (37.5° C) measured rectally. To convert degrees Fahrenheit (F) into degrees Centigrade (C, or Celsius), subtract 32, then multiply by 5, then divide by 9. To convert degrees C into degrees F, multiply by 9, then divide by 5, then add 32. A temperature conversion chart is found on page 459.

Temperature should be measured with a thermometer. Electric (digital) thermometers are easiest to use and require the least time to record a temperature. If you use a mercury or alcohol thermometer, first shake it to pool the mercury or alcohol below the 94° F (35° C) marking. If you suspect the victim to be hypothermic, a special thermometer is necessary (see page 269). To take a temperature by mouth, place the thermometer under the tongue, close the mouth, and take a reading after 3 to 4 minutes. To take a temperature rectally (the more reliable method, and necessary in a case of suspected hypothermia), the thermometer is *gently* placed—ideally lubricated with oil or petroleum jelly—1" (2.5 cm) into the rectum. It is held for at least 2 minutes and then read. Never leave a child or confused adult unattended with a thermometer in the mouth or rectum.

Armpit (axillary) temperatures are far less reliable, because they may underestimate the temperature elevation. However, a high temperature recorded from the armpit may be interpreted to mean that there is some elevation in body temperature. An armpit temperature may be the only one you get in an uncooperative child less than 2 years of age. Since such a temperature tends to read on the low side, add 1.4° F (0.8° C) to obtain the equivalent rectal temperature.

Generally, an infection will not elevate the core (rectal) body temperature higher than 105° F (40.5° C). Anyone with a temperature measured above that level should be examined for heat illness (see page 281), stroke (see page 129), or drug overdose. Vigorous prolonged muscular activity (seizure or marathon running) can raise the core temperature above 107° F (41.7° C).

A child is considered to have a fever if his rectal temperature is greater than 100.4° F (38° C), oral temperature is greater than 100° F (37.8° C), or armpit temperature is greater than 99° F (37.2° C). You should be concerned about a fever greater than 100.4° F (38° C) in an infant less than 3 months of age or greater than 104° F (40° C) in any small child, since this can indicate a severe infection. Prolonged fever in a child should be investigated by a physician. Signs of a serious infection in an infant include lethargy ("floppy baby"), pain (persistent crying), labored breathing, purple skin rash, excessive drooling, a bulging "soft spot" (fontanel) on the top of the head, or a stiff neck.

If a person has a temperature higher than 100.5° F (38° C) that is felt to be due to an infection, he will be made more comfortable (fever lowered) by the administration of aspirin, ibuprofen (Motrin or Advil), or acetaminophen (Tylenol). To avoid Reye's syndrome (postviral encephalopathy and liver failure), *do not use aspirin to control a fever in a child under the age of 17.* Infants and small children with fevers (usually due to ear infections or viral illnesses) should be treated as soon as any elevation of temperature is noted, to prevent febrile seizures. An infant (younger than 6 months) with a fever should be seen as soon as possible by a physician. Sponging a child with cold water doesn't help much to reduce fever and can even be counterproductive if the child struggles or begins to shiver, both of which generate heat. If the fever is greater than 104° F (40° C), however, sponging can be attempted using lukewarm water. Never sponge a child with alcohol, because it can be absorbed through the skin and act as a poison.

If the victim suffers from environmental heat-induced illness (see page 281), he will not benefit from and should not be given aspirin or acetaminophen. Ibuprofen is not as dangerous but is also *not* helpful.

Whether to use an antibiotic for a "fever of unknown origin" (a fever that cannot be definitively linked to a specific site of infection) is a judgment call. If a person has an altered immune system (AIDS, cancer, diabetes, chronic corticosteroid administration) and a high or persistent fever not associated with symptoms suggestive of a particular infection, it is probably wise to administer a "broad-spectrum" antibiotic, such as ciprofloxacin or azithromycin. If there are symptoms that lead you to a specific site of infection (such as cough—pneumonia; burning on urination and flank pain—kidney infection), then the appropriate antibiotic should be started. Finally, any feverish small child can become rapidly debilitated; he will rarely suffer from the initiation of a common antibiotic, such as amoxicillin or trimethoprim-sulfamethoxazole.

Chills are caused by the release of bacteria or viruses (or their toxins) into the bloodstream. The victim will suddenly feel very cold and begin to shiver, with teeth chattering, goose bumps (piloerection), and weakness. The "chill" may actually occur during a temperature spike within a fever.

Coughing Blood

The blood coughed up by a victim may have originated anywhere from the mouth to the lungs. Causes of coughing blood include:

Sore Throat

The victim will complain of an irritated throat and difficulty swallowing, and will cough up whitish phlegm streaked with blood. If the victim is not short of breath and is not in distress, rapid medical attention is not necessary (see page 173). Similarly, if a person has a nosebleed, he may cough and spit a lot of blood (see page 170).

Pneumonia

The victim will complain of fever, chills, chest pain, and shortness of breath. He will cough up green or rust-colored thick sputum (see page 43).

Pulmonary Embolism

The victim will complain of difficult and painful breathing, shortness of breath, agitation, and weakness. Generally, only severely ill persons will cough up small clots of blood (see page 41).

Lung Cancer

The victim will suddenly cough up small pieces of spongy lung tissue or tumor, along with blood clots. Attend to the airway (see page 17) and seek medical attention.

Lung Injury

If a victim is struck in the chest, and particularly if his ribs are broken, the underlying lung can be bruised or torn. The victim will cough up small clots of blood or, if the injury is major, mouthfuls of blood. This is extremely serious and requires constant attention to the airway (see pages 17 and 35).

Dizziness

Dizziness is a feeling of light-headedness, with or without a sensation of spinning (vertigo). It often precedes a fainting episode (see page 150) or may accompany a stroke (see page 129), heart attack (see page 45), low blood sugar (see page 128), heat illness (see page 281), ear infection (see page 157), the bends (see page 357), plant poisoning (see page 368), motion sickness (see page 390), and many other disorders. Frequently, dizziness is caused by an infection or disorder of the middle ear, which controls balance. Indeed, if the external ear canals are blocked by wax, this alone can cause dizziness.

If a victim is dizzy, he should lie on his back and attempt to regain orientation to his surroundings. Examine him for obvious causes and treat accordingly. If the dizziness does not resolve, and particularly if the victim is elderly (in which case it might indicate a stroke), he should be taken to a physician. True vertigo is very distressing to the victim and described by him as "the room spinning around," with nausea and/or vomiting, weakness, ringing in the ears (tinnitus), and occasional slow jerking or fluttering movements of the eyeballs (nystagmus). Inflammation of the inner ear (often associated with a recent cold) is known as labyrinthitis. It is treated with the same medications used for motion sickness (see page 390). This is a diagnosis to be reached by a physician after more serious problems are excluded.

Hiccoughs

Hiccoughs can be extremely annoying. A few tricks for stopping them include immersing the face in ice water, swallowing in a series of 10 sips without interruption, and hyperventilating for a moment. If none of these work, gently sliding a well-greased length of thin, flexible rubber tubing through one nostril to the point where it just barely touches the back of the throat may terminate the hiccoughs. This must be done while taking care not to injure the sensitive interior lining of the nose.

HEAD (ALSO EYE, EAR, NOSE, THROAT, AND MOUTH)

Headache

Tension or fatigue headache is characterized by throbbing pain in the temples, over the eyes, and in the posterior neck and shoulder muscles. It can be treated with rest, sunglasses, and moderate pain medication, such as aspirin or acetaminophen every 3 to 4 hours. Sometimes, applying warm packs or massage to tense muscles relaxes them and helps relieve the pain.

Migraine headache is generally more severe. It is caused by painful dilation and constriction of small arteries in the head. Migraine headaches have many variations, which may include any or all of the following: photophobia (aversion to light), nausea, vomiting, runny nose, and weakness of an arm or leg. Some people experience an "aura" prior to the "classic" migraine headache, in which they may smell strange odors or see flashing lights. Others develop tunnel vision—diminished peripheral vision. The headaches are characterized as excruciating, pounding, or explosive. Migraines require stronger pain medications and may be treated with narcotics. Other medicines that are effective include sumatriptan (Imitrex), zolmitriptan (Zomig), prochlorperazine (Compazine) given with diphenhydramine (Benadryl), and ergotamine drugs (such as dihydroergotamine mesylate [Migranal] nasal spray) that directly constrict arteries; these latter should only be used under the guidance of a physician, since they may worsen the effects of the certain types of migraines. If an oxygen (see page 383) tank is available, the victim may get some relief by breathing 10 liters per minute by face mask. An elderly person with a severe migraine, which may be confused with a stroke (see page 129), should seek immediate medical attention. A migraine headache may be precipitated by lack of sleep, high altitude, emotional stress, cyclical hormone changes, noxious odors, and certain ingested substances (such as caffeine and monosodium glutamate).

Sinus headache is associated with sinus infection (see page 172) and is typified by fever, nasal congestion, production of a foul nasal discharge, and pain produced by tapping over the affected sinus(es). It should be treated with an oral decongestant (pseudoephedrine), nasal spray (Neo-Synephrine ¼% or Afrin 0.05%), an antibiotic (azithromycin, amoxicillin-clavulanate, erythromycin, or ampicillin) if an infection is present, and warm packs applied over the affected sinus(es).

Subarachnoid hemorrhage is bleeding that occurs, usually suddenly, from a leaking blood vessel underneath the thin tissue layer that surrounds the brain and spinal cord. The headache is usually sudden in onset, described as "the worst headache of my life," and may be associated with a fainting spell, altered mental status, seizure, and collapse. If a person suffers a subarachnoid hemorrhage and remains awake, he may complain of a stiff or painful neck with or without back pain about 2 to 4 hours after the bleed. Anyone who complains of a severe headache after extreme physical straining (such as weight lifting or a difficult bowel movement) or who collapses suddenly after reporting a headache should be suspected to have suffered a subarachnoid hemorrhage and be brought rapidly to a hospital.

Meningitis, an infection that involves the lining of the brain and spinal cord, is a true emergency. The headache of meningitis is severe, and often accompanied by nausea, vomiting, photophobia, fever, altered mental status, and weakness. A purplish skin rash indicates meningococcal infection, a particularly fulminant and contagious form of infectious meningitis. The classic signs of meningitis are a stiff neck with a fever. The victim demonstrates extreme discomfort when the chin is flexed downward against the chest. It is important to note that an infant can suffer meningitis without a stiff neck and may present only with poor feeding, fever, vomiting, seizures, and extreme lethargy ("floppy baby"). If meningitis is suspected, the victim must be evacuated rapidly.

A headache that is atypically severe or prolonged may represent a serious problem, such as accelerated (out of control) high blood pressure (hypertension), brain tumor, infection, or hemorrhage. The victim should be evaluated by a physician at the earliest opportunity. If a person develops a severe headache associated with a fainting spell or stiff neck, or is known to suffer from high blood pressure, keep him as calm as possible and urgently seek assistance.

Ear

Earache

An earache may be caused by infection, injury, or a foreign body in the ear. For a discussion of ear squeeze (barotitis) that occurs with scuba diving, see page 358.

Ear Infection

Ear infection can be either internal (otitis media) or external (otitis externa) to the eardrum (tympanic membrane) (see figure 93).

Otitis Media. Infection may occur that reddens and inflames the eardrum and causes blood, serum, or pus to collect behind the drum (see figure 93B). With otitis media (middle ear infection), there is no drainage from the external ear canal (unless the eardrum ruptures, which is unusual in an adult, although more common in a child) and the victim has a fever, often with a sore throat. In many cases, the victim has a history of prior infections. Most often, otitis media occurs in children; when it occurs in an adult, it may be associated with a sinus infection or functional obstruction of the eustachian tube (the pressure-release mechanism from the middle ear into the throat). A young child can rapidly become severely ill from otitis media; an infant may develop meningitis (see page 156) following an ear infection.

If you suspect otitis media, treat the victim with an oral decongestant and an antibiotic. Adults and children should be treated with amoxicillin, trimethoprim-sulfamethoxazole, amoxicillin-clavulanate, cefixime, or clarithromycin for 10 days, or with azithromycin for

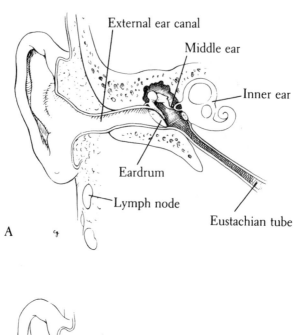

External ear canal

Middle ear

Inner ear

Eardrum

Lymph node

Eustachian tube

A

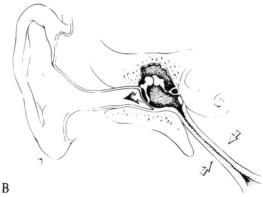

B

Figure 93. Ear infections. (A) Normal ear anatomy. (B) Otitis media (inner ear infection). The eardrum bulges outward as the middle ear fills with fluid. The eustachian tube narrows or closes.

5 days. An additional antibiotic choice for children is erythromycin-sulfisoxazole for 10 days. Aspirin, ibuprofen, or acetaminophen should be used to control fever. *To avoid Reye's syndrome (postviral encephalopathy and liver failure), do not use aspirin to control fever in a child under the age of 17.*

Otitis Externa (swimmer's ear). Ear infection that develops in the external ear canal (often noted in swimmers and divers who do not keep

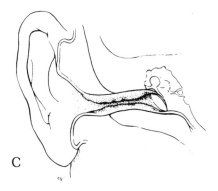

C

Figure 93. (CONT.) (C) Otitis externa (external ear canal infection). The canal becomes swollen and drains pus.

the canal completely dry) rarely involves the eardrum (figure 93C). Symptoms include a white to yellow-green liquid or cheesy discharge from the ear, pain, and decreased hearing. Occasionally, the victim complains of exquisite tenderness when the earlobe is tugged, and has tender, swollen lymph glands in the neck on the affected side. In a severe case, the victim may have a fever and appear toxic.

If the victim has only a discharge without fever or swollen lymph glands, he may be treated with ear drops, such as 2% nonaqueous acetic acid (VōSoL). Household vinegar diluted 1:1 with fresh water or with rubbing alcohol can be used as a substitute. These ear drops should be administered four to five times a day and may be retained with a cotton or gauze wick gently placed into the external ear canal, or by using an expanding foam ear sponge (such as a Speedi-Wick, Shippert Medical Technologies, Englewood, Colorado). To avoid injuring the eardrum, do not attempt to clean out the ear with a cotton swab or similar object.

If the victim has a discharge with fever and/or swollen lymph glands, the ear drops should contain hydrocortisone (VōSoL HC); he should also be given oral ciprofloxacin, erythromycin, or penicillin. A newer ear drop that may be useful is ciprofloxacin with hydrocortisone (Cipro HC otic suspension). Another is ofloxacin otic solution (Floxin otic) 0.3%. These ear drops are used twice a day. Aspirin, ibuprofen, or acetaminophen should be used to control fever. *To avoid Reye's syndrome (postviral encephalopathy and liver failure), do not use aspirin to control fever in a child under the age of 17.*

To prevent swimmer's ear, the external ear canal should be irrigated with VōSoL or diluted vinegar (described above) after each scuba dive or immersion episode in the water.

Referred Pain

"Referred" pain is pain that appears in one body region but actually originates in another. This occurs because different body regions are supplied with nerves that share common central pathways. In the case of ear pain, the cause may be a sore throat, tooth infection, or arthritic jaw. The ear pain will not disappear until the underlying cause is corrected.

Injury to the Eardrum

If something is poked into the ear, a hard blow is struck to the external ear, a diver descends rapidly without equalizing the pressure in his middle ear (see page 358), or a person is subjected to a loud explosive noise, the eardrum may be ruptured. This causes immediate intense pain and possibly loss of hearing, along with occasional nausea, vomiting, and dizziness. If the eardrum is ruptured, cover the external ear to prevent the ingress of dirt, and seek the aid of a physician. If debris has entered the ear, start the victim on penicillin or erythromycin by mouth. Do not put liquid medicine into the ear if you suspect that the eardrum is ruptured. If the dizziness is disabling, administer medicine for motion sickness (see page 390). Use appropriate pain medication.

Foreign Body in the Ear

A foreign body in the ear can be incredibly painful, particularly if it is dancing on the eardrum or resting against the sensitive lining of the ear canal. An inanimate foreign body (a piece of corn, peanut, foxtail, stone, or the like) can be left in the ear until an ear specialist with special forceps can remove it. If a live creature (cockroach, bee) enters the external ear canal and causes pain that is intolerable, the ear should be filled with 2 to 4% liquid lidocaine (topical anesthetic), which will (slowly) numb the ear and drown the bug at the same time. If lidocaine is not available, mineral oil can be used, with the caution that it will frequently cause the insect to struggle, which may encourage a sting or bite and incredible temporary pain. Once the animal is dead (a few minutes), a gentle attempt should be made with small tweezers to remove it. Don't attempt this unless you can

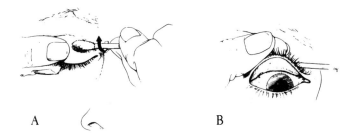

A   B

Figure 94. Eversion of the eyelid to locate a foreign body. (A) The lid is grasped and pulled over a cotton swab or small blunt stick. (B) The underside of the eyelid is inspected for a foreign body while the victim looks downward.

see part of the bug, however. Don't push the bug in farther, or you might rupture the eardrum.

Wax in the Ear

If hearing is diminished in an ear because of a wax plug, the wax must first be softened with a solution such as Cerumenex or Debrox. Put a few drops in the ear (retained by a wick or cotton) four to five times a day for 3 days. This will turn hard ear wax into mush. Then use a forceful stream of luke-warm water to flush out the wax. You can fashion a flushing device by attaching a plastic 18-gauge intravenous catheter (without the needle) to a 8 to 30 ml syringe. Don't try to clean out the ear with a cotton-tipped swab or other rigid object, because you may force the wax down deeper, perfo-rate the eardrum, or scrape and cut the exquisitely sensitive skin that lines the external ear canal.

Eye

Foreign Body Under the Eyelid and Scratched Cornea

If a foreign body lodges on the cornea (the clear surface of the eye) with-out actual penetration of the eyeball, irrigate the eye copiously with an eyewash solution (use water if you do not have eyewash). If this is not suc-cessful, have the victim look downward, grasp his upper lid firmly by the eyelashes, and fold it up and inside out over a cotton swab (figure 94). If you can see the foreign body on the undersurface of the upper eyelid,

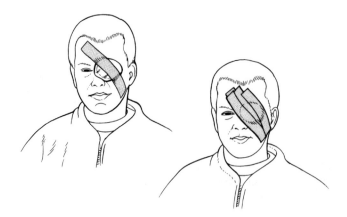

Figure 95. Taping a patch over the eye.

gently wipe it away with a cotton swab or piece of moistened cloth. If you do not see the object, check between the lower eyelid and the eyeball.

Once you have removed the object, if the victim still feels as if something is in his eye, he may have suffered a scratch on the cornea (corneal abrasion). In this case, patch the eye closed for 24 hours. However, *never patch an eye closed if there is any sign of an active infection* (pus or discharge). When the patch is removed, if there is residual pain, a gritty sensation, gooey discharge, or blurred vision, see a doctor as soon as possible. Tiny objects, such as the spine of a horse nettle (sand brier), can become embedded in the cornea and not be visible without the magnification available to an ophthalmologist.

To patch an eye, a ½"- (1.3 cm) thick pad of soft cloth or bandage should be shaped to fit neatly over the eye socket, and affixed snugly to the face with tape or bandages extending across the patch onto the cheek below and the forehead opposite the affected eye (figure 95). Prepackaged sterile elliptical eye pads are available. If only tape is available, the eyelids may be taped closed with a single small piece of tape.

Another way to hold an eye shield, patch, or padding around the eye is with a cravat (see page 244). First, place a strip of cloth approximately 2" (5 cm) wide and 15" (38 cm) long over the top of the head front-to-back, so that the face-side end hangs over the uninjured eye, near the nose. Place the patch, pad, or shield over the eye and hold it in place with a cravat, which should be wrapped horizontally around the head and then tied in position on top of the hanging cloth strip. Make the first tie (single loop or half square knot) in the cravat behind the head and at the base of the

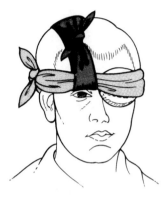

Figure 96. Holding an eye patch in place with a cravat. Hang a cloth strip over the uninjured eye. Hold the patch in place with a cravat. Tie the cloth strip to lift the cravat off the uninjured eye.

skull, and keep wrapping it around, to complete the final tie (square knot) where the ends meet. If the final tie will be over an eye, shift the cravat. Pull up the ends of the hanging cloth strip and tie them at the top of the head; this should lift the cravat up off the uninjured eye (figure 96).

If the eye cannot be patched, sunglasses should be worn.

Injured Eyeball

If the eyeball is perforated, there will be a combination of loss of vision (ranging from hazy vision to blindness), pain, excessive tearing, a dilated pupil, and visible blood in the eye. Do not attempt to rinse out the wound vigorously; remove obvious dirt and debris without placing any pressure on the eye. Close the eyelid gently and cover the eye with a protective shield. This can be fashioned by cutting gauze pads or soft cloth to the proper size, or by fashioning a doughnut-shaped shield with a cloth, cravat bandage, or shirt (see figure 97). Another good way to keep pressure off the eye is to cut an eye-sized hole in a stack of gauze pads and place the stack over the eye, taping or wrapping it in place. An eye shield can also be improvised by cutting off the bottom 2" (5 cm) of a paper cup and taping it over the eye. Metal or plastic preshaped eye shields can be carried.

Do not exert pressure on the eyeball, because this can increase the damage. Instruct the victim to keep both eyes closed, and start him on ciprofloxacin, penicillin, cephalexin, or erythromycin. Seek immediate medical attention.

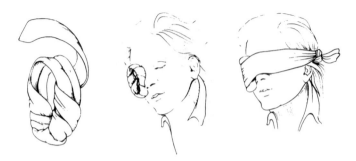

Figure 97. Bandage for the injured eye. A cravat or cloth is rolled and wrapped to make a doughnut-shaped shield, which is fixed in place over the eye.

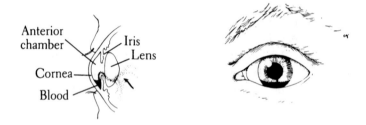

Figure 98. Hyphema. Bleeding into the eye causes an accumulation of blood in the anterior chamber, where it settles into a layer behind the cornea. In severe cases, the pupil is obscured by red blood.

Bleeding into the Eye

If the eyeball has been struck (not torn or ruptured), there may be bleeding from small blood vessels within the eye into the clear liquid that fills the space directly behind the cornea and in front of the lens. Such bleeding is called a hyphema. It first appears as diffuse bloody (red) clouding of the fluid behind the cornea, which settles over the course of 6 to 8 hours into a clearly visible layer of blood (figure 98). If such a condition is noted, the victim should have his eye patched closed (see the previous section) or wear sunglasses; he should be transported to an eye doctor. If possible, keep his head elevated and in an upright position. The victim should avoid straining.

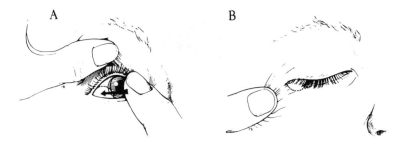

Figure 99. Contact lens removal. (A) Push the lens gently to the lateral (away from the nose) white portion of the eye. (B) A downward and outward pull on the skin at the lateral corner of the eye pops the lens free.

Removing Contact Lenses

If a victim is severely injured and he is wearing contact lenses, they should be removed. Either soft or hard lenses can be removed by the following technique (figure 99):

1. Slide the lens off the clear surface of the eye (cornea) over to the white area away from the nose.
2. Place one finger at the outside edge of the lower eyelid and pull the eyelid taut, while keeping the eye slightly open. This should lift the edge of the lens, so that you can pick it up. If you cannot remove the lens, position it so that as much as possible is over the white (and not on the cornea).
3. Place the lens in a container with contact lens solution, eyewash, or water (if possible, add 1 tsp, or 5 ml, of salt per pint, or 473 ml, of water).
4. A soft contact lens can often be removed by simply pinching it gently between your thumb and index finger.

If you cannot remove a contact lens, it is best to close the eye gently, place a soft cloth or gauze pad patch over it, and tape it closed. Be certain that someone knows why this has been done.

Subconjunctival Hemorrhage

Bleeding into the white of the eye (subconjunctival hemorrhage) may occur spontaneously or after coughing, straining (vigorous exertion), or

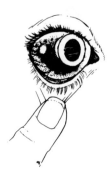

Figure 100. Subconjunctival hemorrhage. The red discoloration does not involve the cornea, which remains clear.

strangulation (figure 100). The bleeding is painless, does not interfere with vision (the cornea is not involved), and does not require any therapy. The blood will absorb over a period of a few weeks, as from any other bruise.

Red Eye

A red or pink, itchy eye is usually caused by a viral infection. Other causes include bacterial infection, allergy, foreign body (see page 161), irritation from chemicals or smoke, snow blindness (see below), or injury (see page 163). If the infection is caused by a virus or bacteria, symptoms include itching, tearing, discharge (runny yellow or greenish pus), crusted eyelashes and lids, and swollen eyelids, which are often stuck together upon awakening in the morning.

If the cause is a known allergy or irritation from smoke, use eyedrops with 0.025% oxymetazoline (OcuClear, Visine L.R.); antazoline phosphate 0.5% and naphazoline 0.05% (Vasocon-A); or tetrahydrolozine (Visine).

If there is much yellowish discharge, suspect a bacterial infection and administer antibiotic eyedrops (sodium sulamyd 10%, or gentamicin); the dose is two drops every 2 hours for 4 to 5 days while the victim is awake. Never use steroid-containing eyedrops unless directed to do so by a physician.

Snow Blindness

Exposure to ultraviolet radiation (UVR) from the sun can lead to a "sunburn" of the cornea (clear surface of the eye). This occurs when proper precautions are not used at high altitudes, where a greater amount of unfiltered (by the atmosphere) ultraviolet radiation is present; the exposure may be compounded by reflection from the snow. The intensity of ultraviolet energy increases by a factor of 4 to 6% for every 1,000' (305 m) increase in altitude above sea level. Snow reflects 85% of ultraviolet B (UVB, the culprit wavelengths that cause snow blindness); dry sand reflects 17%, while grass or sandy turf reflects 2.5%. Water may reflect 10 to 30% of ultraviolet B, depending upon the time of day and location.

The cornea absorbs ultraviolet radiation below 300 nanometers (nm), which includes a fair portion of UVB. Radiation of wavelengths longer than 300 nm is transmitted to the lens and, over time, can cause cataracts.

High exposure to UVB can cause a corneal burn within 1 hour, although symptoms may not become apparent for 6 to 12 hours. Symptoms include excessive tearing, pain, redness, swollen eyelids, pain when looking at light, headache, a gritty sensation in the eyes, and decreased (hazy) vision. Similar symptoms occur when the surface of the eye is physically scratched (corneal abrasion). Treatment consists of patching the eye closed (see page 162) after instilling a few drops of ophthalmic antibiotic solution (such as sodium sulamyd 10%, or gentamicin), because the surface of the cornea will regenerate spontaneously in 24 to 48 hours. It is important to check the eye first for a foreign body (see page 161). After patching, the eye must be rechecked in 24 hours. If the eye appears infected with pus, then it should be left unpatched; administer a topical antibiotic solution (see page 166) three to four times a day, and have the victim wear sunglasses. Pain medicine should be used as appropriate. If both eyes are involved, then only the more severely affected eye should be patched, so that the victim can continue to make his way.

Some people recommend topical steroid solution to hasten the resolution of snow blindness. In a situation in which the diagnosis is certain and such medication is available, instillation may indeed improve things. However, if a topical steroid is applied to a misdiagnosed bacterial or viral infection—particularly herpes virus—the effect can be to worsen the situation. Since snow blindness is self-limited, the application of a topical steroid is not imperative and best left to an ophthalmologist.

Protective Eyeglasses (Sunglasses)

The wavelengths of sunlight that appear to be most damaging to the eye are blue (400 to 500 nm), ultraviolet A (320 to 400 nm), and ultraviolet B (290 to 320 nm). Ultraviolet C (200 to 290 nm) is filtered out by the ozone layer of the atmosphere. Standards for ultraviolet protection in nonprescription sunglasses are set by the American National Standards Institute (ANSI). These state that such lenses should block 99.8% of ultraviolet B light. Lenses advertised for mountaineering or specifically for ultraviolet protection also block out considerable ultraviolet A light.

Sunglasses should be equipped with side protectors and, if necessary, optional nose guards. Frames should be prepared with wraparound temples and retaining straps or lanyards. Polycarbonate lenses, which are lightweight, scratch resistant, and shatterproof, can be manufactured to absorb 99% of ultraviolet light. Most recreation supply companies manufacture or carry sunglasses and wraparound goggles that meet ANSI standards.

In general, amber, yellow, orange, brown, and rose lenses filter out blue light and increase the perception of contrast. Green and gray lenses soften glare and transmit a spectrum that does not increase contrast. Glass ambermatic or photochromic lenses (darker in bright sunlight), which contain millions of silver halide crystals, darken when exposed to ultraviolet light close to the visible spectrum.

Improvised sunglasses can be made by cutting small slits or puncturing pinholes in cardboard or two layers of a strip of duct tape whose adhesive sides you have stuck together. Fashion a shape that will fit across the eyes like a pair of sunglasses; tie in the back with a string attachment. The opening should be just large enough to allow adequate vision. This serves two purposes: limitation of ultraviolet transmission and creation of crude refraction to improve focus.

Injury to the Retina

The retina is the thin inner posterior-surface tissue layer of the eye, the "screen" upon which images are transmitted by light. From the retina, nerves from the eye carry signals to the brain. The retina can be injured by the transmission of unrestricted infrared rays (wavelengths of light beyond the red end of the visible spectrum). Usually, this occurs when someone views the sun directly during an eclipse or when a person stares at the sun while under the influence of hallucinogenic drugs. Symptoms include pain and blindness. If such an injury is suspected, sunglasses should be worn or the eye should be patched. The victim should be transported to an eye doctor.

Occasionally, the aging process or a blow to the eye will cause the retina to become separated from the back of the eye (retinal detachment). Early symptoms include flashes of light and persistent floating spots in the field of vision ("floaters"). As the retina peels off farther, a person loses vision painlessly, as if a curtain were descending. Retinal detachment is a serious condition and requires emergency repair.

Glaucoma

Glaucoma is a condition in which the pressure of the fluid within the eye is elevated. If this happens suddenly, the pressure can injure the nerves within the eye that record vision; blindness can result. Symptoms of an acute attack of glaucoma include severe pain, blurred vision or "halos" around lights, clouding of the cornea, intense reddening of the white of the eye, a dilated pupil that doesn't react to light, nausea, vomiting, and headache. The victim of acute glaucoma is truly miserable. If an attack occurs, the victim should be kept in a sitting or standing position and rushed to an ophthalmologist. If the victim is carrying medication, instill a drop of pilocarpine in the affected eye.

Injured Eyelid

If the eyelid is injured, wash the eye carefully and then patch the eye closed (see page 162). If the eye cannot be covered with eyelid, apply a thick layer of bacitracin or mupirocin ointment to the eyelid and exposed eyeball and patch the eye. Seek immediate medical attention.

Sty

A sty is a small abscess (see page 212) that develops in one of the glands at the base of an eyelash. The infection causes the eyelid to swell, redden, and become painful. The victim may notice increased tear production and the sensation of a foreign body in the eye. Usually, the sty comes to a head on the outside of the lid, but occasionally it will come to a head inside. If a sty begins to develop, the victim should hold warm, moist compresses to his eyelid for 30 minutes four times a day to soften the abscess. It will either disappear or enlarge and come to a head. *Never squeeze an abscess on the face.* If the sty enlarges, comes to a head, and is extremely painful or interferes with vision, but will not open spontaneously, it can be carefully lanced with a sharp blade or needle to drain the pus. A physician should perform this procedure, unless the victim is more than 48 hours from medical attention and the infection has worsened to the extent that there is progressive swelling of the eyelid that impedes vision, or of the cheek or forehead. In this event, also administer dicloxacillin, erythromycin, or cephalexin. After the sty is incised, the pus can be expressed gently by pressing on opposite lateral sides with two cotton-tipped applicators.

Periorbital Cellulitis

Redness and swelling of the eyelid and "soft" tissues around the eye (eyebrow, upper cheek) caused by infection (see page 166) is known as periorbital (around the orbit, or eye) cellulitis. This is extremely serious and must be treated aggressively, because the infection can spread to create an abscess in the brain. Treatment consists of administration of an antibiotic (amoxicillin-clavulanate, dicloxacillin, cephalexin, or erythromycin) and immediate evacuation to a hospital. To differentiate periorbital cellulitis from the swollen eyelids associated with an allergic reaction, note that with cellulitis, the onset will have been more gradual (typically associated with a less severe eye infection, such as conjunctivitis, or a local infection such as a sty or pimple), the affliction is only on one side, there are fever and chills, the soft tissues are painful, there is headache, and there is often a purulent (with pus) discharge from the eye. With an allergy, the eye is more "puffy," the onset is sudden, the eye is itchy and watering, there is no purulent discharge, and there are associated signs and symptoms of allergy (skin rash, generalized itching, swollen lips, and so on.) (see page 58).

Nose

Nosebleed

Nosebleed is classified as anterior or posterior, depending on where it originates within the nose. Generally, anterior nosebleed is less serious, because the victim will usually drain blood outward through the nostrils. Posterior nosebleed is more difficult to control, and the victim often drains blood back into the throat, with coughing and potential choking. Anterior nosebleed is more common and can usually be managed outside of the hospital. *If you suspect a posterior nosebleed* (bleeding from the nose accompanied by brisk bleeding into the throat, so that a lot of blood is continually swallowed, particularly after the anterior bleeding has been controlled), *immediately evacuate the victim to a hospital.*

The most frequent cause of a nosebleed is a small bleeding blood vessel or cut on the inner surface of a nostril. This is more common at high altitudes and in cold weather, because the drying effect causes the skin to become irritated and crack. One way to prevent nosebleeds is to keep the inside of the nose lubricated with an ointment such as bacitracin, or to spray regularly with saline solution (such as Ocean saline mist or drops with 0.65% sodium chloride). A more serious cause of nosebleed is high blood pressure that has risen out of control. People on prescription anticoagulant drugs are prone to nosebleeds.

To control an anterior nosebleed, attempt simple maneuvers first. Have the victim blow his nose to remove all clots. Keep him upright (sitting leaning forward) and calm, and firmly press both nostrils closed against the nasal septum (middle cartilage). Hold this position for 15 minutes without release; letting go prior to this time will only restart the bleeding, because it takes the small blood vessels and scratched surface a while to stop oozing. After 15 minutes, let go and see if the bleeding has stopped. If not, gently but firmly pack both nostrils with a gauze or cotton roll soaked with phenylephrine 0.25% (Neo-Synephrine ¼%) and repeat the pinching maneuver for 20 minutes. Generally, this does the trick; if it doesn't, repeat the packing without the phenylephrine. After the bleeding has stopped, leave the packing in place for 2 hours and then gently remove it. Cold compresses applied to the bridge of the nose or a roll of gauze or cotton placed beneath the upper lip are of limited help when dealing with a brisk nosebleed. A useful device for packing the nose to stop a nosebleed is the Rhino-Rocket (Shippert Medical Technologies, Englewood, Colorado), which is a compressed medical-grade foam sponge with applicator. The foam is guided into place, where it swells on contact with moisture (blood) to 8 to 10 times its compressed size. A string is attached to the sponge so that it can be easily removed.

Broken Nose

A fractured nose may or may not be deformed. If the nose is obviously depressed or deformed to one side, and the victim is having difficulty breathing through his mouth, the nose can be relocated, but this is quite painful. Grasp the bridge of the nose firmly and crunch it upward and back over to the midline. In the wilderness, it can be difficult to improvise an external splint. A malleable soft-aluminum nasal splint with adhesive ventilating foam is available as The Denver Splint (Shippert Medical Technologies, Englewood, Colorado). Treat any nosebleed as previously discussed. *The only reason to relocate the injury is to improve breathing if mouth breathing is inadequate.* The nasal bones won't begin to set solidly for 5 to 7 days; cosmetic manipulation can easily be performed after such a delay. If the skin is cut deeply over a broken nose, start the victim on an antibiotic (penicillin, cephalexin, or erythromycin).

Another risk from a broken nose is the formation of a blood clot under the skin that lies over the nasal septum (cartilage) between the nostrils. If such a clot is not promptly drained, its resolution can cause collapse of the cartilage, infection, or erosion through the septum, leaving a hole through the septum. Anyone who has suffered a broken nose needs to be examined by a physician within 3 to 5 days of the injury, in order to avoid erosion of the nasal septum by a blood clot.

Foreign Body in the Nose

A small child will occasionally stuff a foreign object, such as a pebble or bead, into a nostril, where it will become stuck. Signs and symptoms include pain, a foul-smelling drainage, and sometimes fever. This can be a tough problem away from the hospital, because once the sensitive skin inside the nostril becomes irritated, it swells and traps the foreign object within a matrix of mucus, and sometimes blood or pus. If the object can't be easily seen and extracted without forcing it farther into the nostril or torturing the child, seek a physician's assistance. If you are carrying a flashlight and a small nasal speculum (a device for gently widening the nostril in order to facilitate access to the inside of the nose—Disposable Nasal Speculum, Bionix, Toledo, Ohio), you can attempt to look up the nose, but most small children will be extremely uncooperative, because this is pretty uncomfortable for them. If fever is present, start the child on dicloxacillin or erythromycin.

Sinusitis

The sinuses are spaces filled with air and lined with mucus-producing tissues found in the front of the skull and in the bones of the face (figure 101). Sinusitis is a blockage and infection/inflammation of the lining of the sinuses, usually caused by bacteria, and characterized by headache, fever, and tenderness in and over the involved sinus, with or without foul yellow or green discharge from the nose. Occasionally, the pain radiates to the eyes, bridge of the nose, and upper teeth. A person with sinusitis can become quite ill and suffer from excruciating headache, nausea, vomiting, and chills. Treatment involves the administration of an antibiotic (trimethoprim-sulfamethoxazole, amoxicillin-clavulanate, ciprofloxacin, trovafloxacin, azithromycin, ampicillin, clarithromycin, cefuroxime axetil,

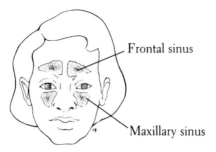

Frontal sinus

Maxillary sinus

Figure 101. Location of the sinuses.

or erythromycin) and decongestants (oral pseudoephedrine and a nasal spray: phenylephrine 0.25% [Neo-Synephrine ¼%] or oxymetazoline 0.05% [Afrin]), as well as warm packs over the affected area(s). Don't use a topical decongestant for more than 3 or 4 consecutive days, to avoid "rebound" swelling of the inside of the nasal passages from chemical irritation and sensitization to the drug. A person suffering from sinusitis should avoid rapid changes in ambient external pressure (such as scuba diving or air travel in unpressurized aircraft).

Throat

Sore Throat and Tonsillitis

Sore throat (pharyngitis) is a common complication of viral infections (the common cold, infectious mononucleosis), breathing dry air ("altitude throat"), or primary bacterial throat infection (strep throat). Symptoms of an infection include pain with swallowing, fever, swollen lymph nodes ("swollen glands") in the anterior neck, red throat, swollen tonsils, and pus over the tonsils and throat (see figure 102).

Because the symptoms of a viral throat and tonsil infection and a bacterial strep throat are frequently identical, it is hard to make the differentiation without a throat-swab "rapid strep test" or bacterial culture. Because the potential complications (kidney or heart disease) of an untreated strep throat in a young person outweigh the complications of antibiotic use, it is advisable to treat with penicillin, cefadroxil, or erythromycin for a full 10-day course, or with azithromycin or clarithromycin for 5 days. Even if the victim improves after 2 to 3 days, the antibiotic should be taken for the full course.

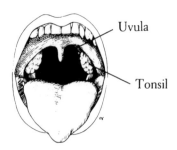

Figure 102. Inflamed tonsils.

Adjuncts to care include saltwater gargles (½ tsp, or 2.5 ml, of salt in 1 cup, or 237 ml, of warm water), throat lozenges, warm fluids (to moisten and soothe the throat), and aspirin or acetaminophen to control fever. To avoid Reye's syndrome (postviral encephalopathy and liver failure), do not use aspirin to control fever in a child under the age of 17.

If a person develops an acute sore throat that rapidly becomes extremely uncomfortable (severe pain, difficulty swallowing), a single dose of dexamethasone or its equivalent (see page 449) may be given along with an antibiotic, assuming the victim can swallow the medications. This may help decrease inflammation, but should not be given routinely for a "nontoxic," or run-of-the-mill, sore throat. *If someone with a sore throat has a high fever associated with difficult or noisy breathing, muffled voice ("like talking with a potato in his mouth"), drooling, stiff neck, or any visible swelling (bulging) in the back of the throat, he should be made as comfortable as possible and transported immediately to a hospital.* Such a condition may indicate an abscess (see page 212) in the back of the throat or next to a tonsil, infection and inflammation of the epiglottis (epiglottitis), or massively swollen tonsils. Any of these may rapidly obstruct the airway.

If a person develops tender swelling under the tongue and/or under the chin, particularly associated with swollen lymph glands in the neck, fever, difficulty swallowing, and foul breath, this may indicate an infection in the floor of the mouth. Treat the victim with an antibiotic as for a strep throat and seek an immediate physician consultation.

Infectious Mononucleosis

Mononucleosis ("mono") is a viral disease characterized by low-grade (less than 101° F, or 38.3° C) fever, sore throat, swollen lymph glands (mostly in the neck, but occasionally in the armpits or in the groin), headache, fatigue, and, occasionally, skin rash, dark urine, muscle aching, and an enlarged spleen. Treatment consists of increased rest (it sometimes requires weeks for a normal energy level to return) and elimination of any physical activity that requires heavy exertion or risks abdominal injury (and thus rupture of the spleen). The diagnosis is confirmed by a blood test; until that can be performed, the victim should be treated for a possible strep throat (see page 173). Because infectious mononucleosis can be spread via saliva, infected people should avoid sharing eating utensils and towels.

Common Cold

See page 179.

Mouth

Fever Blisters (Cold Sores)

Crops of blisters on the face, mouth, and lips that break out in times of stress (viral illness, emotional crisis, intense sun exposure) are often caused by reactivated herpes simplex virus. The blisters often weep and may become infected (see page 211). Unfortunately, there is little to do for these when they first appear except keep them clean and dry. If the skin cracks and becomes painful, the blisters may be lubricated with bacitracin or mupirocin ointment. Anesthetic ointment can be used if it is helpful. Further sun exposure should be prevented with an adequate lip sunscreen (see page 201) of SPF 20 or greater.

Untreated, the lesions will disappear spontaneously in 10 to 15 days. Acyclovir (Zovirax) ointment applied thinly five times a day for a week can hasten resolution of the blisters. Alternately, a person may be prescribed acyclovir 200 mg five times a day, or 400 mg three times a day, for 5 days.

All herpes viruses are contagious. During times of visible blisters, eating and drinking utensils should not be shared. To maximize prevention, use a high-SPF sunscreen and consider taking acyclovir (Zovirax) (400 mg twice daily by mouth) the day before and during intense ultraviolet light exposure.

Canker (Mouth) Sores

These painful white patches with reddened edges form inside the mouth and may be associated with viral infections or an immune response to an infection or disease. Usually they are a chronic problem. Untreated, they last for 10 to 14 days. They may be treated with a topical application of anesthetic lidocaine ointment 2.5% for a minute or two prior to eating, in order to kill the pain temporarily. Another useful topical anesthetic is 20% benzocaine (Hurricaine), which can be conveniently applied from a prepackaged dry handle swab. One recommendation is to apply a pinch of powdered alum (as in a styptic pencil) to initiate healing. In order to hasten resolution, a physician might prescribe a mixture of fluocinonide 0.05% ointment (Lidex) and Orabase to be laid over the ulcer six to eight times per day, or triamcinolone dental paste (Kenalog in Orabase) to be administered similarly. The inside of the mouth should be rinsed thoroughly after eating to prevent food from becoming trapped in the sores. Any new sore in the mouth of an elderly person or frequent user of tobacco should be seen by a physician, who must consider a precancerous lesion or oral cancer.

Toothaches and Tooth Infections

Toothaches occur in teeth that are decayed or have lost fillings. In this manner, the central pulp, which carries nerves and blood vessels, becomes inflamed (pulpitis). Symptoms of tooth inflammation include pain in the tooth and jaw that occasionally travels into the neck and ear, pain on contact with cold or hot liquids, and headache. Sometimes it is difficult to localize the problem to a specific tooth, since it may not be sensitive when it is tapped. To identify the culprit tooth, apply an ice cube sequentially to each tooth until you elicit a painful reaction. Pain medication appropriate for the degree of suffering should be administered. Have the victim keep his head elevated.

If it hurts to bite down on a tooth, but nothing is obvious upon inspection of it, there may be inflammation of the supporting structures. In this case, the victim can point to the affected tooth, or feel pain when you tap on a particular tooth. Treatment is a soft diet, pain medication, and something like a strip of leather to bite down upon positioned on the non-painful (opposite) side, to create a space and prevent pressure on the affected tooth.

If an abscess (infection) (see page 212) develops in the root of the tooth or in the gum, there may be associated fever; swelling of the gum, jaw, or palate; and swollen lymph glands under the jaw and in the neck. If the abscess extends, the cheek and side of the face may swell. The victim should be started on penicillin, metronidazole, cephalexin, or erythromycin, and given appropriate pain medication. If there is a soft, pointing abscess in the gum adjacent to a tooth and the victim is suffering, the abscess can be

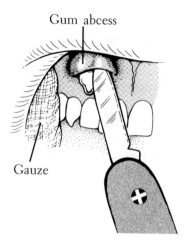

Gum abcess

Gauze

Figure 103. Incision and drainage of a gum abscess.

punctured with a scalpel or knife and drained (figure 103). Hold snow or ice against the gum to provide some anesthesia prior to the incision. A gauze or cotton wick should be placed into the abscess cavity for a day or two (see page 212). After this procedure, the area should be rinsed with salt water after each meal, at least four times a day.

To temporarily treat a cavity (decay) or site of a lost filling, dry the affected tooth carefully with cotton. Next, apply a cotton pad moistened with oil of cloves (eugenol) to the tooth cavity. In a pinch, you can use vanilla extract. Take care to keep eugenol off the gums, lips, and inside surfaces of the cheeks. Alternately, Anbesol can be applied to the gums. The patient needs to be taken to a dentist to have the tooth repaired or removed.

Another remedy for a cavity caused by decay or a lost filling is to fill the cavity with temporary filling material from a dental kit. Such materials include Cavit (Premier Co., Norristown, Pennyslvania), which requires no mixing. It is applied directly to the tooth, using a wetted toothpick or cotton-tipped applicator as a packing and shaping instrument. Intermediate Restorative Material (IRM, from L. D. Caulk Co., Milford, Delaware) is prepared by adding a few drops of clove oil to powdered zinc oxide to make as dry a "dough" as possible. Zinc oxide—eugenol combination cements are advantageous in that they have an anesthetic effect and can be mixed to different consistencies, depending upon whether they are to be used as filling material or adhesives. However, the liquid can leak from its container, and the cement is sticky and more difficult to work with than Cavit.

Such fillings set after exposure to saliva and usually have to be replaced every few days. Another improvised filling is softened candle wax mixed with a few strands of cotton fiber, applied over a drop or two of eugenol.

If the gum line is inflamed or appears infected adjacent to a tooth, you can try to "break up" the infection by flossing vigorously or running a toothpick (probe) down into the space between the tooth and gum line. Administer an antibiotic, such as penicillin or metronidazole.

Pericoronitis is an infection of the gum flap that overlies a tooth that has only partially advanced ("erupted") into the mouth. This is most common with a lower third molar and usually indicates an infection with *Streptococcus* bacteria. The treatment is to scrape and clean underneath and around the flap, initiate warm saltwater rinses every 2 hours, and begin the victim on dicloxacillin, cephalexin, or erythromycin.

Broken or Lost Tooth

If a tooth is cracked (with the root still present and in place), there is little for the victim to do other than keep his mouth clean and avoid contact with extremes of temperature. If air coming into contact with an exposed nerve causes intolerable pain, a temporary cap (shield) can be created by mixing melted paraffin (candle wax) with a few strands of cotton. When the mixture begins to harden but can still be easily molded, press a wad onto the tooth, using the teeth on either side as anchors. A cap can also be fashioned from Cavit or IRM (see the discussion above).

If a crown falls off, apply a little eugenol to the tooth and see if the crown will hold without cement. If not, apply a dab of Cavit and use it as a fastener, scraping away the excess. If all else fails, cover the tooth with paraffin or dental wax.

If a tooth is knocked cleanly out of the socket, it can sometimes be replaced successfully if the victim can reach a dentist within the first hour. After 2 hours, there is little hope for salvage of that particular tooth. The best treatment for a tooth that has been out of the socket for 15 minutes or less is to gently rinse it clean (do not scrub the root of the tooth) and reinsert it with firm pressure into the socket to the level of the adjacent tooth. Try to splint the tooth in place with a paraffin bridge or a cap to the adjacent tooth. A better material for this purpose is Express Putty, which hardens within 4 minutes after equal amounts of the putty base and catalyst are mixed.

The best storage solution for a tooth that will be carried to a dentist is pH (acid-base) balanced (Hank's balanced salt solution) and accompanied by a cushion to prevent injury to the microscopic ligament cells that hold the tooth in place and must reattach for the tooth to "take." The Save-A-Tooth storage device (3M Health Care) is recommended.

Alternately, the tooth can be placed in a container and covered with a small amount of cool, pasteurized whole milk (not yogurt, low-fat milk, or powdered milk) for transport. Do not carry the tooth on a dry cloth or paper. Do not soak the tooth in tap water. A tooth can also be rinsed and carried by the victim in the space between his lower lip and lower gum (taking care not to swallow the tooth), although saliva is not particularly good for the periodontal ligament. *Do not place a tooth back into the socket unless an antibiotic (penicillin 500 mg four times a day for 2 weeks) can be administered to avoid an infection, and tetanus toxoid given if necessary.*

Temporal-Mandibular Joint (TMJ) Syndrome

The temporal-mandibular joint—where the jaw hinges into the face—can become tender if the jaw is struck, from forceful chewing or yawning, or from grinding the teeth at night. If this joint becomes irritated, the pain can be extremely distracting. Therapy consists of a nonsteroidal inflammatory drug such as ibuprofen, warm packs, and avoiding foods (like beef jerky) that are difficult to chew. Don't chew gum or open the mouth excessively wide.

Mouth Ulcer (Canker Sore)

See page 175.

UPPER RESPIRATORY DISORDERS

Common Cold

Most "colds" are upper respiratory tract infections caused by one of a host (at least 200) of viruses. It is not true that exposure to a cold climate ("catching a chill") causes a cold. Symptoms include runny nose, cough, sore throat, headache, muscle aches, fever, fatigue, weakness, and occasional nausea with vomiting and/or diarrhea. Unfortunately, there is no cure for the common cold. The best medicine is rest, increased fluid intake to prevent dehydration and loosen secretions, and acetaminophen or aspirin for fever. To avoid Reye's syndrome (postviral encephalopathy and liver failure), do not use aspirin to control fever in a child under the age of 17.

Keep the victim warm and dry. Treat nasal congestion with an oral decongestant and nasal spray (use the latter for 3 days maximum). Be aware that an oral decongestant can make a child hyperactive. For an infant, use saline nose drops (¼ tsp, or 1.3 ml, of table salt in 1 cup, or 237 ml, of water) in a dose of two to three drops in each nostril a few times a day; the child will sneeze, or the drops can drain via gravity or be sucked out with a "baby bulb" syringe.

A person who breathes steam (which has not been proven to improve a common cold) must be careful to avoid burns. There is no scientific evidence to support the use of chest rubs or megavitamins (specifically, vitamin C) in the prevention or amelioration of viral illnesses. Probably the most important factor in rehabilitation is adequate rest.

Do not attempt to "sweat out" a cold with vigorous exercise. Such harmful behavior causes worsened fever, debilitation, and dehydration. It is a method guaranteed to convert a common cold into pneumonia. A person with a cold should see a doctor if he is ill for more than 3 weeks, his temperature elevation becomes extreme (see page 151), he develops a cough productive of yellow-green or darkened phlegm (see pages 43 and 181), or he develops chest pain associated with breathing, shaking chills, a severe earache, or a headache with a stiff neck (see page 157). Since colds are spread by contact, take particular care to wash your hands after contact with an infected person.

The most common complication of a cold in a child is a middle ear infection. If a child with a runny nose and cough begins to pull at his ear(s) or if a fever returns near the end of the course of a cold, consider treating the child for otitis media (see page 157). Pneumonia can also be a complication (see page 43). It should be suspected in a child who appears short of breath (respiratory rate above 30 per minute in a child, or 40 per minute in an infant).

A cold can be differentiated from seasonal allergies on the basis of the following: cold—fever, chills, yellowish or green nasal discharge, sore throat, diarrhea, muscle aches; allergies—clear nasal discharge, repetitive sneezing, watery and itchy eyes.

Someone who has a chronic (lasts longer than 3 weeks) cough not clearly associated with a cold or other viral infection of the respiratory tract, who is coughing up blood, or who has another known problem such as pneumonia or lung cancer should seek the attention of a physician. The most common causes of a chronic cough are cigarette smoking, postnasal drip (often stimulated by seasonal allergies), unsuspected asthma, chronic sinus infection, or acid reflux from the stomach into the esophagus. In addition, those who take a certain category of medicine (ACE inhibitors) to treat high blood pressure may develop a cough; this usually disappears a few days after the medicine is discontinued.

Influenza

The influenza virus is responsible for seasonal epidemics of the flu, a predominantly respiratory disease. The illness is recognized by sudden high fever, sore throat, cough, headache, muscle aches, weakness, and occasional nausea with vomiting and/or diarrhea. It is distinguished from a common cold by its intensity, particularly of the headache and muscle aches.

Elderly or infirm individuals are at greatest risk for becoming severely debilitated or developing complications, such as pneumonia. General therapy is the same as that for a cold: rest, adequate nutrition, increased fluid intake, and medicine for fever. Vaccines are prepared each year that are somewhat effective in the prevention of types A and B influenza (see page 402). During an epidemic, elderly or infirm people may benefit from the administration of the oral drug amantadine hydrochloride, which is available by prescription for the prevention and treatment of type A influenza (it is ineffective against type B).

Bronchitis

Bronchitis is an infection of the air passages (bronchi), characterized by cough, production of sputum (yellow or green phlegm, or "secretions"), fever, and fatigue. Pneumonia is much more intense than bronchitis, and involves severe progressive pulmonary deterioration; bronchitis is a less debilitating infection. Cigarette smokers are prone to recurrent bouts of bronchitis, because they suffer from scarred lungs and continually paralyze the defense mechanisms of the nose, throat, and lungs with cigarette smoke.

Treatment consists of an oral antibiotic (amoxicillin, amoxicillin-clavulanate, trimethoprim-sulfamethoxazole, doxycycline, erythromycin, or azithromycin), copious fluid intake, inhalation of humidified warm air (taking care to avoid steam burns) in order to loosen secretions and ease coughing, and acetaminophen or aspirin (not for children under the age of 17 years) for fever. It is best to allow the victim to cough up secretions; however, if coughing fits become intolerable, a cough medicine (see page 449) should be used. If pneumonia is suspected (see page 43), treat appropriately and seek immediate medical attention.

Hay Fever

Hay fever ("rose fever," "catarrh") is an allergic reaction, often seasonal, to dust, animal dander, plant (usually ragweed, sage, trees, and grasses) pollens, or other compounds found in the air. The victim suffers from red, itchy, and watery eyes; a runny nose with large amounts of clear mucus (allergic rhinitis); sneezing; and general misery. In a severe case, a victim may suffer asthma, sinusitis, loss of smell, and fatigue. In most cases, the symptoms can be relieved by taking an antihistamine medication—although some of these have side effects, the most troublesome of which is drowsiness. Antihistamines that cause drowsiness include triprolidine (Actifed), diphenhydramine (Benadryl), and chlorpheniramine (Chlor-Trimeton). Newer prescription antihistamines, such as fexofenadine (Allegra, which replaces terfenadine [Seldane]), loratadine (Claritin), cetirizine (Zyrtec), and astemizole (Hismanal), cause much less or no sedation. A nasal decongestant (such as oxymetazoline [Afrin]) will clear out the nose, but does not halt the allergic reaction. Furthermore, a nasal decongestant should not be used for more than 5 consecutive days, to avoid "rebound" nasal congestion from drug-induced inflammation. An allergy doctor can use skin tests to evaluate a victim for desensitization injections. If allergies are debilitating and a change in environment is impossible, the victim will almost certainly benefit from a tapering dose of prednisone (see page 100). Nasal steroid sprays (such as fluticasone propionate 0.05% [Flonase] or beclomethasone diproprionate [Beconase]) are a new method for treating nasal irritation from allergies, but usually require approximately 3 days of continual use before a beneficial effect is noted. Cromolyn sodium nasal spray (Nasalcrom), as recommended by some allergists, is another useful adjunct. This requires administration of up to four to six doses per day, and it may be 1 to 4 weeks before any benefit is noted.

Nonsteroidal eyedrops for ocular allergy manifestations (seasonal allergic conjunctivitis) include 4% cromolyn sodium, ketorolac tromethamine 0.5% (Acular), lodoxamide 0.1% (stabilizes the cells that release histamine), and levocabastine hydrochloride 0.05% (histamine antagonist). While each of these is effective, it remains to be proven if any is more effective than cold soaks, artificial tears, and/or topical antihistamine eyedrops. Eye symptoms usually respond to oral medications used to treat systemic allergies.

Pleuritis

The lining of the lung, or pleura, is two layers of tissue separated by a thin film of lubricating fluid, which allows the lung to expand with a gliding motion when the chest wall moves outward during inhalation. When the pleura is irritated by an infection, most often caused by a virus, the inflammation may allow fluid to accumulate in this space and cause pain with breathing, localized to the area of irritation. The pain is sharp and worsened by a cough or deep breath. The treatment for viral pleuritis is rest and aspirin. Encourage the victim to breathe deeply. If he is weak or has a high fever, suspect deterioration into pneumonia (see page 43).

DISORDERS OF THE GASTROINTESTINAL TRACT

Diarrhea

Although diarrhea is included here in the "minor problems" section, severe diarrhea can be devastating. Diarrhea can be due to a number of causes, which include bacterial infection, viral infection, protozoal infection, food poisoning from toxin(s), unusual parasites (such as *Cyclospora cayetanensis*, which can contaminate fresh berries), inflammatory bowel disease, allergies, and anxiety. It is not always easy to determine the cause of loose bowel movements, but there is a general approach to therapy that ordinarily suffices until a precise diagnosis can be made.

In all cases of diarrhea, a common discomfort is the irritated anus (particularly one that has been wiped with leaves or newspaper). Every traveler should carry a roll of toilet paper and 1% hydrocortisone lotion or steroid ointment for an irritated bottom. Desitin diaper cream and A&D ointment also work well.

General Therapy for Diarrhea

Diet. If nausea and vomiting do not prevent eating, adjust the diet:
   1. When diarrhea is severe, stick to clear fluids such as mineral water, soda, Kool-Aid, or broth. Electrolyte-containing sports beverages are fine. Apple and grape juices are good, but orange, tomato,

pineapple, and grapefruit juices may irritate the stomach. Avoid milk products, tea, coffee, raw fruits and vegetables, and fatty foods. Do not take aspirin.

2. As soon as there is improvement (less frequent bowel movements, decreased cramping, increased appetite), begin solid foods, starting with broth, crackers, toast, gelatin, and hard-boiled eggs.

3. As the diarrhea subsides, add applesauce, mashed bananas, rice, boiled or baked potatoes, and plain pasta.

4. When stools begin to harden, add cooked lean meat, cooked vegetables, yogurt, and cottage cheese. Avoid alcohol, spicy foods, and stewed fruit.

Dehydration can be estimated as follows:

1. Mild dehydration: thirst, dry mucous membranes (mouth, eyes), dry armpits, dark urine, decreased sweating, normal pulse rate.

2. Moderate dehydration: the above plus sunken eyes, doughy skin, weakness, scant darkened urine, rapid and weak pulse rate.

3. Severe dehydration: the above plus altered mental status, elevated body temperature, no urine, no tears, no sweating, collapse, shock (see page 54).

In a baby, dehydration is manifest as dry diaper (decreased urine output), sunken eyes, sunken "soft spot" (fontanel) on the top of the head, dry tongue and mouth, rapid pulse, poor skin color (blue or pale), lethargy ("floppy baby"), and fast breathing (greater than 30 breaths per minute in a small child, or 40 per minute in an infant). For purposes of estimation, a normal pulse rate (per minute) in a newborn averages 120; at 2 years, 110; at 4 to 6 years, 100; and at 8 to 10 years, 90.

Fluid replacement. If fluid losses are significant (more than five bowel movements per day), begin to replace liquids as soon as you can.

1. Mild diarrhea/dehydration: Drink soda water, clear juices, tea, broth, and electrolyte-containing sports beverages.

2. Moderate diarrhea/dehydration: Drink diluted (by half, with water) electrolyte-containing sports beverages, mineral water (bottled), or a homemade solution (1 quart or liter of disinfected water plus ½ to 1 tsp, or 1.3 to 2.5 ml, of sodium chloride [table salt], ½ tsp of sodium bicarbonate [baking soda], ¼ tsp, or .6 ml, of potassium chloride [salt substitute], and glucose [6 to 8 tsp, or 30 to 40 ml, of table sugar; or 1 to 2 tbsp, or 15 to 30 ml, of honey]). Take care not to oversweeten (exceed 2 to 2.5% glucose) the solution with sugar, because this may worsen the diarrhea; too high a sugar concentration inhibits water absorp-

tion through the gastrointestinal tract. Each quart of this "home brew" should be alternated with ½ to 1 quart of plain disinfected water.

Oral Rehydration Salts (ORS) that meet World Health Organization standards are available in a dry mix; use one packet per quart (liter) of water. One packet contains sodium chloride 3.5 g, potassium chloride 1.5 g, glucose 20 g, and trisodium citrate 2.9 g (or sodium bicarbonate 2.5 g). Cera Lyte 70 oral rehydration salts are based on a rice solution. One packet is mixed with a quart (liter) of water.

Try to get the victim to ingest a quart per hour until the frequency of urination begins to increase and the urine color turns light or clear. A child should be given 1 ½ oz (44 ml) of ORS per pound (.45 kg) of body weight over the first 4 hours, then 1 oz (30 ml) of ORS per pound of body weight per 8-hour period until the diarrhea resolves. For an infant with diarrhea, decrease the amount of milk in the diet, and add more water, diluted juices, half-strength sports beverages, and ORS. If the child is breast-fed, keep nursing (offer the breast more often). If the child is formula-fed, stick with it for a few days, then change to a soy-based formula or ORS if the diarrhea persists.

If premeasured salts are not available with which to supplement water, you can alternate glasses of the following two fluids, as recommended by the U.S. Public Health Service:

GLASS ONE—8 oz fruit juice with ¼ tsp (a "pinch") salt and ½ tsp honey or corn syrup (237 ml juice, 1.3 ml salt, 2.5 ml honey or corn syrup)

GLASS TWO—8 oz disinfected water with ¼ tsp baking soda (sodium bicarbonate) (237 ml water, 1.3 ml baking soda)

Another homemade fluid mixture is 1 teaspoon (5 ml) table salt and 1 cup (275 ml) rice cereal in a quart (liter) of water; this must be used within 12 hours or discarded. If only fruit juice (without supplementation) is available, remember to cut it to half strength with water. Otherwise, the sugar content will be too high and may contribute to continued diarrhea. Estimation techniques to measure powdered ingredients (such as a "pinch" of salt) are notoriously inaccurate, and can even be dangerous if you add excessive amounts. Use a proper measuring implement whenever possible.

3. Severe diarrhea/dehydration: Same as moderate. After a certain

point, as with cholera, intravenous hydration may be lifesaving. See
a physician as soon as possible.

Antimotility (decreased bowel activity) drugs. If fever, severe cramping, and
bloody diarrhea are absent, it is safe to use antimotility drugs,
although they should be immediately discontinued if diarrhea lasts for
more than 48 hours. If diarrhea lasts longer than 3 days, if the victim
has a fever greater than 101° F (38.3° C), if he cannot keep liquids
down because of vomiting, if there is blood in or on the stool, if the
abdomen becomes swollen, or if there is no significant pain relief after
24 hours, seek a physician immediately.

The antimotility drug of choice is loperamide (Imodium AD) (see
page 445). The initial adult dose is 4 mg (two 2 mg capsules, or 4 tsp—
20 ml—of the liquid), followed by 2 mg after each loose bowel movement, not to exceed 16 mg (eight capsules) per day or 2 days of
administration. With uncomplicated (no fever or blood in stools),
watery diarrhea, this drug can be given to children age 2 years and
older. Give children 0.2 mg per kg (2.2 lb) of body weight dose every 6
hours. The liquid preparation contains 1 mg per tsp (5 ml).

For adults, diphenoxylate (Lomotil) (see page 445) is an alternative, but has side effects of dry mouth and urinary retention. Pepto-
Bismol is another, less effective choice (see page 446).

Kaopectate (kaolin plus pectin) is of limited value; it does not
shorten the course of diarrheal illness, and acts only to add a little consistency to stools. Lactobacillus preparations (acidophilus beverages or
yogurt) do not shorten the course of acute diarrheal illness.

In foreign countries, drugs are on occasion recommended for diarrhea without a specific diagnosis. These drugs include chloramphoeni-
col (Chloromycetin), Enterovioform, MexaForm, Intestopan, clio-
quinol, and iodoquinol. This may be dangerous, because these drugs
can have certain adverse direct effects or side effects. Therefore, they
should not be taken without a specific diagnosis for which they are felt
to be indicated.

Antibiotics. These should be used if diarrhea is moderate to severe (more
than eight bowel movements per day), particularly if it is bloody and
associated with severe cramping, vomiting, and fever.

1. Administer ciprofloxacin (Cipro) 500 mg twice a day, or trimethoprim-
sulfamethoxazole (Bactrim or Septra) one double-strength pill twice
a day for 3 days. These will treat *E. coli* and *Shigella,* may be of use for
Salmonella, and will not adversely affect the course of viral, *Staphylococcus,* or *Campylobacter* infections. The duration of cholera caused by
Vibrio cholerae may be shortened by treating with ciprofloxacin (1 g
single dose) or doxycycline (300 mg single dose) for adults, or

trimethoprim-sulfamethoxazole for children (5 mg per kg, or 2.2 lb, of body weight, based on the trimethoprim component, for 3 days). Enteric fever caused by *Salmonella typhi* (typhoid fever) is best treated in adults with ciprofloxacin.

Alternative drugs include norfloxacin (Noroxin) 400 mg twice a day for 3 days, ofloxacin (Floxin) 200 or 300 mg twice a day for 3 days, or fleroxacin 400 mg once a day for 3 days. Another alternative drug is doxycycline (Vibramycin) 100 mg twice a day. Children younger than 12 years of age should not be given doxycycline, because it may cause discoloration of the permanent teeth. Because ciprofloxacin may affect bone growth in children, it should only be given to adults.

2. If the clinical picture clearly points to *Giardia lamblia* (see page 190), administer metronidazole (Flagyl) 250 mg three times a day for 7 days. (A woman who is possibly pregnant should not use this drug except under the advice of her physician.)

Traveler's Diarrhea

Traveler's diarrhea ("turista") is caused by waterborne or food-borne pathogens, most commonly produced by forms of the bacterium *Escherichia coli*, which is introduced into the diet as a fecal contaminant in water or on food. When caused by *E. coli*, symptoms usually occur 12 to 36 hours after ingesting the bacteria, and include the gradual or sudden onset of frequent (four to five per day) loose or watery bowel movements, rarely explosive, and far less violent than diarrhea associated with classic food poisoning (see below). Fever, bloating, fatigue, and abdominal pain are of minor to moderate severity. Nausea and vomiting are less frequently found than with viral gastroenteritis.

The affliction will resolve spontaneously in 2 to 5 days if untreated, but may be hastened to a conclusion if an antibiotic is administered. The current recommendation is to treat adults with ciprofloxacin (Cipro) 500 mg twice a day for 3 days or a single dose of 1 g, norfloxacin 800 mg in a single dose, or trimethoprim-sulfamethoxazole (Septra or Bactrim DS) in a dose of one double-strength tablet twice a day for 3 days. For known traveler's diarrhea, the addition of loperamide (Imodium AD) (see page 445) to the antibiotic regimen can be of significant benefit, with the precaution that it should be used only in the absence of high fever or bloody diarrhea. Alternately, the diarrhea can be treated with bismuth subsalicylate (Pepto-Bismol); give two 262 mg tablets (or the liquid equivalent) every 30 minutes for five doses, which may be repeated the second day.

To prevent traveler's diarrhea, a person traveling to high-risk regions with questionable hygiene and municipal water-disinfection standards (developing countries of Latin America, Africa, the Middle East, and Asia) can take prophylactic trimethoprim-sulfamethoxazole (Septra or Bactrim) one double-strength tablet a day, or ciprofloxacin 500 mg (or norfloxacin 400 mg or ofloxacin 200 mg) once a day, during the journey. Southern Europe (Spain, Greece, Italy, Turkey) and parts of the Caribbean pose a lesser risk. Another drug that can be used is doxycycline (Vibramycin) 100 mg twice a day. This should be done under the guidance of a physician, who will explain the risks (allergic reactions, blood disorders, antibiotic-associated colitis, vaginal yeast infection, skin rashes, photosensitivity) versus the benefits (particularly for those prone to infectious diarrhea or who would suffer unduly from an episode of severe diarrhea). Ingesting lactobacilli may improve certain aspects of digestion, but does not prevent traveler's diarrhea.

Alternately, it has been recommended that you can drink 4 tbsp (60 ml) of Pepto-Bismol (bismuth subsalicylate) four times a day; this necessitates carrying one 8 oz bottle for each day. The tablets (two 262 mg tablets four times a day) are less palatable. However, this prophylaxis is not intended to substitute for dietary discretion. In addition, large doses of bismuth subsalicylate can be toxic, particularly to people who regularly use aspirin. Anyone with an aspirin allergy should not use bismuth subsalicylate.

People who would be advised to consider taking a drug to prevent infectious diarrhea include those with a significant underlying medical problem (such as AIDS, inability to produce stomach acid, inflammatory bowel disease) and those with an itinerary rigid enough that it would be catastrophic to the mission to be laid up with diarrhea.

In general, it is safe to brush your teeth with foreign or mountain water, so long as you spit and don't swallow. Salads, raw vegetables, raw or undercooked meat (particularly hamburgers), raw seafood, unpeeled fruits and vegetables, cold sauces, ice cream, fresh cheese, spicy sauces in open containers, tap water, and ice are risky business. Fruits and leafy vegetables should be washed in iodinated water, washed with dilute soap and previously boiled water, or immersed in boiling water for 30 seconds. In some underdeveloped countries, melons are injected with contaminated water to increase their weight prior to sale. Be cautious with the salads served on flights that originate from third world countries.

Water disinfection is discussed on page 385. Stick to boiled water, food that is served steaming hot, dry foods (bread), bottled carbonated beverages, and reputable food establishments. Alcohol in mixed drinks does not disinfect water. Packaged butter and packaged processed cheese are usually safe to eat. Unpasteurized dairy products should be avoided. With regard to seafood, raw or undercooked products, particularly shellfish, are especially hazardous. *Vibrio* organisms—which cause, among other problems, cholera—frequently reside in crabs and oysters. Cook all shellfish for a minimum of 10 minutes of boiling, or 30 minutes of exposure to full steam.

Viral Diarrhea

Viral gastroenteritis includes diarrhea as a symptom. It is often associated with nausea and vomiting, fever, stomach cramps, copious rectal gas, and a flulike syndrome. The diarrhea is typically watery, frequent (up to 20 movements per day), and often foul smelling, discolored (green to greenish brown), and without significant mucus or blood. Generally, the victim will have cyclic waves of lower-abdominal cramps, relieved by bowel movements.

Therapy requires continual oral hydration with clear liquids such as apple juice or broth. If they are available, drink electrolyte-containing sports beverages. It is critical to keep the victim from becoming dehydrated. What comes out below should be replaced from above.

The cramps can be controlled with propantheline bromide (Pro-Banthine), loperamide (Imodium AD), or diphenoxylate (Lomotil), which will also help limit the diarrhea (see page 183). It should be noted, however, that these drugs will slow down the activity of the bowel and allow any toxins that are in the gut to remain in contact with the bowel wall. With certain bacterial infections, these drugs may prolong the carrier state and actually increase the severity and duration of the disease. Therefore, it is prudent to avoid the use of Imodium AD or Lomotil unless the intake of fluids cannot keep pace with the diarrhea, and dehydration is becoming a real concern. *Never give an antimotility agent to an infant.* Imodium AD can be used in children age 2 years and older if the diarrhea is clear (no blood) and watery, there is no associated fever, and diarrhea is leading to debilitating dehydration. Give a child a 0.2 mg per kg (2.2 lb) of body weight dose every 6 hours. The liquid preparation contains 1 mg per tsp (5 ml).

Food Poisoning

Food poisoning is caused by toxins that are produced by a number of bacteria, with the most common being *Staphylococcus*. Improper preservation (generally, lack of refrigeration) of food allows bacterial proliferation, which is not corrected by cooking. Typically, the symptoms occur 2 to 6 hours after eating and consist of severe abdominal cramps with nausea and vomiting. Diarrhea may be delayed by an hour or two, or may occur simultaneously with the nausea and vomiting. The diarrhea is often explosive. As with viral gastroenteritis, the bowel movements may be foul smelling and blood tinged. The disease is self-limited, and generally subsides after 6 to 12 hours. Treatment consists of rehydration with clear liquids. Antimotility drugs, such as loperamide (Imodium AD) or diphenoxylate (Lomotil), may prolong the disorder, and should not be used unless the victim cannot replenish fluid losses.

E. coli O157:H7

Escherichia coli O157:H7 is a bacterium that has been transmitted in raw or undercooked hamburger meat, fruit juices, and other food with fecal contamination. It has also been transmitted in recreational-swimming-pool water. It causes a syndrome of fever, abdominal pain, vomiting, and non-bloody diarrhea, followed in a few days by bloody diarrhea, dehydration, anemia, and kidney failure. There is not yet an effective treatment with antibiotics. In fact, therapy with some antibiotics may contribute to more severe illness. Prevention means cooking ground beef until it is no longer pink. Fruit juices prepared from crushing processes may require boiling or pasteurization.

Giardia lamblia

Giardia lamblia is a flagellate protozoan (one-celled organism) that has become a worldwide problem, particularly in wilderness settings in the western United States, Nepal, and the Soviet Union. It is transmitted as cysts in the feces of many animals, which include humans, elk, beavers, deer, cows, dogs, and sheep. Dormant *Giardia* cysts enter water, from which they are ingested by humans. Cysts can live for up to 3 months in cold water.

If more than 10 to 25 cysts are swallowed, the organisms establish residence in the duodenum and jejunum (first parts of the small bowel), and after an incubation period of 7 to 20 days emerge in another form (trophozoite) to cause stomach cramps, flatulence, a swollen lower abdomen, often explosive and foul-smelling watery ("floating") diarrhea, "rotten" (sulfurous) belching, and nausea. Fever and vomiting are unusual except in the first few days of illness. Foul flatus and abdominal cramping are common. Because of the delay in onset after ingestion of the cysts, many a backpacker develops "backpacker's diarrhea" or "beaver fever" after he returns to civilization, and he does not make the mental connection to his recent journey. If the diarrhea becomes chronic, the victim can lose appetite, lose weight, and become weak. Diagnosis is made by a physician who recognizes trophozoites or microscopic cysts in the stool of the victim, takes a sample of mucus from the duodenum, or is confident with a clinical diagnosis.

Untreated, the illness usually resolves after about 6 weeks. However, the diarrhea can go on for months. Therapy for *Giardia* infestation is the administration of metronidazole (Flagyl) 250 mg three times a day for 7 days. An alternate prescription drug is quinacrine hydrochloride (Atabrine) 100 mg twice a day for 7 days; the pediatric dose is 7 mg per kg (2.2 lb) of body weight per day in three divided doses for 7 days. Unfortunately, this drug has side effects (which occur in 1 to 4 out of every 1,000 people) that include making the person psychotic (lose touch with reality) for up to a few weeks. A good drug that is available in Nepal and some other foreign countries is tinidazole (Tiniba, Fasgyn), which is taken in one 2 g dose; the pediatric dose is 50 mg per kg (2.2 lb) of body weight in a single dose. A good drug for children is furazolidone (Furoxone) 6 mg per kg of body weight in four divided doses for 7 days. There have been mixed reports of success with albendazole, given in a dose of 400 mg per day for 5 days. Particularly when an expedition will not reach civilization for 3 to 4 weeks, there is no reason to withhold treatment awaiting a definitive diagnosis. If the field diagnosis is correct, in most cases drug therapy will cause dramatic relief from symptoms within 3 days. There is no prophylactic drug that is recommended to prevent infestation.

Other Infectious Diarrheas

Diarrhea can be caused by a number of parasites and other infectious agents, which include *Campylobacter, Shigella, Salmonella, Yersinia, Vibrio,* and *Entamoeba histolytica* (and other amoebae). Each pathogen may cause a constellation of fever, chills, nausea, vomiting, diarrhea (with or without mucus and blood), weakness, and abdominal pain. Because the clinical picture can be similar with infection from all of these organisms, the differentiation frequently relies on examination of the stool under the microscope and/or culture of the stool to identify the specific pathogen. For the sake of the brief expedition, the treatment is the same: rehydration with copious amounts of balanced electrolyte solutions, and antimotility agents only when essential to prevent severe dehydration. If the victim suffers from high fever with shaking chills, has persistent bloody or mucus-laden bowel movements, or is debilitated by dehydration, he should seek the care of a physician. Meanwhile, the administration of ciprofloxacin (Cipro) 500 mg two times a day or trimethoprim-sulfamethoxazole (Bactrim or Septra) one double-strength tablet two times a day for 3 days will treat *E. coli* and *Shigella,* may eradicate *Salmonella,* and will not adversely affect other infections. As soon as the victim of persistent diarrhea returns to civilization, he should visit a physician for a thorough evaluation. If the ova or parasitic forms of amoebae are seen during microscopic examination of stool, other drugs, such as tinidazole, metronidazole, diloxanide furoate, paromomycin, or diiodohydroxyquin, may be prescribed. If the ova or parasitic forms of worms are seen, drugs such as mebendazole or pyrantel pamoate may be prescribed.

Emotional Diarrhea (Colitis)

Emotional diarrhea, or irritable colon, is a manifestation of anxiety, often otherwise unmanifested, that is characterized by abdominal distention, the passage of flatus, cramping, and mucus-laden diarrhea. This can be debilitating. Occasionally, the sufferer will also complain intermittently of constipation. Many sufferers carry their own medication, such as clidinium bromide with chlordiazepoxide (Librax). Irritable colon is a diagnosis of exclusion that should be made by a physician. If a person is known to suffer from irritable colon, he should be encouraged to eat adequate fiber (bran, steamed vegetables) and avoid coffee.

Constipation

If a person becomes constipated (difficult bowel movements with hard stools), the retention of stool and discomfort can be severe. The greatest contributing factors to constipation are improper diet, dehydration, and lack of exercise. During outdoor activities, take care to drink fluids at regular intervals. In addition, sufficient fiber (bran, whole-grain cereals, vegetables, fruits) must be maintained in the diet. The "city backpacker" diet of chocolate bars, peanuts, and cheese sandwiches will turn the most irascible bowels into mortar. Regular, preemptive doses of a stool softener such as docusate sodium (Colace), or a bulking agent such as psyllium seed hydrophilic mucilloid (Metamucil), must be ingested with at least two glasses of water in order to be effective.

In order to relieve the victim of mild constipation:
1. Force fluids.
2. Adjust the diet (more for prevention than treatment).

3. Consider the use of stool softeners (mineral oil, Colace [docusate sodium]), bulking agents (Metamucil), or gentle laxatives (prune juice, milk of magnesia, mineral oil). Peri-Colace is a combination of the stool softener docusate sodium and casanthranol, a laxative. In general, it is best to avoid the use of repetitive enemas or potent laxatives, because they can cause large fluid losses. A useful enema is a Colace 5 ml (200 mg) "microenema." A child may benefit from a glycerin suppository. Other drugs are listed on page 446.

4. If a victim becomes impacted (has not had a bowel movement for 5 to 10 days due to constipation), using stool softeners will probably be ineffective, and piling on an ingested load of bulky fiber is just dumping more backfill behind the dam. Unfortunately, to break the roadblock, you may have to perform the physical removal of stool from the rectum, using a softening enema first and then a gloved finger for the extraction. This should be done gently, to prevent injury to the anus and walls of the rectum.

On a prolonged expedition, you can carry the oral drug bisacodyl (Dulcolax). This is administered in oral (5 mg) or suppository (10 mg) form, with onset of effect in a few hours. Bisacodyl causes the bowel to contract, which can be extremely uncomfortable in someone with a large fecal impaction.

An elderly person with any significant change in bowel habits should see a physician upon return to civilization.

Hemorrhoids

Hemorrhoids are enlarged veins that are found outside (external) or inside (internal) the anal opening (figure 104). They cause problems that range from minor itching and skin irritation to excruciating pain, inflammation, and bleeding. The bleeding is noticed as bright red blood either on the outside of the stool (not mixed in with the excrement), in the toilet water, or on the toilet paper. Bleeding is usually sporadic, associated with difficult bowel movements (constipation) with straining, and passage of hard stools. To avoid problems, keep your stools soft. If hemorrhoids flare, the treatment is sitz (sitting) baths in warm water for 30 minutes three times a day, and the application of medication in the form of cream, ointment, or suppositories (Preparation H [essentially a petrolatum lubricant]; Anusol or Tronolane [with pramoxine 1% for pain and itching] or Anusol HC-1 [without pramoxine, but with hydrocortisone 1% for inflammation]; Nupercainal [1% dibucaine]; pramoxine hydrochloride 1% with hydrocortisone acetate 1% [proctoCream-HC]). Unless bleeding is severe, it can

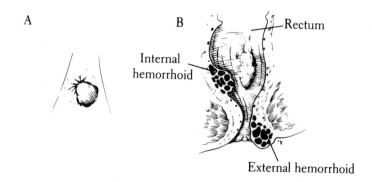

Figure 104. Hemorrhoids. (A) External view of the anus with an enlarged external hemorrhoid. (B) A cross-sectional view of the anus and rectum shows dilated veins that protrude into the rectum (internal hemorrhoids) and externally from the anus.

be managed with sterile pads and gentle pressure. If the victim develops a fever associated with severe rectal pain or cannot pass a bowel movement, a physician should be sought.

A thrombosed hemorrhoid is one in which the blood has clotted within the dilated vein and formed a visible and palpable enlarged, hardened, and dark blue-purple knot. Pain is generally severe, and the victim may be unable to complete a bowel movement. The treatment usually involves incision through the wall of the vein and removal of the clot. Until the victim can be brought to a physician, warm soaks may ease the discomfort. Generally, all elderly people with rectal bleeding should be fully evaluated by a physician, to be sure that there is not another, more serious, cause.

Flatus

The rectal passage of bowel gas offers relief and occasional embarrassment. If stomach cramps are due to excessive gas production, the drug of choice is simethicone (Mylicon or Mylicon-80), which causes dissolution of large gas collections and eases the passage of flatus. Charcoal Plus tablets and Flatulex tablets contain simethicone combined with activated charcoal, an absorbent. Beano food enzyme dietary supplement contains the enzyme alpha-galactosidase, which is advertised to be effective in preventing gas formation from vegetables, beans, and grains that contain indigestible sugars that ferment in the bowel to create gas. Because intestinal gas (methane) can be flammable, do not attempt to ignite rectal gas or direct the stream of gas into a campfire. Backflashes and minor burns are a real risk.

Heartburn

Heartburn is a manifestation of esophageal reflux, in which stomach contents containing acid and food travel backward from the stomach into the esophagus. This causes irritation and pain, which is typically sharp or burning and located under the breastbone and/or in the upper abdomen. It may be associated with belching, a sour taste in the mouth, and/or near-vomiting. When severe, the pain may be confused with angina (see page 44). Heartburn is best managed with antacids, particularly Gaviscon, which forms a "foam" that floats upon the stomach contents and protects the esophagus from refluxed acid. Metoclopramide hydrochloride (Reglan) helps control muscle tone at the sphincter (junction) between the stomach and the esophagus, and thus helps prevent reflux. Nizatidine 75 mg (Axid AR ["acid reducer"]) is an H2-blocker drug (see page 197) that inhibits gastric acid secretion. It is swallowed 30 to 60 minutes prior to eating, and can be used up to twice in 24 hours. Cimetidine (Tagamet) 200 mg can be used in a similar manner. Famotidine (Pepcid) 20 mg twice a day for up to 6 weeks is another therapy. Omeprazole (Prilosec) is a drug that suppresses gastric acid secretion. It can be prescribed by a physician for a 4- to 8-week period for severe erosive inflammation of the esophagus.

Keep meals small, and do not eat them immediately prior to reclining (no bedtime snacks). Known gastric irritants (alcohol, cigarettes, pepperoni sandwiches) should be avoided. If possible, sleep with the head of your bed or sleeping bag elevated. Occasionally, it is necessary to sleep in the sitting position, to counteract the forces of gravity and a loose esophageal sphincter.

Nausea and Vomiting

Nausea and vomiting may arise from causes as simple as anxiety, or may represent a serious problem such as appendicitis, ingestion of a poisonous plant, or response to a head injury. When vomiting is secondary to a serious underlying disorder, the basic problem must be remedied. Any victim with nausea and vomiting who suffers from altered mental status, uncontrollable high fever, extreme abdominal pain, or chest pain that might represent heart disease—or who is either very young or very old—should be evacuated promptly. Anyone who vomits blood should be taken to a hospital immediately. Vomiting in children is particularly worrisome if it accompanies head trauma (see page 55), abdominal trauma (see page 105), or lethargy or confusion (which might represent an infection or poisoning); severe vomiting (which might represent a bowel obstruction [see page 114] or appendicitis [see page 112]) is also of concern.

If nausea and vomiting due to gastroenteritis become excessive, they can be managed with an antiemetic. The drug of choice is prochlorperazine (Compazine), which can be administered orally or as a suppository. An alternative is promethazine (Phenergan), which comes in suppository form. Yet another is trimethobenzamide (Tigan), which can be taken orally or by suppository. If the victim is so ill that he cannot keep anything in his stomach, it makes no sense to administer an oral medication, so an injection or suppository must be used. A person who requires medication to control vomiting should see a physician. After multiple episodes of vomiting, the victim may suffer from dehydration (see page 184), particularly if there is associated diarrhea as part of a gastroenteritis. Fluid replacement is essential. The diet should be advanced slowly as the victim's hunger returns.

Nausea and vomiting due to motion sickness are discussed on page 390.

Vomiting Blood

Bleeding from the gastrointestinal tract can cause the victim to vomit blood (either bright red or dark brown "coffee grounds"). If the blood is not vomited, it passes through the bowels and emerges as dark black tarry stools (melena) or occasionally as maroon clots or bright red blood. Brisk bleeding in the stomach or bowels may be painless; any bleeding should be considered serious. Even if the bleeding episode is brief (except for bleeding from known hemorrhoids), the victim should be evacuated immediately to a hospital. If the victim is known to have ulcer disease and ceases vomiting, antacids should be given by mouth.

Persistent retching can cause the stomach wall to tear and begin to bleed. For this reason, persistent nausea and vomiting from any cause should be controlled with medications, if possible.

Ulcer Disease

A gastric ulcer is an erosion into the stomach. A peptic ulcer is an erosion into the duodenum (first portion of the small bowel) that is worsened by the constant assault from gastric acid and digestive juices. Many ulcers are caused by infection of the inner lining of the stomach and bowel with the microorganism *Helicobacter pylori,* which can be eradicated with an intensive course of multiple antibiotics. Such therapy should not be undertaken in the field, but rather under the supervision of a physician.

The major symptom of ulcer disease is burning, sharp, or aching pain in the upper abdomen that is usually relieved by the ingestion of food or antacids, although the latter alone may be therapeutic. Classically, the pain occurs when the stomach is empty, particularly during times of emotional stress. Because the greatest amounts of acid are secreted following meals and between the hours of midnight and 3 A.M., these are times when pain is most frequent.

If the victim is strongly suspected or known to have an ulcer, and can control the pain readily with medications, the journey can continue. Make every attempt to keep on a regular meal schedule and to take medication properly during waking hours. As noted below, cigarette smoking and alcohol ingestion are strictly prohibited. If pain is not immediately controlled, or if there is any suggestion of bleeding or perforation, rapid transport to a hospital is indicated.

Therapy

1. *Antacids.* These are the traditional mainstay of therapy and should be taken in a dose of 2 to 3 tbsp (30 to 45 ml) 1 and 3 hours after meals, at bedtime, and as necessary to control pain. Liquids are generally more effective than tablets. Solid food and milk are not recommended as antacids. While they may decrease pain briefly, they actually stimulate the secretion of acid.

2. *Drugs to inhibit the secretion of acid.* Medications used to decrease acid secretion (antagonists to histamine H2 receptors [H2RAs] and proton [acid] pump inhibitors [PPIs]) decrease bowel activity and cramping.

3. *Drugs to protect the lining of the gastrointestinal tract.* Sucralfate (Carafate) is a drug that binds with the ulcer and protects the bowel lining from further erosion. Because it requires the presence of acid in the ulcer crater to be activated, it should not be given at the same time as antacids.

4. *Avoidance of alcohol, tea, coffee, tobacco, and known gastric irritants.*

5. *Do not use household baking soda to neutralize acid in the stomach.* Baking soda (bicarbonate) reacts with the acid to liberate heat and gas.

Hepatitis

Hepatitis is inflammation of the liver that is caused by viral infection or parasitic infestation, drugs, toxic chemicals, alcohol abuse, or autoimmune disease. Type A infectious (short-incubation) hepatitis is the more commonly encountered viral form. The virus is excreted in urine and feces and contaminates drinking water and food products (such as raw shellfish). Type B infectious (long-incubation) hepatitis is caused by a virus found in many body fluids (blood, saliva, semen) and is spread by direct person-to-person contact. Type C infectious hepatitis (formerly non-A, non-B hepatitis) is caused by at least one virus and is most commonly associated with blood transfusions. Multiple other forms of viral hepatitis have been discovered by medical researchers.

Hepatitis causes the victim to have a constellation of signs and symptoms, which include yellow discoloration of the skin and eyes (from the buildup of bilirubin pigment, which the diseased liver cannot process properly), nausea and vomiting, fatigue, weakness, fever, chills, darkened urine, diarrhea, pale-colored bowel movements (which may precede the onset of jaundice by 1 to 3 days), abdominal pain (particularly in the right upper quadrant over the swollen and tender liver), loss of appetite, joint pain, muscle aching, itching, and red skin rash. A young child may suffer from Type A infection, yet show only a mild flulike illness.

Anyone suspected of having hepatitis should be placed at maximum rest and transported to a physician. Avoid medication and alcohol ingestion, because the metabolism of many drugs is altered in the victim with a diseased liver. He should be encouraged to avoid dehydration and should maintain adequate food intake. If the cause of hepatitis is viral, the victim's disease may be contagious for his first 2 weeks of illness. Do not share eating utensils or washrags. Body secretions (saliva and waste products) frequently carry the virus; therefore, pay strict attention to hand washing. Sexual contact should be avoided during the infectious period. In no case should a needle used for injection of medicine into one person be reused for another individual.

Protection against hepatitis is best accomplished by prevention of virus transmission through good hygiene. Hepatitis A vaccine is available (see page 401). In countries of high hepatitis incidence (poor sanitation, infested water or food), pooled immune serum globulin (ISG, or gamma globulin) injections are advised (see page 401); these protect unimmunized people against hepatitis A, and diminish symptoms in infected people. Hepatitis B vaccine (see page 401) is intended for health care workers or those who will visit or reside in regions of high endemicity. It is of little benefit against hepatitis A.

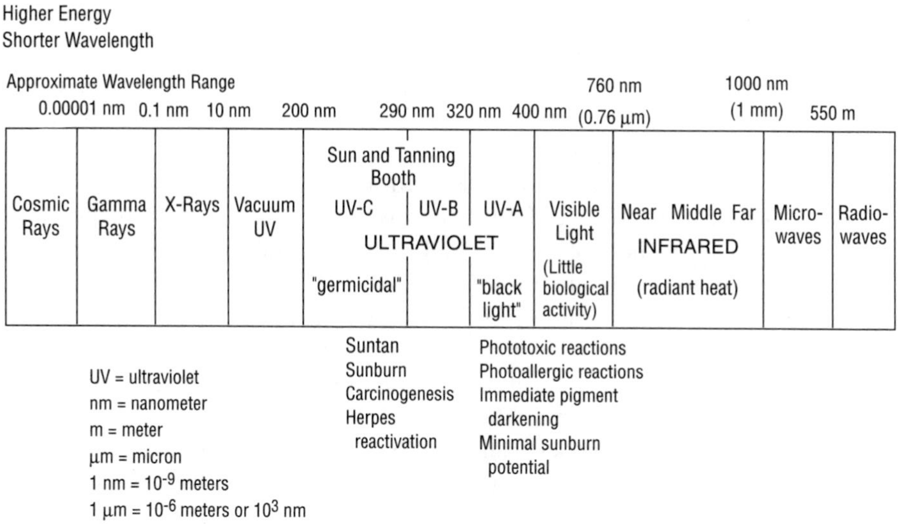

Higher Energy
Shorter Wavelength

Approximate Wavelength Range

0.00001 nm	0.1 nm	10 nm	200 nm	290 nm	320 nm	400 nm	760 nm (0.76 μm)	1000 nm (1 mm)	550 m

Cosmic Rays	Gamma Rays	X-Rays	Vacuum UV	Sun and Tanning Booth			Visible Light	Near Middle Far INFRARED	Micro-waves	Radio-waves
				UV-C	UV-B	UV-A				
				ULTRAVIOLET						
				"germicidal"		"black light"	(Little biological activity)	(radiant heat)		

UV = ultraviolet
nm = nanometer
m = meter
μm = micron
1 nm = 10^{-9} meters
1 μm = 10^{-6} meters or 10^{3} nm

Suntan
Sunburn
Carcinogenesis
Herpes
  reactivation

Phototoxic reactions
Photoallergic reactions
Immediate pigment
  darkening
Minimal sunburn
  potential

Figure 105. Solar radiation.

SKIN DISORDERS

Sunburn

The solar radiation that strikes the earth includes 50% visible light (wavelength 400 to 800 nanometers), 40% infrared (1,300 to 1,700 nm), and 10% ultraviolet (UV) (10 to 400 nm) (figure 105). Sunburn is a cutaneous photosensitivity reaction caused by exposure of the skin to ultraviolet radiation (UVR) from the sun. There are three types of UVR: UVA is 320 to 400 nm, UVB is 290 to 320 nm, and UVC is 100 to 290 nm. UVC is filtered out by the ozone layer of the atmosphere. UVB is the culprit in the creation of sunburn. UVA is of less immediate danger but is a serious cause of skin aging, drug-related photosensitivity, and skin cancer.

Ultraviolet exposure varies with the time of day (greatest between 9 A.M. and 3 P.M. because of increased solar proximity and decreased angle of light rays), season (greater in summer), altitude (4 to 6% increase per each 1,000', or 305 m, of elevation above sea level), location (greater near the equator), and weather (greater in the wind). Snow or ice reflects 85% of UVR, dry sand 17%, and grass 2.5%. Water may reflect 10 to 100% of UVR, depending upon the time of day, location, and surface. Most clothes reflect (light-colored) or absorb (dark-colored) UVR. However, it is important to note that wet cotton of any color probably transmits considerable UVR.

Skin darkening occurs immediately upon UVA exposure, as preformed melanin is released, and lasts for 15 to 30 minutes. Tanning occurs after 3 days of exposure, as additional melanin is produced. If the skin is not conditioned with gradual doses of UVR (tanning), then a burn can be created. A person's sensitivity to UVR depends on his skin type and thickness, the pigment (melanin) in his skin, and weather conditions. Well-hydrated skin is penetrated four times as effectively by UVR as is dry skin, because the moist skin does not scatter or reflect UVR as well.

Depending upon the exposure, the injury can range from mild redness to blistering and disablement. Rapid pigment darkening from immediate melanin release is followed by the redness with which we are all familiar, caused by dilatation of superficial blood vessels. This begins 2 to 8 hours after exposure and reaches its maximum (the "burn") in 24 to 36 hours, with associated itching and pain.

Wind appears to augment the injury, as do heat, atmospheric moisture, and immersion in water. "Windburn" is not possible without UVR or abrasive sand. Since windburn is due in part to the drying effect of low humidity at high altitudes, it can be helpful to protect the skin with a greasy sunscreen or barrier cream.

People may be more sensitive to UVR after they have ingested certain drugs (such as tetracycline, doxycycline, vitamin A derivatives, nonsteroidal anti-inflammatories, sulfa derivatives, thiazide diuretics, and barbiturates) or have been exposed to certain plants (such as lime, citron, bitter orange, lemon, celery, parsnip, fennel, dill, wild carrot, fig, buttercup, mustard, milfoil, agrimony, rue, hogweed, Queen-Anne's-lace, and stinking mayweed).

For a mild sunburn in which no blistering is present, the victim may be treated with cool liquid compresses, cool showers, a nonsensitizing skin moisturizer (such as Vaseline Intensive Care), and aspirin to decrease the pain and inflammation. Topical anesthetic sprays, many of which contain benzocaine, should be avoided, because they can cause sensitization and an allergic reaction. Menthol-containing lotions may be helpful. Topical steroids do not diminish a sunburn.

If the victim is deep red ("lobster") without blisters, then a stronger anti-inflammatory drug, such as ibuprofen, may be given. A 5-day course of prednisone (80 mg on the first day; 60 mg the second; 40 mg the third; 20 mg the fourth; and 10 mg the fifth) works wonders to decrease the discomfort of "sun poisoning," which is the constellation of low-grade fever, loss of appetite, nausea, and weakness that accompanies a bad total-body sunburn. Corticosteroids should always be taken with the understanding that a rare side effect is serious deterioration of the head ("ball" of the ball-and-socket joint) of the femur, the long bone of the thigh. An extensive nonblistering first-degree sunburn can make the victim nauseated and weak, with low-grade fever and chills. He should be forced to drink enough balanced electrolyte liquids to avoid dehydration (see page 184).

Topical steroid creams, such as pramoxine with hydrocortisone (Pramosone cream or lotion) may be used if blisters are not present. Pramoxine alone (Prax) is a nonsensitizing topical anesthetic. Topical steroid preparations should not be applied to blistered skin, because wound healing may be delayed and infection made likelier. On the other hand, aloe vera lotion or gel may be soothing and promote healing. Vitamin E is an antioxidant that, when mixed with aloe vera, may soothe the skin. However, this hasn't been proven to promote healing any better than aloe vera alone.

With a severe sunburn in which blistering is present, the victim has by definition suffered second-degree burns (see page 98) and should be treated accordingly. Gently clean the burned areas and cover with sterile dressings. Administer appropriate pain medication.

Sunscreens

Sunscreens (available as lotions or creams) either absorb light of a particular wavelength, act as barriers, or reflect light. Choose sunscreens based on your estimated exposure and on your own propensity to tan or burn. Remember, there is no such thing as a "safe tan," because sun exposure is directly linked to skin cancer. In addition, long-term exposure to ultraviolet radiation from sunlight causes premature skin aging and loss of skin tone. The term photoaging refers to these effects— increased wrinkles, loose skin, brown spots, a leathery appearance, and uneven pigmentation.

Dermatologists classify sun-reactive skin types (based on the first 45 to 60 minutes of sun exposure after winter or after a prolonged period of no sun exposure) as follows:

Type I. Always burns easily, never tans.
Type II. Always burns easily, tans minimally.
Type III. Burns moderately, tans gradually and uniformly (light brown).
Type IV. Burns minimally, always tans well (moderate brown).
Type V. Rarely burns, tans profusely (dark brown).
Type VI. Never burns, is deeply pigmented (black skin).

In all cases it is wise to overestimate the protection necessary and to carry a strong sunscreen. To protect hair from sun damage, wear a hat.

Para-aminobenzoic acid (PABA) derivatives, which are water soluble, are sunscreens that absorb UVB (not UVA) and that accumulate in the skin with repeated application. The most commonly used PABA derivative is padimate O (octyl dimethyl PABA). The most effective method of application is to moisturize the skin (shower or bathe) and then apply the sunscreen. For maximum effect, this should be done at least 15 to 30 minutes prior to exposure, and the skin should be kept dry for at least 2 hours after sunscreen application. When PABA itself is used, a recommended preparation is 5 to 10% PABA in 50 to 70% alcohol. However, PABA is now used infrequently because its absorption peak of UVB at 296 nm is too far from 307 nm, where UVB exerts its greatest effect. Furthermore, it causes skin irritation—a stinging sensation—and can stain cotton and synthetic fabrics. PABA derivatives are less problematic.

Benzophenones are sunscreens that are more effective against ultraviolet A. These should be used in 6 to 10% concentration. Because they are not well absorbed by the skin, they require frequent reapplication. Photoplex broad-spectrum sunscreen lotion contains a PABA-ester combined with a potent UVA absorber, Parsol 1789. This is an excellent sunscreen for sensitive people, particularly those at risk for drug-induced photosensitivity.

Sunscreens come in different concentrations (such as PreSun "8" or "15") (see page 453). A higher sun protection factor (SPF) number (range 2 to 50) indicates a greater degree of protection against UVB. The SPF number assumes a liberal (approximately 1¼ oz, or 37 ml, per adult) application of the sunscreen. In general, a sunscreen with an SPF number of 8 or less will allow tanning, probably by ultraviolet A exposure. Those with sensitive or unconditioned skin should use a sunscreen with an SPF number of 10 or greater. Fair-skinned people who never tan or who tan poorly (Types I, II, or III) or mountain climbers (there is more UV exposure at higher altitudes, and more is reflected off snow) should always use a sunscreen with an SPF number of 15 or greater.

Substantivity refers to the ability of a sunscreen to resist water wash-off. Good waterproof choices include Vaseline 15, PreSun 29, Sundown 30, Bullfrog 36, Sawyer Products Bonding Base 45, Solbar 50, and Aloegator 40. Layering sunscreens doesn't work well, because the last layer applied usually washes off.

Sunscreens are first applied to cool, dry skin for optimal absorption; wait 10 minutes prior to water exposure. Reapply them liberally after swimming or heavy perspiration. Although many sunscreens are designed to bond or adhere to the skin under adverse environmental conditions, there are certain situations in which any sunscreen should be reapplied at 3- to 4-hour intervals:

Continuous sun exposure, particularly between the hours of 10 A.M. and 3 P.M.

Exposure at altitude of 7,000' (2,135 m) or higher

Exposure within 20 degrees latitude of the equator

Exposure during May through July in the Northern Hemisphere, and December through February in the Southern Hemisphere

Frequent water immersion, particularly with toweling off

Preexisting sunburn or skin irritation

Ingestion of drugs, such as certain antibiotics, that can cause photosensitization

Some authorities recommend using sunscreens of at least SPF 29, with the rationale that most people underapply or improperly apply them. Bald-headed men should protect their domes. All children should be adequately protected. However, avoid PABA-containing products in children less than 6 months old. Those sensitive to PABA can use Piz-Buin, Ti-Screen, Sawyer Products Bonding Base 45, Uval, and Solbar products. Eating PABA does not protect the skin.

For total protection against ultraviolet and visible light, a sunblock can be prepared from various mixtures of titanium dioxide, red petrolatum, talc, zinc oxide, kaolin, red ferric oxide (calamine), and icthammol. These preparations or similar commercial products ("glacier cream") are used for lip and nose protection. Micronized titanium dioxide can be prepared in an invisible preparation (such as Ti-Screen Natural 16 and Neutrogena Chemical Free 17) that does not cause skin irritation. Sunblocks that prevent infrared transmission may help prevent flares of fever blisters caused by herpes virus. An improvised sunscreen can be prepared by preparing a sludge of ashes from charcoal or wood, or from ground clay. In a pinch, axle grease will work to some degree.

Substances that are ineffective as sunscreens and that may increase the propensity to burn include baby oil, cocoa butter, and mineral oil.

Although "tanning tablets" or "bronzers" induce a pigmentary change in the skin that resembles a suntan, they provide minimal, if any, true protection from the effects of ultraviolet exposure. Like the sun, tanning machines may induce skin changes that lead to premature skin aging and cancer.

Taking aspirin or a nonsteroidal anti-inflammatory drug (such as ibuprofen) at 6-hour intervals three times prior to sun exposure may help protect the sun-sensitive person.

Many effective sunscreens, particularly those advertised to stay on in the water, are extremely irritating to the eyes, so take care when applying these to the forehead and nose. Near the eyes, avoid sunscreens with an alcohol or propylene glycol base. Instead, use a sunscreen cream.

There are also newer sunscreen/insect repellent combinations, such as Coppertone Bug & Sun and Banana Boat Bite Block. Bug Guard contains Skin-So-Soft (mostly mineral oil) in combination with citronella, enhanced by a sunscreen.

A new line of medical clothing, Solumbra by Sun Precautions, is advertised to be "soft, lightweight and comfortable," and offers 30-plus SPF protection. A recent phone number for the company was 1-800-882-7860. Frogskin, Inc. (1-800-845-9531), also manufactures high-SPF protective clothing. Sunday Afternoons (1-888-874-2642) manufactures comfortable broad-brimmed hats with neck shields advertised to provide 97% UV block.

Melanoma

Melanoma is a type of skin cancer that can be caused by ultraviolet B light exposure. Indeed, regular use of a sunscreen with sun protective factor (SPF) of at least 15 during the first 18 years of life may reduce the lifetime risk of developing melanoma by more than 75%. People with white skin and a tendency to burn rather than tan are at increased risk for the development of melanoma.

Although you wouldn't self-treat a melanoma, it is important for those who spend a great deal of time outdoors to recognize the features of skin cancer. Regularly inspect existing moles, birthmarks, and other skin lesions. Since melanoma is often found on a person's back or other area that cannot be easily inspected, it is important to have a knowledgeable person (such as a dermatologist) inspect all suspicious skin lesions from time to time.

Warning signs within a skin lesion include:

1. Irregular, ragged, jagged, notched, or blurred border.
2. Asymmetrical appearance (one portion different than the rest, with respect to color, darkness, or texture).
3. Change in appearance or features (size, color, texture, sensation); onset of pain in a lesion; rapid growth of a lesion.
4. Recent growth, bleeding, itching, scaling, or tenderness.
5. Discoloration (black, dark brown, blue, red, white, mottled).

If you note any of these features, see a dermatologist for a proper evaluation.

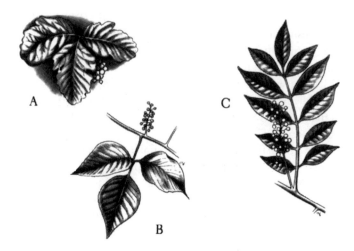

Figure 106. (A) Poison oak. (B) Poison ivy. (C) Poison sumac.

Poison Ivy, Sumac, and Oak

The rashes of poison ivy, poison sumac, and poison oak are caused by a resin (urushiol) found in the resin canals of leaves, stems, berries, and roots (figure 106). The resin is not found on the surface of the leaves. The potency of the sap does not vary with the seasons. In its natural state, the oil is colorless; on exposure to air, it turns black. Because the plant parts have to be injured to leak the resin, most cases are reported in spring, when the leaves are most fragile. Dried leaves are less toxic, because the oil has returned to the stem and roots through the resin canals. However, smoke from burning plants carries the residual available resin in small particles and can cause a severe reaction on the skin and in the nose, mouth, throat, and lungs.

The poison oak group does not grow in Alaska or Hawaii. Other plants or parts of plants that contain urushiol include the india ink tree, mango rind, cashew nut shell, and Japanese lacquer tree. Because the resin is long lived, it can be spread by contact with tents, clothing, and pet fur.

Sensitivity to the resin varies with each individual. The first exposure produces a rash in 6 to 25 days. Subsequent exposures can cause a rash in 8 hours to 10 days, with a 2- to 3-day interval most common. Unless the resin is removed from the skin within 10 minutes of exposure, a reaction is inevitable in extremely sensitive individuals; other people may have up to 4 hours to wash it off, although it is generally accepted that the resin binds to the skin in 30 minutes and is thereafter extremely difficult to remove with soap and water. After exposure, it is usually most convenient to remove the resin with soap and cool water, but to be effective, washing must occur within 30 minutes. Rubbing alcohol is a better solvent for the resin than is water. Technu Poison Oak-N-Ivy Cleanser (alkane and alcohol) works quite well when applied soon after exposure, rubbed in for 2 minutes, and rinsed off, with a repeat of the entire sequence. Another wash designed to remove urushiol is Dr. West's Ivy Detox Cleanser, which contains magnesium sulfate.

For treatment of the skin reaction, shake lotions such as calamine are soothing and drying, and they control itching. A good nonsensitizing topical anesthetic is pramoxine hydrochloride 1% (Prax cream or lotion); Caladryl contains calamine and pramoxine. Avoid topical diphenhydramine, benzocaine, and tetracaine. Antihistamines (such as diphenhydramine [Benadryl]) control itching and act as sedatives. Nonsedating antihistamines, such as fexofenadine (Allegra), may also diminish itching. A soothing bath in tepid (not hot) water with half a 1-lb box of baking soda, 2 cups (551 ml) of linnet starch, or 1 cup (275 ml) Aveeno oatmeal is excellent. If Aveeno is not available, a woman's nylon stuffed with regular (not instant) oatmeal can be thrown in the tub. Soothing aluminum acetate (1:20) soaks may help. Topical steroid creams are generally of little value. Alcohol applications are painful and do not hasten resolution of the rash.

If the reaction is severe (facial or genital involvement or intolerable itching), the victim should be treated with a course of oral prednisone (60 to 80 mg each of the first 3 days, then decreased by 10 mg every 2 days until the final dose is 10 mg—80, 80, 70, 70, 60, 60, and so on). Corticosteroids should always be taken with the understanding that a rare side effect is serious deterioration of the head ("ball" of the ball-and-socket joint) of the femur, the long bone of the thigh.

Once the resin has been removed from the skin, the rash and blister fluid are not contagious. However, if the resin is still present, touching the involved skin will allow resin to be transferred to other areas. All clothes, sleeping bags, and pets should be washed with soap and water, because the resin can persist for years, particularly on woolen garments and blankets.

For prevention, there are few commercially available topical chemical preparations that act as effective barriers, although it appears that activated charcoal, aluminum oxide, and silica gel may work. Ivy Shield (Interpro, Haverhill, Massachusetts), which contains fatty acids, is a protective agent for sensitive individuals. It should be applied over any sunscreen, and must be washed off carefully after use according to instructions. Stokogard Outdoor Cream is a linoleic acid dimer barrier cream preparation that is advertised to provide up to 8 hours of skin protection. Hollister Moisture Barrier and Hydropel may prove useful as barriers.

Other Irritating Plants

Some plants produce fluids or crystals that act as primary irritants to the skin, in a nonallergic reaction. These plants include buttercup, croton bush, spurge, manchineel, beach apple, daisy, mustard, radish, pineapple, lemon, crown-of-thorns, milkbush, candelabra cactus, daffodil, hyacinth, stinging nettle, itchweed, dogwood, barley, millet, prickly pear, snow-on-the-mountain, primrose, geranium, meadow rue, narcissus, oleander, opuntia cactus, mesquite, tulip, mistletoe, wolfsbane, and horse nettle.

The skin should be thoroughly washed with soap and water. If barbs are embedded in the skin, removal may be easiest if you apply the sticky side of adhesive tape to the skin, then peel the barbs off with the tape.

Small cactus spines can be removed by applying the sticky side of adhesive (duct) tape and peeling it off, or spreading a facial gel (mask or peel) or rubber cement, allowing it to dry, and peeling it off. Large spines can be removed with forceps, which may be necessary if the barbs on the cactus spine inhibit easy removal with the adhesive-tape method. A single cactus thorn can be as sharp as a needle and penetrate easily through the skin without leaving an external mark.

Medicated soaks recommended by dermatologists for plant-induced skin irritation include aluminum acetate solution (1:20) or Dalibour (Dalidane) solution (copper and zinc sulfate and camphor). Administration of corticosteroids (such as prednisone) is not useful for a primary (nonallergic) skin irritation.

Rashes Incurred in the Water

Seaweed Dermatitis

There are more than 3,000 species of alga, which range in size from 1 micron to 100 meters in length. The blue-green algae *Microcoleus lyngbyaceus* is a fine, hairlike plant that gets inside the bathing suit of the unwary aquanaut in Hawaiian and Floridian waters, particularly during summer months. Usually, skin under the suit remains in moist contact with the algae (the other skin dries or is rinsed off) and becomes red and itchy, with occasional blistering and/or weeping. The reaction may start a few minutes to a few hours after the victim leaves the water. Treatment consists of a vigorous soap-and-water scrub, followed by a rinse with isopropyl (rubbing) alcohol. Apply hydrocortisone lotion 1% twice a day. If the reaction is severe, oral prednisone may be administered in a dose similar to that for a severe poison oak reaction (see page 205).

Swimmer's Itch

Swimmer's itch (clamdigger's itch) is caused by skin contact with cercariae, which are the immature larval forms of parasitic schistosomes (flatworms) found throughout the world in both fresh and salt waters. Snails and birds are the intermediate hosts for the flatworms. They release hundreds of fork-tailed microscopic cercariae into the water.

The affliction is contracted when a film of cercaria-infested water dries on exposed (uncovered by clothing) skin. The cercariae penetrate the outer layer of the skin, where itching is noted within minutes. Shortly afterward, the skin becomes reddened and swollen, with an intense rash and, occasionally, hives. Blisters may develop over the next 24 to 48 hours. If the area is scratched, it may become infected and the victim develop impetigo (see page 211). Untreated, the affliction is limited to 1 to 2 weeks. Those who have suffered swimmer's itch previously may be more severely affected on repeated exposures, which suggests that an allergy might be present.

Swimmer's itch can be prevented by briskly rubbing the skin with a towel immediately after leaving the water, to prevent the cercariae from having time to penetrate the skin. Once the reaction has occurred, the skin should be lightly rinsed with isopropyl (rubbing) alcohol and then coated with calamine lotion. If the reaction is severe, the victim should be treated with oral prednisone as if he suffered from poison oak (see page 205).

Because the cercariae are present in greatest concentration in shallow, warmer water (where the snails are), swimmers should seek to avoid these areas.

Sea Bather's Eruption

Sea bather's eruption, often misnamed sea lice (which are true crustacean parasites upon fish), occurs in seawater and more often involves bathing-suit-covered areas of the skin, rather than exposed areas. The skin rash distribution is very similar to that from seaweed dermatitis, but no seaweed is found on the skin. The cause is stings from the nematocysts (stinging cells) of the larval forms of certain anemones, such as *Linuche unguiculata,* and thimble jellyfish. The victim may notice a tingling sensation under the bathing suit (breasts, groin, cuffs of wet suits) while still in the water, which is made much worse if he takes a freshwater rinse (shower) while still wearing the suit. The rash usually consists of red bumps, which may become dense and confluent. Itching is severe and may become painful. Treatment is often not optimal, because application of vinegar or rubbing alcohol to stop the envenomation may not be very effective. An agent that may work

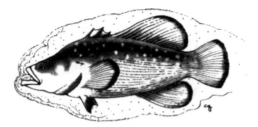

Figure 107. A soapfish enveloped by a cloud of irritant mucus that it secreted.

better is a solution of papain (such as unseasoned meat tenderizer), which is also available via a saturated abrasive pad in the product Wipe-Out! (Wipe-Out Distributors Inc., Laguna Niguel, California; (800)859-1520). After the decontamination and a thorough freshwater rinse, apply hydrocortisone lotion 1% twice a day to treat the inflammatory component of the skin reaction. If the reaction is severe, the victim may suffer from headache, fever, chills, weakness, vomiting, itchy eyes, and burning on urination, and should be treated with oral prednisone as if he suffered from poison oak (see page 205). Topical calamine lotion with 1% menthol may be soothing.

The stinging cells may remain in the bathing suit even after it dries, so once a person has sustained a sea bather's eruption, his clothing should undergo a machine washing or be thoroughly rinsed in alcohol or vinegar, then be washed by hand with soap and water.

To prevent sea bather's eruption, an ocean bather or diver should wear, at a minimum, a synthetic nylon-rubber (Lycra [DuPont]) "dive skin."

Soapfish Dermatitis

The tropical soapfish *Rypticus saponaceus* (figure 107) is covered with a soapy mucus. When exposed to this slime, the victim's skin becomes red, itches, and undergoes mild swelling. Treatment involves a thorough wash with soap and water, followed by cool compresses, application of calamine lotion, and treatment for a mild allergic reaction similar to that for hives (see page 210).

Fish Handler's Disease

When cleaning marine fish or shellfish, the handler frequently creates small nicks and scrapes in his skin, usually on his hands. If these become

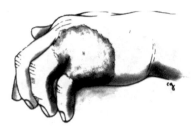

Figure 108. Typical rash of fish handler's disease.

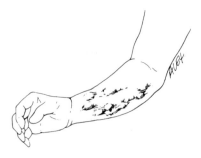

Figure 109. Hives.

infected with the bacteria *Erysipelothrix rhusopathiae,* a skin rash may develop within 2 to 7 days. The rash appears as a red to violet-colored area of raised skin surrounding the small cut or scrape, with warmth, slight tenderness, and a well-defined border (figure 108). The sufferer should be treated with penicillin, cephalexin, or ciprofloxacin for 1 week.

Hives

Hives are one skin manifestation of an allergic reaction. They appear as raised, red, and irregularly bordered welts or thickened patches of skin (figure 109). Often, the victim will also complain of itching and/or fever. The treatment is to administer an antihistamine (such as diphenhydramine [Benadryl]) at 6-hour intervals until the rash has begun to subside and the itching is relieved, and to observe the victim closely for progression to a serious allergic reaction. Hives can appear in moments, yet take days to completely resolve. If the victim complains of shortness of breath or wheezing, or has a swollen tongue (muffled voice) or lips, anticipate a more serious allergic reaction (see page 58). Be prepared to administer epinephrine.

Hives can also be induced by exposure to cold or during rewarming of cold skin (cold urticaria). Accompanying the skin lesions can be fatigue, headache, shortness of breath, rapid heart rate, and rarely, full-blown anaphylaxis (see page 58). Avoidance of cold may not be totally preventive, since the rate of cooling seems to be as important a factor as the environmental temperature. Avoidance of sudden temperature changes and cold exposure are advised. Certain drugs, such as cyproheptadine (Periactin) may be prescribed by a physician as treatment.

Heat Rash

Heat rash is a skin irritation composed of small raised spots that coalesce to form large areas of redness, particularly in the groin, under the arms, in the creases of the elbows, over the chest, under the neck, and under the breasts. It is rarely itchy; more often, it becomes irritated, particularly with rubbing. It should be treated with cool compresses; with light cotton clothing that will absorb sweat; and, if painful, with thin applications of 0.5 to 1% hydrocortisone lotion twice a day.

Impetigo

Impetigo is a skin infection caused by the bacteria *Streptococcus* and/or *Staphylococcus*. It is seen as discrete weeping sores, with honey yellow crusted scabs (with or without yellow pus) of the sort often associated with infected insect bites, small scrapes, or areas frequently scratched. The rash may start as pinhead-sized blisters filled with white or yellow pus. Once a few sores have become infected and ruptured, they coalesce and crop up all over the body (particularly in children), and can cause fevers, fatigue, and swollen regional lymph glands.

Treatment involves the administration of oral penicillin, cephalexin, or erythromycin for 1 week, and improved skin hygiene. Alternative antibiotics include dicloxacillin and azithromycin. The skin should be washed twice a day with pHisoHex (not for infants and children under the age of 2 years) scrub, a half-strength solution of hydrogen peroxide, or soap and water, and the sores covered with a thin layer of mupirocin ointment or cream, or bacitracin ointment.

If a person is prone to impetigo, he may be a chronic carrier of *Staphylococcus* bacteria inside his nose. This can be controlled for up to 3 months by an intranasal application, using a cotton-tipped swab, of mupirocin calcium ointment 2% (Bactroban Nasal) twice a day for 5 days.

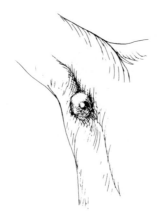

Figure 110. External appearance of an abscess in the armpit.

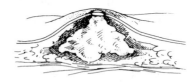

Figure 111. Cross section of a pus pocket, with a soft cap.

Abscess

An abscess (boil) is a collection of pus. Although it can occur anywhere on or in the body, it is most frequently noticed on the skin, particularly in an area of high perspiration, friction, and bacterium (particularly *Staphylococcus*) accumulation, such as associated with hair follicles under the arm (figure 110) or in the groin. The early abscess first appears as a firm, tender red lump, which progresses over the course of a few days into a reddish purple, soft, tender, raised area, occasionally with a white or yellowish cap ("comes to a head") (figure 111). The surrounding skin is reddened and thickened, and regional lymph glands may be swollen and tender. Fever, swollen lymph glands, and red streaking that travels in a linear fashion from the infected site toward the trunk indicate the spread of infection into the lymphatic system (figure 112).

Treatment involves drainage of the pus and dead tissue from within the core of the soft abscess. This is performed by taking a sharp blade and cutting a line into the roof of the abscess at its softest point (figure 113). The incision must be large enough (generally, at least half the size of the soft

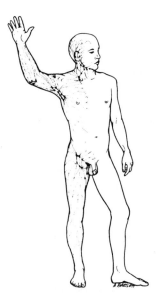

Figure 112. Location of lymph nodes within the lymphatic system. Tenderness and enlargement of the nodes mark inflammation in the lymph nodes; red streaking can sometimes be appreciated.

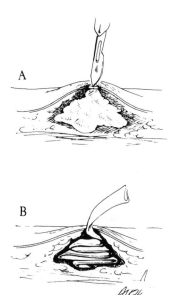

Figure 113. (A) To drain an abscess, a stab wound is made in the center of the softest area. (B) After the pus is removed and the cavity is rinsed, a gauze wick is layered into the cavity.

area) to allow all of the pus to run out. After the pus is allowed to drain, the cavity should be rinsed well and then packed snugly with a small piece of gauze to prevent the skin from sealing closed over the created empty space (and thus merely reaccumulating pus, rather than healing). Each day, the packing is removed (yank it out quickly to minimize pain), and the wound irrigated and then repacked until the cavity shrinks to a small size. If the abscess is adequately drained, there is no need to begin antibiotic administration.

Do not squeeze an abscess to cause rupture, particularly not on the face. This may force bacteria into the bloodstream and create a much more serious infection elsewhere (such as behind the eye or in the brain). After you make an incision into the top of an abscess and it is draining freely, it is all right to push the sides gently in order to express the pus.

If the abscess has not yet softened, but is still red, painful, and hard, begin the victim on warm soaks and administer dicloxacillin, erythromycin, or cephalexin. Continue the soaks until the abscess softens and a white or yellow cap becomes apparent. If the abscess is soft, but there is evidence of lymphatic infection (see above), administer an antibiotic.

Ingrown Toenail

An ingrown toenail occurs when the lateral edge of a nail penetrates into the skin alongside or outside the groove in which it advances during growth. This can be caused by an injury to the nail or toe, improperly fitting footwear, or improper trimming. Redness, pain, and swelling are common, and an infection may develop.

Treatment involves relieving the pressure created by the toenail on the soft tissues that surround it. Soak the affected toe for 30 minutes in a basin or bucket of warm water, preferably with a squirt of disinfectant such as povidone iodine solution. Using a blunt, stiff tweezer, needle driver (see page 235), scissors, or nail clipper, rotate (extract) the ingrown portion of the nail out of the nail bed, and clip (cut) it off (figure 114). If this is impossible because of pain, which is common when there is an infection, you may need to first administer pain medication. To prevent the nail from growing back into the groove and once again becoming ingrown, layer (pack) the groove with cotton or strips of gauze or clean cloth. Change the packing every few days until the nail has grown back correctly or you can no longer keep the packing in place.

If you don't have any tools to trim the nail and wish to relieve the pressure, try taking a piece of tape and placing one edge on the soft tissue of the toe against, but not touching, the edge of the ingrown nail

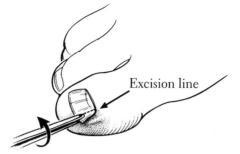

Figure 114. Removing an ingrown toenail.

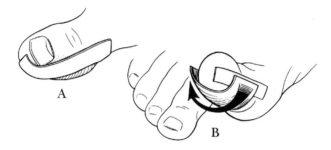

Figure 115. Relieving the pressure on an ingrown toenail. (A) Place a strip of tape next to the painful ingrown toenail. (B) Wrap the tape under the toe to separate the tissue from the nail.

(figure 115). Wrap the tape underneath the toe while pulling, to separate the soft tissue from the nail and relieve the pressure. This is a temporary measure at best.

If there are signs of an infection (see page 247), administer dicloxacillin, cephalexin, or erythromycin for 5 to 7 days and continue the warm- or hot-water soaks two or three times a day.

Fingertip Cracks

Annoying superficial fingertip skin cracks occur in cold, dry climates or after repeated exposure to salt water and abrasion. They can be prevented by using skin moisturizers and limiting hand washing. Healing can be accelerated by applying a greasy (petrolatum-based) ointment and covering with a bandage. If the crack is resilient, it can be closed with a small amount of

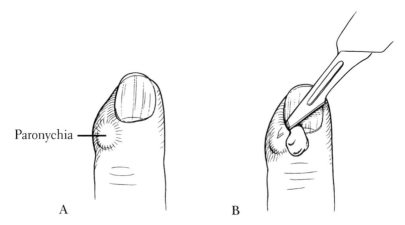

Figure 116. (A) Paronychia. (B) Draining a paronychia.

superglue (ethyl-2-cyanoacrylate). Medicinal tissue adhesives that should be used, if available, in preference to ethyl-2-cyanoacrylate are n-2-butyl-cyanoacrylate (Histoacryl Blue or GluStitch) or 2-octyl-cyanoacrylate (Dermabond). After you apply the glue and let it set, apply a fingertip bandage to keep the wound dry for 2 to 3 days. As the crack heals, the shed skin carries away the residual glue. If the glue is dislodged by accident before the crack heals, it should be reapplied.

Paronychia

A paronychia is a small abscess (see page 212) at the base of a nail (just beyond the cuticle) in the space between the soft tissue and the nail. It commonly appears as a red or yellowish, soft, and tender swelling in one corner at the base of the nail (figure 116A).

To treat a paronychia, soak the affected finger in nonscalding hot water with a squirt of disinfectant (such as povidone iodine) for 30 minutes. To drain the collection of pus, you need to slide the tip of a #11 scalpel blade underneath the cuticle, holding the blade flat against the nail, to puncture the pocket and allow drainage (figure 116B). If you don't have a scalpel, you can use a clean, small knife blade, or even the prong of a fork. The abscess will be no more than ¼" (0.6 cm) below the margin of the cuticle; if you have penetrated that far without the obvious release of pus, cease your digging, start the victim on dicloxacillin, cephalexin, or erythromycin, and continue with hot-water soaks three times a day. If pus is released, jam a 1" (2.5 cm) wick of gauze into the pocket, if the victim

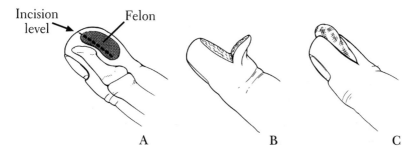

Incision level → Felon

A   B   C

Figure 117. (A) Felon. (B) Fish-mouth incision for drainage of a felon. (C) Packing a small wad of gauze in the incision site to allow drainage.

will tolerate it; with or without the wick, continue the soaks for a few days to keep the pocket draining.

Felon

A felon is a severe infection of the pulpy tip of a finger (figure 117), usually caused by infection with *Staphylococcus* bacteria. It can arise from a nick in the skin, extension of a paronychia, infected hangnail, or puncture wound. The finger becomes swollen and extremely tender, with throbbing pain. Occasionally, there is extension of the infection via the lymphatic system (see page 212), with swollen lymph glands behind the elbow and in the armpit. It is possible to develop a fever with a felon.

Soaking the felon in hot water will not help much. The victim should be started on dicloxacillin, cephalexin, or erythromycin.

The definitive treatment is drainage, but this can be extremely painful. An incision needs to be made that allows extensive drainage from the fingertip. This is usually performed by a physician completely through the finger, with placement of a gauze or rubber "drain," or involves flaying the fingertip pad down from the bony tip of the finger ("fish-mouth incision") (figures 117B and C).

Blisters

Blisters are the bane of hikers. These clear fluid- or blood-filled vesicles have probably ended more outings than all major illnesses combined. They can be prevented by keeping feet dry, wearing adequate and properly fitting socks, wearing thin liner socks (polypropylene or polyester)

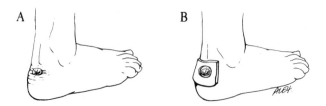

Figure 118. (A) Blister on the heel. (B) A cushion of Moleskin protects the area from further irritation.

under heavier wool-blend hiking socks, breaking in footgear prior to the expedition, and padding all rough edges within hiking boots. If an area is known to rub, prevent a blister by applying a nonwrinkled layer of mole-skin, Molefoam, or athletic tape over the skin before a "hot spot" develops.

If a blister is caused by pressure (ill-fitting boots), you have a couple of choices. If the blister site can be padded with moleskin or other adhesive foam, so that rubbing no longer occurs, the blister should be ringed with a doughnut of padding and left intact (figure 118). For a better cushion, a piece of Spenco 2nd Skin (an inert gel consisting of polyethylene oxide and water) can be laid into the doughnut hole and the entire area covered with a second layer of moleskin or an absorbent bandage, such as a Spenco Adhesive Knit Bandage. If no such padding is available, if contin-ued rubbing will rupture the blister, or if the blister interferes with walk-ing, then you can drain it of fluid by using a "sterile" needle (heat a sewing needle to red hot and allow it to cool) to punch a small hole at its edge. If the blister appears infected, it should be unroofed entirely, an appropriate dressing applied, and the victim treated with dicloxacillin, erythromycin, or cephalexin for 5 days or until the skin appears normal.

Blisters or reddened skin may also be caused by an allergic ("contact") reaction to chemicals such as formaldehyde or rubber. If a rash is confined to the soles of the feet (shoe inserts) or top of the feet (shoe tongue dye), suspect this problem. In this case, the footgear must be changed.

If a blister is caused by a thermal burn, it should be immediately immersed in cold water (*do not* apply ice directly to the burn) for 10 to 15 minutes, in order to relieve pain and lessen the ultimate injury. Then dry the wound and apply a soft, sterile dressing. Unless there is a reason to sus-pect infection (cloudy fluid or pus, fever, redness and swelling beyond the blister edges, swollen lymph glands), burn blisters should be left intact (see page 101). Opening an uninfected blister or sticking a needle into it risks introducing bacteria that can cause an infection. Topical antibacterial creams such as silver sulfadiazine or mupirocin, or ointments such as mupirocin or bacitracin, should be applied if the blister is broken, or to prevent the dressing from sticking to the wound. Alternately, apply a layer of Spenco 2nd Skin or Aquaphor gauze underneath a sterile gauze dressing.

Athlete's Foot, Ringworm, and Jock Itch

Athlete's foot, ringworm, and jock itch are all caused by fungal infections. These more commonly develop in warm, moist areas, such as between the toes and in the groin. Athlete's foot (tinea pedis, or "foot") can be recognized as a red rash, moist or scaling, with small blisters and frequent weeping. Itching is the major symptom. Ringworm (tinea corporis, or "body") appears as one or more ring-shaped red areas on the torso. The rash spreads outward in an enlarging circle; the central area may clear slightly as the fungus in the center dies. There is scaling and itching, and occasionally tiny blisters at the expanding margin. Jock itch (tinea cruris, or "groin") is a red rash with a well-demarcated border that causes itching and irritation in the groin and occasionally over the genitals.

These rashes are more common in summer, particularly among those who do a lot of sweating and bathe infrequently. They are managed with antifungal cream (ketoconazole 2% [Nizoral] or miconazole [Micatin]) and antifungal powder, such as tolnaftate (Tinactin) or clotrimazole 1% (Lotrimin), applied two or three times a day. Because a fungal infection is contagious, socks and underwear should not be shared. If possible, wear cotton underclothing that absorbs sweat.

Tinea Versicolor

Tinea versicolor is a fungal infection that causes skin discoloration with minimal itching or scaling. It appears as multiple discolored (white, pink, or darkened [like a tan]) spots or patches on the shoulders, arms, chest, and back. It is treated with topical applications of selenium sulfide (Selsun) solution for 15 minutes a day for 10 days. If that is ineffective, it may be treated with topical antifungal preparations (see above) or an oral dose of ketoconazole (Nizoral) prescribed by a dermatologist.

Onychomycosis

Onychomycosis is a fungal infection under a nail, most commonly a toenail. This causes the nail to become discolored and deformed. The condition may be associated with chronic fungal infection in the skin, either as an itchy, scaling, or moist rash, or as recurrent blisters between the toes and on the sole of the foot.

Topical medications are not very effective. A physician may prescribe the antifungal medication itraconazole 200 mg twice a day for 1 week per month for 3 consecutive months, or terbinafine 250 mg per day for 3 months. Because these medications can induce side effects—such as headache, liver and gastrointestinal disturbances, and skin rash—and because they may interact adversely with certain drugs (such as astemizole, terfenadine, cisapride, midazolam, triazolam, cimetidine, and rifampin), their administration should strictly be guided by a physician. Newer topical therapies, such as amorolfine, ciclopirox nail laquer, and tioconazole, may be effective in cases where less than half of the nail is involved.

Prevention involves excellent foot hygiene and avoidance of fungal infection between the toes (athlete's foot) (see page 219). If possible, wash and dry your feet each day. To control foot sweating—which leads to blisters, fungal infections, and foot odor—spray your feet daily with an aluminum chlorhydrate antiperspirant, unless a fissure or crack appears in the skin, in which case spraying must be discontinued until the skin is healed. An alternative is to use a drying, deodorant foot powder. Each day, gently massage your feet and apply antifungal powder. Keep your nails trimmed. When hiking, use two pairs of socks—an inner thin liner sock of polypropylene or polyester and a thicker outer sock densely woven from a wool (or similar material) blend.

Diaper Rash

If a baby develops a diaper rash, keep the diaper area clean and dry. For redness alone, apply Desitin diaper cream or A&D ointment. If a fungal infection is suspected, as evidenced by a more intensely red rash, raised bumps, and faint whitish discharge in the groin creases, add an antifungal cream, such as miconazole (Micatin). Do not apply steroid cream or ointment preparations, which can cause an infant's skin to atrophy.

Lice

In a situation of poor hygiene and shared living quarters, particularly overseas, you may acquire head and/or body lice, which make their homes predominantly in hair-covered areas of the body. The overwhelming symptom is itching. To search for head lice, inspect the scalp carefully. Upon close inspection, you may discover nits (white, ovoid 0.5 mm eggs) attached to the hair shaft, or tiny crawling forms, particularly in the scalp, on the eyelashes, and in the pubic hair. A common finding is swollen lymph glands behind the ears or running down the back of the neck. Body lice and their nits live in the seams of clothing. The bites are most abundant on the shoulders, trunk, and buttocks. The pubic louse, or "crab" louse, prefers to reside in pubic hair, but may also appear on the eyebrows, on the eyelashes, or under the arms. Bites are hard to find, but if the infestation has been present for a few weeks, peculiar steel gray spots may be seen on the trunk and thighs.

Fortunately, lice cannot leap or fly. The treatment is to lather the body and scalp vigorously with lindane 1% (Kwell) shampoo or crotamiton 10% (Eurax) lotion, leave the lather in place for 10 minutes, and then rinse. Children may be treated with 5% permethrin (Elimite) cream in a single application; this is safe for infants over 2 months of age. Rub the cream into the skin and scalp, and wash it off after 8 to 12 hours. Comb the hair thoroughly in a direction toward the scalp to remove all nits. To be most effective, the process should be repeated in 1 week.

Another treatment for head and body lice is pyrethium and piperonyl butoxide (R and C shampoo, or RID) applied to all affected areas and washed off after 10 minutes.

One percent permethrin (Nix) is less effective for the general eradication of lice and not recommended for treatment, but is good for removing lice nits from the hair. Apply it after the hair has been washed and towel-dried, leave it on for 10 minutes, then rinse it off. Repeat the treatment in 7 days to eliminate emerging lice. For pubic lice, it may be necessary to rub crotamiton lotion into the affected area daily for several weeks to destroy hatching ova.

All clothing and bedding (including sleeping bags) should be washed thoroughly with laundry soap in hot water or dry-cleaned. All people in close contact should be treated.

Scabies

Scabies is caused by the human scabies mite *Sarcoptes scabiei* var. *hominis,* which completes its entire life cycle on the skin of a human. It is usually acquired during sexual contact, but can also be acquired from clothing and bedding. The usual manifestations are severe nocturnal itching, which is provoked by body warming, such as occurs from the heat of a fire. A serpentine burrow is seen on the surface of the skin, which is created as an impregnated adult female burrows into the skin and deposits eggs along a path that usually does not exceed ⅕ to ⅓" (5 to 10 mm) in length. Common sites for infestation are the web spaces between fingers, sides of fingers, wrists, elbows, buttocks, feet and ankles, and belt line. Infants may be infested on the scalp and soles of the feet.

Untreated, the disorder can persist indefinitely. A cure can be effected with a single overnight application of 1% gamma benzene hexachloride (Kwell) lotion or cream. Symptoms may persist (up to a month) after the mites have been killed, until the uppermost layer of skin is shed. The chemical should also be applied beneath the fingernails, where mites may be deposited during scratching. Permethrin cream 5% (Elimite) is an alternative therapy and is approved for use in infants over 2 months of age. Other therapies are crotamiton ointment or cream 10% for 2 consecutive nights, or sulfur in petrolatum (5 to 10%) for 3 consecutive nights.

Creeping Eruption

Creeping eruption is the common term for cutaneous larva migrans, which is caused by the larvae of hookworms that infest cats and dogs. Humans pick up the larvae upon exposure to dirt, particularly moist, sandy soils following a rainfall. The larvae invade the skin, most commonly on the feet, lower legs, hands, and buttocks (from sitting). The larvae tunnel through the top layer of skin, leaving a serpentine, threadlike trail of inflamed (red) tissue, which itches and may be slightly painful. Treatment is with topical thiabendazole four times a day for 2 weeks. If the topical medication is not available, thiabendazole can be administered in an oral form in a dose of 22 mg per kg (2.2 lb) of body weight, not to exceed 1.5 g per dose, twice a day for 2 days. If the rash doesn't completely resolve within 48 hours after therapy, repeat the treatment.

Shingles

Shingles is the common name for herpes zoster, a skin eruption with activation often related to stress. Individuals carry the varicella virus (the same agent that causes chicken pox in children) "silently" in nerve roots. Upon stimulation, it causes the outcropping of a series of blisters in patterns that correspond with skin areas served by particular nerve roots originating from the spinal cord (figure 119). Classically, the victim will have a day or two of unexplained itching or burning pain in the area that is going to break out, and then will notice the onset of the rash. The discomfort can be tremendous and may necessitate liberal use of pain medication. The rash itself should be kept clean and dry, and covered with a light, dry dressing to prevent further irritation from rubbing or the sun.

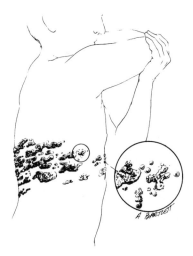

Figure 119. Shingles (herpes zoster) eruption.

The disorder is self-limited, and will resolve spontaneously over the course of approximately 10 days to 3 weeks. If the victim becomes moderately ill (fever, chills, severe headache) or if the rash involves the eyes, mouth, or genitals, see a physician, who may prescribe acyclovir (Zovirax) 800 mg five times a day, valacyclovir (Valtrex) 1 g three times a day, or famciclovir (Famvir) 500 mg three times a day for 5 to 7 days.

Fever Blisters

See page 175.

MINOR BRUISES AND WOUNDS

Bruises

A bruise is a collection of blood that develops in soft tissue (muscle, skin, or fat), caused by a direct blow to the body part, a tearing motion (such as a twisted ankle), or spontaneous bleeding (ruptured or leaking blood vessel). With trauma, tiny blood vessels are torn or crushed and leak blood into the tissue, so that it rapidly becomes discolored. Pain and swelling are proportional to the degree of injury. People on anticoagulants (such as Coumadin) and hemophiliacs tend to develop larger bruises; elders and those taking steroid medications tend to bruise easily, often spontaneously.

The immediate (within the first 48 hours) treatment of a bruise is to apply cold compresses or to immerse the injured part in cold water (such as a mountain stream). This decreases the leakage of blood, minimizes swelling, and helps reduce pain. Cold applications should be made for intermittent 10-minute periods until a minimum total application time of 1 hour is attained. Do not apply ice directly to the skin (to avoid frostbite). Rather, wrap the ice in a cloth before application.

If the swelling progresses rapidly (such as with bleeding into the thigh), an elastic bandage can be wrapped snugly to try to limit the swelling. Continue cold applications over the wrap. It is important to keep the wrap loose enough to allow free circulation (fingertips and toes should remain pink and warm; wrist and foot pulses should remain brisk). Elastic wraps are indicated only if pain and swelling will not allow the victim to extricate himself in order to seek medical attention.

Elevation of the bruised and swollen part above the level of the heart is essential, in order to allow gravity to keep further swelling to a minimum.

Never attempt to puncture or cut into a bruise in order to drain it. This is fraught with the risk of uncontrolled bleeding and the introduction of bacteria that cause infection. The exception to this rule is a tense and painful collection of blood under the fingernail (see page 225).

After 48 to 72 hours, the application of moist or dry heat will promote local circulation and resolution of the swelling and discoloration. Heat ointments or liniments are ineffective; they only irritate nerve endings in the outermost layers of the skin and give a false impression of warmth.

People who have prolonged blood-clotting times and/or who have large bruises should avoid products that contain aspirin, which might cause increased bleeding. A hemophiliac who sustains an expanding bruise will likely need to be transfused with a blood-clotting "factor" to promote coagulation; transport to a medical facility should be prompt.

A severe bruise, usually caused by a direct blunt force, can on rare occasion develop into a compartment syndrome (see page 64).

Black Eye

A black eye is a darkened blue or purple discoloration in the region around the eye. It can be caused by a direct blow (bruise) or by blood that has settled into the area from a broken nose, skull fracture, or laceration of the eyebrow or forehead. If it is due to a direct injury (with swelling and

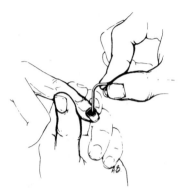

Figure 120. Hot paper-clip technique to drain blood from under the finger-nail.

pain), first examine the eyeball for injury (see page 163). The skin discoloration may be treated with intermittent cold compresses for 24 hours.

Blood Under the Fingernail

When a fingertip is smashed between two objects, there is frequently a rapid blue discoloration of the fingernail, which is caused by a collection of blood underneath the nail. Pain from the pressure may be quite severe. To relieve the pain, it is necessary to create a small hole in the nail directly over the collection of blood, to allow the blood to drain and thus relieve the pressure. This can be done during the first 24 to 48 hours following the injury by heating a paper clip or similar-diameter metal wire to red-hot temperature in a flame (taking care not to burn your fingers while holding the other end of the wire; use a needle-nose pliers, if available) and quickly pressing it through the nail (figure 120). Another technique is to drill a small hole in the nail by twirling a scalpel blade, sharp knife, or needle. As soon as the nail is penetrated, blood will spurt out, and the pain will be considerably lessened. Before and after the procedure, the finger should be washed carefully. If the procedure was not performed under sterile conditions, administer dicloxacillin, erythromycin, or cephalexin for 3 days.

Puncture Wounds

Puncture wounds are most frequently caused by nails, tree branches, fish-hooks, and the like. Because they do not drain freely, these wounds carry a high risk for retained bacteria and subsequent infections. A puncture wound should be irrigated copiously with the cleanest solution that is available and left open to heal. Bleeding washes bacteria from the wound, so a small amount of bleeding should be encouraged. *Never* suture or tape a puncture wound closed, unless necessary to halt profuse bleeding; doing so promotes the development of infection. Similarly, do not occlude the opening of a puncture wound with a "grease seal" or plug of medicinal ointment; apply any antiseptic sparingly. If the wound is more than ¼" (0.6 cm) at its opening, you can leave a piece of sterile gauze in the wound as a wick for a day or two, to allow drainage and prevent the formation of an abscess cavity (see page 212). If the wound becomes infected (see page 247), apply warm soaks four or more times a day. Treat the victim with dicloxacillin, erythromycin, or cephalexin for 4 days.

Impaled Object

See page 52.

Scrapes

Scrapes (abrasions) are injuries that occur to the top layers of the skin when it is abraded by a rough surface. They are generally very painful, because large surface areas with numerous nerve endings are involved. Bleeding is of an oozing, rather than free-flowing, nature.

An abrasion should be scrubbed until every last speck of dirt is removed. Although it hurts just to think about this, scrubbing is necessary for two reasons. The first is the infection potential when such a large area of injured skin is exposed to dirt and debris. The second is that if small stones or pieces of dirt are left in the wound, these in essence become like ink in a tattoo, leaving the victim with permanent markings that require surgical excision. Soap-and-water scrubbing with a good final rinse should be followed with an antiseptic ointment such as bacitracin or mupirocin, or cream such as mupirocin, and a sterile nonadherent dressing or Spenco 2nd Skin. You can also place Hydrogel occlusive dressing over an abrasion; it will absorb up to 2½ times its weight in fluid weeping from the wound. It should be covered with a dry, light dressing. This technique is useful for burns as well. If the surface area is not particularly large or is on a difficult-to-bandage area, such as the nose or ears, the bandage (not the ointment) may be omitted.

The pain of cleansing can be relieved by applying pads soaked with lidocaine 2.5% ointment to the abrasion for 10 to 15 minutes prior to scrubbing. To avoid lidocaine toxicity, don't do this if the surface area of the abrasion exceeds 5% of the total body surface area (an area approximately five times the size of the victim's fingers and palm). In some cases, particularly when there is deeply embedded grime that will be extremely painful to remove, it is useful to inject the wound with a local anesthetic (see page 228).

Cuts (Lacerations)

Remove all clothing covering a wound so that you may determine the origin and magnitude of any bleeding.

1. *Control bleeding.* This can be done in almost every instance by direct pressure (see page 48). Apply firm pressure to the wound using a wadded sterile compress, cloth, or direct hand contact (wearing latex gloves, if possible; if you are allergic to latex, use other nonpermeable gloves, such as nonlatex synthetic). Hold the pressure for a full 10 to 15 minutes without release. If this does not stop the bleeding, apply a sterile compress and wrap with an elastic bandage, taking care to not wrap so tightly as to occlude the circulation (check for warm and pink fingers and toes). During all of these maneuvers, keep the victim calm and elevate the injured part as much as possible.
2. *Clean the wound.* After you have controlled the bleeding, the wound(s) should be properly cleansed. Wear latex gloves or, if you are allergic to latex, other nonpermeable gloves. Examine the wound and remove all obvious foreign debris.

   The best way to clean a wound is to irrigate away the dirt and bacteria. The irrigating stream should be forceful enough (approximately 8 to 12 pounds per square inch) to dislodge the foreign material without injuring the tissues beneath the stream or forcing harmful material deeper into the wound. Use the cleanest disinfected water available. The best irrigants are "normal" saline (0.9% NaCl) solution (add 1½ level tsp, or 9 g of salt, per quart or liter), or a quart of disinfected saline or water into which you have added 1 fluid oz (30 ml) of povidone iodine (Betadine) solution (not soapy "scrub"). Don't use a povidone iodine solution to irrigate eyes, and don't drink this stuff.

   Use a syringe (10 to 20 ml is best) with a 16- to 20-gauge (18-gauge is best) plastic catheter or steel needle attached to draw up the irrigating fluid and act as a "squirt gun." This creates a stream of the appropriate

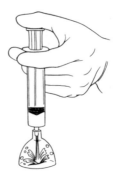

Figure 121. Using a Zerowet Splashield attached to a syringe to irrigate the open wound.

force. Another way to obtain the appropriate stream diameter and force is to attach a Zerowet Splashield (P.O. Box 4375, Palos Verdes Peninsula, CA 90274) to a plastic syringe (figure 121). A complete wound irrigation system (Klenzalac) with a 10-ml syringe, fill stem, and Splashield is also available. This technique protects the operator from splash exposure to blood and tissue fluid. If you don't have these supplies, you can fill a small (as sturdy as possible) plastic bag with the irrigating solution, punch a tiny hole in the bag, and squeeze out the liquid. Irrigate the wound until it appears clean, usually with at least a pint to a quart (½ to 1 liter) of liquid. Take care to avoid splashing yourself.

Sometimes irrigation isn't enough to remove all of the dirt from the wound, or you won't be carrying irrigation equipment. In that case, the wound needs to be scrubbed out with a gauze or cloth, using a disinfectant solution or hand soap and the cleanest disinfected water available. This can be painful, so get everything ready in advance and then try to accomplish the task as quickly as possible. Remember to rinse the wound thoroughly when you are finished.

Scrubbing and irrigation will often cause a wound to begin bleeding again as blood clots are dislodged from tiny blood vessels. Stop this bleeding by holding absorbent gauze with pressure against the wound.

Do not pour tincture of iodine, rubbing alcohol, merthiolate, mercurochrome, or any other over-the-counter antiseptic into the wound (except for potentially rabid animal bites—see page 364). These preparations inhibit wound healing and are extremely painful. Although recommended by healers in ancient civilizations, herbal doctors, and professional woodsmen, the use of butter, pine sap, ground charcoal, hard liquor, or wine as an antiseptic is not recommended.

3. *Anesthetize (numb) the wound.* Most laypeople will never be called upon to sew (suture) or staple a wound closed. However, for the benefit of rescuers who might need to practice advanced skills, here are the basics:

Local anesthesia of a wound can be achieved by injecting sterile 1% lidocaine or 0.25% bupivacaine solution into the edges of the wound using a 25-, 27-, or 30-gauge needle attached to a 10 ml syringe. There will be less stinging sensation with injection if you add 1 ml of 8.4% sodium bicarbonate solution to each 10 ml of the lidocaine solution prior to using it. Bicarbonate should not be added to bupivacaine, because it causes precipitation if the solution is not used immediately. Once bicarbonate has been injected, the shelf life of the multidose vial of anesthetic decreases considerably, so this maneuver may not be practical in the field. Whenever possible, use a new ampoule or vial of anesthetic for each episode (event, or victim). This minimizes the risk of injecting a contaminated (with bacteria) product and causing a wound infection. *Never* share needles between victims.

To draw up medication into a syringe, follow the instructions given for subcutaneous injection on page 419. The onset of anesthesia from injection of lidocaine or bupivacaine is 2 to 5 minutes, with duration of action 1 hour for lidocaine and 4 hours for bupivacaine. The maximum safe adult dose (volume) of 1% lidocaine is 30 ml; for 0.25% bupivacaine, it is 70 ml. For a child, the maximum safe dose for 1% lidocaine is 0.4 ml per kg (2.2 lb) of body weight, up to 30 ml; the maximum safe dose for 0.25% bupivacaine is 1 ml per kg, up to 70 ml. Of course, it is best to stay as far as possible below the maximum safe dose.

The wound should be cleansed of all major debris and dirt before injecting an anesthetic, so as not to plunge the needle through the grime. Inject through the open (cut or torn) portion of the wound, rather than through the surface of the skin, unless this is necessary to avoid gross contamination. One useful technique is to insert the short needle up to its hub, and then inject while you slowly withdraw the needle back out from the skin, rather than injecting during entry. As with any other medical intervention, it is important to have practiced ahead of time before attempting to numb a wound by injecting it with an anesthetic.

Numbing a wound can be done before it is definitively cleansed and irrigated, particularly if the cleansing process will be extremely painful (as when an abrasion needs to be scrubbed). In order to not have to reinject the wound because the anesthetic has worn off, have all of your supplies gathered and your helpers ready to assist before you inject.

4. *Reapproximate the anatomy (close the wound) as best possible.* Most cuts do not involve tissue loss, so that edges fit together like a jigsaw puzzle. *Because of the infection risk away from the hospital or doctor's office (a relatively germ-free*

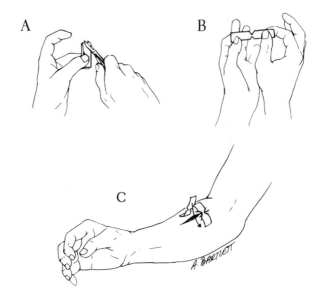

Figure 122. Fashioning a butterfly bandage. (A) Fold a piece of tape (however, don't let the tape stick together) and cut off both corners at the crease. (B) The straightened tape reveals the "butterfly." (C) The bandage is used to hold the wound edges close together.

environment), do not close a wound tightly with stitches of thread (sutures) unless absolutely necessary. Instead, bring the wound edges together with paper tape with adhesive specifically made for wound closure (such as elastic or nonelastic Steri-Strips) or with butterfly bandages (see also page 233—"Taping a Wound Closed"). The latter can be fashioned from regular surgical adhesive tape (figure 122). A small scar is preferable to a wound infection caused by tight closure that requires hospitalization for surgical management of a wound infection. If nothing else is available to hold together the edges of a widely gaping wound that prevents the victim from seeking help, use a safety pin(s).

No matter what method you use to close a wound, the best way to make the opposite sides match up properly, and to take tension off the wound while the remainder of the closure is completed, is to place the first piece of tape, staple, or suture (thread) at the midpoint of the wound ("halve the wound") (figure 123). The second fastener should then "halve the halves" (figure 124), so that the wound is now quartered, and so forth until the closure is complete. A final long locking strip can be placed over the ends of the crossing strips to complete the closure (figure 125).

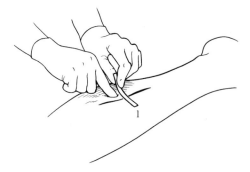

Figure 123. "Halving" a wound for the first act of closure.

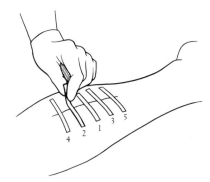

Figure 124. Halving a half, or "quartering the wound." This helps keep the wound in alignment and prevent mismatched sides (of different lengths).

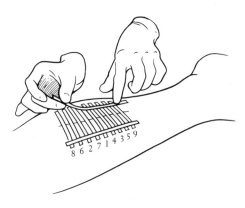

Figure 125. Completed wound closure using tape.

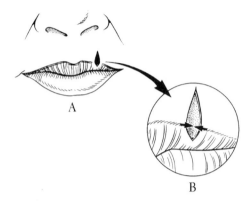

Figure 126. Matching the vermilion border of the lip.

When aligning the two sides of a cut lip, be sure to match the vermilion border perfectly (figure 126). The same concern holds for aligning a laceration of the eyebrow. Never shave an eyebrow, because it might not grow back! In fact, there is no absolute need to shave hair from the skin around any wound. Shaving hair may increase the risk for infection, because you create micro-nicks in the skin with your razor or knife edge.

Regardless of which technique you choose to close the wound, it is useful to splint the repair (see page 65) for at least a few days, to allow healing to begin without the wear and tear of motion, particularly across a joint.

Skin Flaps and Avulsions

If a cut occurs at an oblique angle to the skin, so that a very thin layer of skin is "shaved" away, the wound should be cleaned carefully and the flap repositioned and held in place with tape (see below). If the flap is extremely thin or if its base of attachment is small, the blood supply may not be sufficient to allow survival of the tissue. In this circumstance, it will turn dusky blue and then blacken, harden, shrivel, and fall away. Unless there is an underlying infection—in which case the obviously dead or dying tissue should be removed—the flap may provide a biologic covering, much like a skin graft, to allow the underlying tissue to proliferate and heal. Since it is difficult to tell which dusky flaps will survive and turn pink and which will deteriorate and "mummify," it is best to give the flap at least a few days before trimming to see which way things are headed.

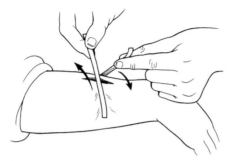

Figure 127. Using opposite-facing tape strips to pull a wound closed.

If a large chunk of skin is cut away entirely, or avulsed, then the wound must either be closed, allowed to fill in as it heals with new tissue, or covered with a skin graft. The first two options are available to you in the field. If fat or muscle are showing and the wound edges will not easily pull together for field closure, then the wound should be cleaned carefully, a sterile bandage (see below) applied, and the victim transported to definitive medical care.

Taping a Wound Closed

To apply tape to a wound, prepare the skin surrounding the cut by drying it thoroughly. Next, apply a thin layer of tincture of benzoin using a cotton-tipped swab, taking care not to get any into the open wound (it will sting like crazy). Push the two sides of the wound together so that they are perfectly opposed, then lay the first adhesive strip across the wound at the midpoint of its length. Continue to apply strips perpendicular to the long axis of the wound until it is closed. Use diagonal or crisscross strips for extra strength.

If you don't have an assistant and it is difficult to hold the wound edges together and lay down an adhesive strip at the same time, you can fix a strip to one side of the wound, fix a second strip immediately next to the first one on the opposite side, and then use the two loose ends to pull the wound together (figure 127). If the strips keep popping off the skin because it is slippery or too much tension is required to keep the edges together, you can run a strip of adhesive tape or duct tape longitudinally along the wound edges on either side of the gash about ¼" (0.6 cm) away from the opening, and use these as anchors for the crossing strips (see figure 128).

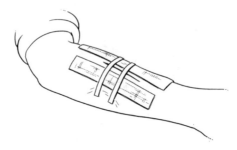

Figure 128. Longitudinal tape strips used as anchors for the cross (closing) pieces.

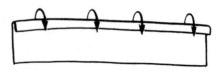

Figure 129. Folding a longitudinal piece of tape to prepare for a suture anchor strip.

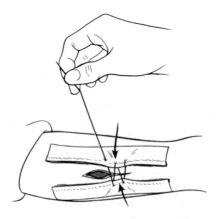

Figure 130. Sewing the tape suture strips together to close the wound.

Another method of wound closure using tape, which may be more appropriate for a longer wound, is to cut two strips of adhesive tape 1" (2.5 cm) longer than the wound. Fold one-quarter of each strip of tape over lengthwise (sticky to sticky) to create a long nonsticky edge on each piece (figure 129). Attach one strip of the tape on each side of the wound, ¼" to ½" (0.6 to 1.3 cm) from the wound, with the folded (nonsticky) edge toward the wound. Using a needle and thread, sew the folded edges together, cinching them tightly enough to bring the wound edges together properly (figure 130). The tape will stick much better if you first apply a thin layer of benzoin to the skin.

Sewing (Suturing) a Wound Closed

In general, it is best to avoid sewing (suturing) a wound closed outside of the sterile environment of the hospital. However, sometimes this is necessary, particularly if the wound is large and cannot be closed with taping methods.

Sutures come in a variety of sizes attached to many different types of needles, depending upon their purpose. For an expedition kit intended for use by a layperson, I recommend carrying 3/O monofilament nylon suture (such as Ethilon, Dermalon, or Prolene) attached ("swaged on") to a large curved "cutting" needle, and 4/O monofilament nylon suture attached to a large curved cutting needle. The 3/O suture is larger in diameter, and should be used to close large wounds on the scalp, trunk, and limbs. The smaller-diameter 4/O suture is used to close smaller wounds on the trunk, limbs, hands, and feet. Although there are other suture types (such as nonabsorbable silk and absorbable synthetics), sizes (thick to so fine [ophthalmic] that it requires a magnifying glass to see them), and needles (such as small curved, and straight), these two suture setups will suffice for most situations in which a layperson might wish to stitch a wound. Ideally, you would use 5/O and 6/O (smaller diameter) suture material on the face, but this is more difficult to manipulate and tie if you're inexperienced.

The instrument used to push the needle through the skin is a needle holder (Webster-style "needle driver"). It has finger handles like a scissors, and clamps open and shut with finger pressure to hold the needle firmly in its finely grooved jaws. It is held in a certain way to allow the wrist rotation that forces the curved needle through the skin.

The goal of stitching a wound is to bring the skin edges neatly together without excessive tightness, which would be manifested by a wound that is puckered up, and stitches that become buried. Most wounds swell a bit; thus, it is not necessary to cinch them closed with too much tension. After a wound is stitched, it should lie flat.

Wear latex surgical gloves if they are available. If you are allergic to latex, use other (such as nonlatex synthetic) nonpermeable gloves. The needle should be placed into the jaws of the needle driver so that it can be clamped just behind (toward the suture) the midpoint of the curve

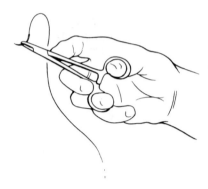

Figure 131. Gripping a suture needle with a needle driver.

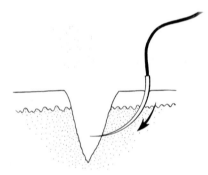

Figure 132. Pushing the needle through the skin and out into the base of the wound.

(figure 131). The needle should be oriented perpendicular to the skin and pushed through using a gentle rotating motion at the wrist; this pushes it out into the base of the wound (figure 132). Then release the needle, reach down into the wound and regrip the needle that has exited into the wound, and pull the needle and suture through the wound until a 2" (5 cm) tag is left outside the skin (figure 133). The needle is once again grasped with the needle driver as before, pushed into the opposite side of the base of the wound at exactly the same depth as it entered into the wound on the other side (figure 134), and rotated out through the external skin surface on the same side (see figure 135). Now you once again release the needle from the needle driver. The ideal suture placement is square or bottle shaped (see figure 136). As shown in this figure, the suture ideally crosses the wound close to its deepest point; slightly above (figures 133–135) or below (see figure 136) is acceptable.

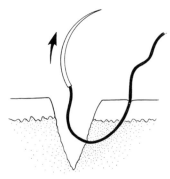

Figure 133. Pulling the suture through the first side of the wound.

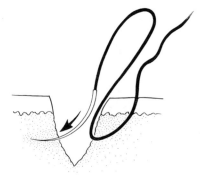

Figure 134. Pushing the needle into the base of the opposite side of the wound.

To tie a modified square knot, the long end (with the needle) of the suture is looped around the needle holder twice (see figure 137); then the short end of the suture—which was left as a 2" (5 cm) tag—is grasped and lock-clamped tightly in the jaws of the needle driver (see figure 138). Holding the needle in one hand and the needle driver in the other, lay the double loop down flat against the skin to pull the wound together (see figure 139). To complete the knot, a single loop is thrown around the needle driver in the direction opposite the first (clockwise versus counterclockwise, or "over" versus "under") (see figure 140), the short end of the suture once again grasped with the needle driver (see figure 141), and the knot pulled tight; cross your hands properly to lay the second loop-tie down flat ("square") against the first (see figure 142). This process should be repeated three more times for a total of five "throws" in order to assure that the knot won't unravel. Cut the long ends ¼" (0.6 cm) from the knot.

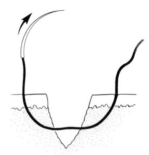

Figure 135. Rotating the needle out through the second (final) side of the wound.

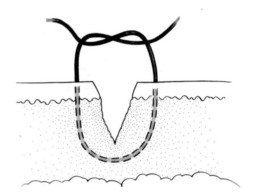

Figure 136. The U shape of proper suture placement.

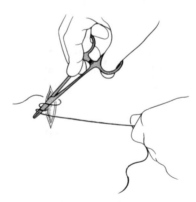

Figure 137. To tie a suture, first loop it around the needle driver twice.

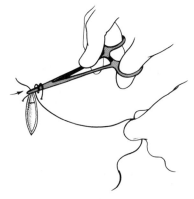

Figure 138. Grab the short end of the suture with the needle driver.

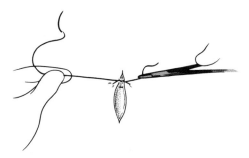

Figure 139. Laying down first loop of a knot.

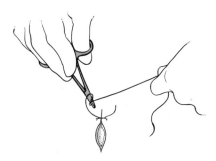

Figure 140. Creating the second loop of a square knot over the needle driver.

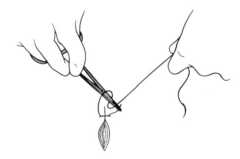

Figure 141. Once again, grab the short end of the suture with the needle driver.

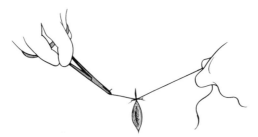

Figure 142. Completing the first square knot.

Place the stitches close enough together (approximately ¼" [0.6 cm]) so that the wound is closed and there is no fat showing from underneath the skin. A nice way to close a wound is to place enough stitches to bring the wound edges into reasonable approximation and support the tension, then close the remainder with cloth or paper adhesive strips. Remember, put the first stitch at the midpoint of the wound, then at the midpoints of the remaining segments, and so forth. If you begin stitching at one end and work your way to the other, you run a much greater chance of misaligning the wound edges and ending up with a tear-shaped "dog-ear" that can't be easily closed; this might force you to remove all of the stitches and begin all over again.

After you stitch a wound, it may ooze blood from the needle holes or the center of the wound. Apply firm, direct pressure with a gauze bandage or cloth for 10 to 15 minutes. To dress the wound, apply a thin layer of bacitracin or mupirocin ointment and an absorbent sterile bandage. Inspect the wound daily for signs of infection (see page 247). If an infection develops, remove a few stitches over the worst area to see if any pus is released. Allowing the wound to drain in one area may allow you to keep the other stitches in place for the normal duration of

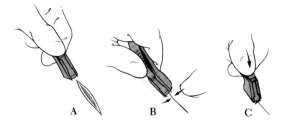

Figure 143. (A) Preparing to staple a wound. (B) Pressing the surgical tissue stapler against the skin while pushing the wound edges together. (C) Squeezing the stapler in order to discharge the staple into the skin.

healing. When in doubt, however, take all of the stitches out and let the wound heal open or under loose approximation with adhesive strips.

Try to keep the wound dry for at least 4 days. Stitches are left in place for 14 days across the joints of the finger and hand, 10 days on the arms and legs, 7 days on the trunk and scalp, and 4 days on the face. After you remove a stitch, you can reinforce a wound with adhesive strips for a week to allow a margin of safety for healing.

If you are going to carry sutures with the intention of sewing a wound, you should have a physician teach you how to suture before you need to do it yourself. You can practice the technique on a pig's foot, a chicken leg, or even a thick-skinned orange.

To remove a stitch from a healed wound, wash the wound carefully, then cut the stitch on one side only of the visible knot. (If you cut on both sides of the knot, you may not be able to retrieve the buried portion of the stitch.) Grasp the knot with a tweezer and pull the stitch out of the skin. If a crust has formed over the stitch, soften it up by applying moist compresses for 30 minutes prior to removing it.

Stapling a Wound Closed

An excellent technique for closing relatively straight lacerations on the arm, leg, trunk, and scalp is stapling. A disposable surgical stapler, such as the Precise 5-, 15-, or 25-staple Disposable Skin Stapler from 3M Medical-Surgical Division (St. Paul, Minnesota), allows precise placement of stainless-steel staples. The proper technique takes practice! Hold the skin edges together and press the business end of the stapler against the wound closure line, then squeeze the stapler to discharge a staple into the skin (figure 143). The recipient feels a quick pinprick. The closure is rapid and sturdy. The staples are left in place for 7 days on the

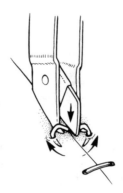

Figure 144. Removing a surgical staple.

scalp and trunk, and 10 days on the arm or leg. A disposable scissors-handle staple remover or smaller pinch-handle-style staple remover (Precise SR-1, 3M) is used to painlessly remove the staples (figure 144).

If you are going to carry surgical staples with the intention of stapling a wound, you should receive proper instruction before the journey.

Gluing a Wound Closed

Tissue adhesives ("glue"), which can be applied in a thin layer on top of a wound (*not* within the wound) to bond the edges together, have been recommended for superficial cuts. Two examples are n-2-butyl-cyanoacrylate (Histoacryl Blue, B. Braun Melsungen AG, Germany; GluStitch, GluStitch, Inc., Delta, B.C., Canada) and 2-octyl-cyanoacrylate (Dermabond, Ethicon, Inc., Sommerville, New Jersey). This technique appears to create a wound closure that, while not initially as strong, ultimately results in a similar outcome to sewing the skin together. It cannot be used on the eye, inner moist surfaces of the mouth and lips, or areas with dense body hair. Superglue should not be used to close full-thickness wounds, because it liberates heat and causes an intense inflammatory reaction.

5. Dress the wound. This is generally done in layers. The first layer is antiseptic cream or ointment, which should be sparingly applied to the surface of the wound, provided that there is good drainage and there are no large, open (deep) pockets in the wound. A thick antiseptic grease seal that prevents drainage may actually promote the development of a deep-space infection. Antiseptic ointment may soften and weaken a tissue glue closure.

A nonadherent next (inner) layer of a bandage keeps the overlying dressing from sticking. This should be nonstick (preferably sterile) Telfa, Metalline, or an impregnated (with petrolatum, for instance) gauze. If an antiseptic ointment or cream will prevent adhesion of the bandage, a prepackaged square of fine-mesh gauze can be used, but be advised that the ooze from a wound usually negates the lubricating features of most creams, and allows bandages to stick.

Special wound coverings include Spenco 2nd Skin, an inert hydrogel composed of water and polyethylene oxide. It absorbs fluids (so long as it doesn't dry out), which wicks serum and secretions away from the wound and promotes wound healing. Other occlusive hydrogel-type dressings are NU-GEL (preserved polyvinyl pyrrolidone in water) and Hydrogel, which can absorb up to 2½ times its weight in fluids exuded from the wound.

The next layer is composed of absorbent sterile dressings, such as dry gauze pads (see "Bandaging Techniques," page 244). If these are not available, use clean white cloth (the more absorbent, the better). Apply the entire bandage assembly snugly enough to control bleeding, but not to impede circulation (as judged by warm and pink fingers and toes). Keep dressings in place with conforming rolled gauze, which can also allow some air circulation. All dressings should be changed as frequently as they become soaked; if there is no significant drainage, they should be changed daily. If the skin is becoming macerated (wrinkled and pale colored; kept perpetually moist), lighten up on the ointment or cream, and apply a less occlusive dressing, while still keeping the wound protected.

Another technique for relatively "dry" wounds (nonseeping and nonbleeding) is to apply a layer of Tegaderm—a thin, semitransparent dressing material that a wound can "breathe" through. This is also available as a small patch packaged with a short (2⅜") Steri-Strip in a Wound Closure System (3M, St. Paul, Minnesota).

If you use tape to secure a dressing, you can apply tincture of benzoin to increase the stickiness of the skin. Do not let any benzoin run into the wound—it really stings. When dressings are applied, keep the body part in the position of function (normal resting position) (see figure 32). Check all dressings daily for soaking, a snug fit, and underlying infection. If you wish to remove a dressing that is stuck to a wound, soak it off by moistening it with warm water or a brief application of hydrogen peroxide. Bandaging techniques are addressed in the next section.

6. Splint the wound (see page 65). For instance, if the injury involves the hand, also place the arm in a sling to minimize motion of the injured part. Movement delays healing and promotes the spread of infection.

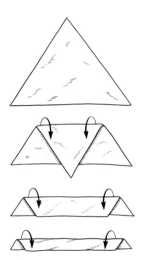

Figure 145. Making a cravat from a triangular bandage.

7. There is always the risk of infection. If the wound is an animal bite, is in the hand or foot, is a puncture wound, has inadequate drainage, has resulted from a crush injury, or is very dirty—or if you are more than 24 hours from medical care—the situation carries a high-risk for infection and the victim should be treated with an oral antibiotic (dicloxacillin, erythromycin, or cephalexin) until the wound is healed or help is reached. This is also true for any large wound. For a cat (feline) bite, use penicillin or tetracycline.

8. Seek appropriate medical attention. Field cleansing and dressing are no substitute for proper irrigation, trimming, and wound management undertaken in a medical facility. Small nicks do not require fancy intervention, but if you are in doubt as to the seriousness of the injury, get good advice.

Bandaging Techniques

Bandage application is an art form. The only way to become proficient is to practice. There is no inviolable rule other than to avoid excessive tightness, which might compromise circulation. Use square knots to tie bandage ends securely.

A triangular bandage is a three-cornered bandage, usually approximately 42" (1 m) across the base. A cravat is a triangular bandage folded two or three times into a long strap (figure 145).

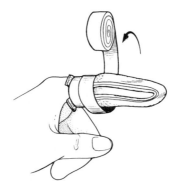

Figure 146. To begin a finger bandage, place layers of gauze over the fingertip.

The following tips should prove useful:

Finger bandage. Fold a 1" (2.5 cm) rolled gauze back and forth over the tip of the finger to cover and cushion the wound (figure 146). Then wrap the gauze around the finger until the bandage is snug and not overly bulky. On the last turn around the finger, pull the gauze over the top of the hand, so that it extends beyond the wrist. Split this tail lengthwise. Tie a knot at the wrist, and wrap the two ends around the wrist; tie again to secure the bandage. Another technique involves not splitting the tail, wrapping it around the wrist twice, then bringing it up over the top of the hand around the base of the finger from the side opposite where it originated, looping it over the hand back to the wrist, and tying it off (see figure 147).

Hand bandage. The hand should be bandaged as if for a fracture, in the position of function (see figure 32). Take care to place gauze or cotton padding between the fingers to separate and cushion them. Use a simple figure-of-eight wrap across the palm.

Arm or leg bandage. Cover the wound(s) with a gauze pad(s). Overwrap the wound using simple spiral turns of rolled gauze or a figure-of-eight pattern. Secure the bandage with adhesive tape in a spiral pattern (see figure 148) to avoid a tourniquet effect. Whenever possible, don't apply tape directly to the skin.

Foot bandage. The foot should be bandaged as if wrapped for an ankle sprain, using gauze instead of elastic wraps (see page 254).

Shoulder bandage. To make a shoulder bandage (see figure 149) from a triangular bandage, lay the base over the shoulder at a downward diagonal across the chest (front and back) with the apex pointed down the

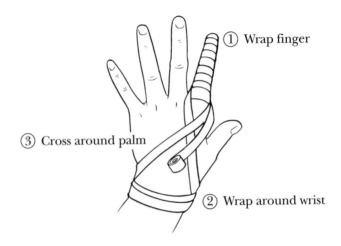

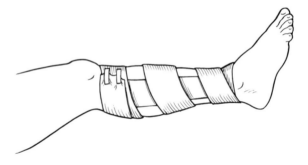

Figure 147. To complete a finger bandage, wrap the gauze around the finger, then bring it across the palm and around the wrist to tie it off.

Figure 148. Spiral leg bandage.

arm. Roll or fold the apex back down a few turns to create the beginning of a cravat; tie this just in front of the opposite armpit. Roll or fold the apex up the arm in the same manner until the bandage achieves the desired coverage, and then tie off this smaller cravat segment with the knot visible on the outside of the arm.

Chest bandage. To wrap the chest with gauze, circle the chest and upper abdomen for a few turns. To keep the bandage from slipping toward the hips, bring it up over the shoulder every third or fourth turn. Secure with adhesive tape.

Head bandage. Place the base edge of a triangular bandage just over the eyes (see figure 150). Fold the base edge 1" (2.5 cm) under to create a hem. Allow the bandage to fall back over the top of the head, with the

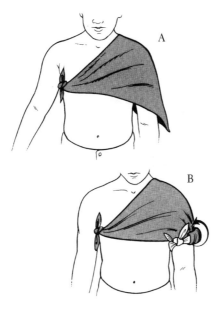

Figure 149. Shoulder bandage. (A) Drape a triangular bandage over the shoulder. Begin to form a cravat and tie off in front of the opposite armpit. (B) Complete the bandage.

apex point (tail) dropping over the back of the head. Then cross the other two free corners (at the ends of the hem) over the tail and tie them in a single turn (half of a knot). Continue to bring them around to the forehead and tie a complete square knot. Tuck the hanging tail over and into the half knot behind the head. If more pressure is necessary, tie a cravat directly over a gauze or cloth bandage.

Another way to secure a bandage to the side of the head, ear, or chin is to lay a cravat over the wound at the cravat's midpoint, then wrap it vertically over the head and under the chin (see figure 151). Cross the cravat on the side of the head at ear level, and wrap the ends in opposite directions horizontally so that one side loops across the forehead. Tie the knot behind the ear.

Eye bandage. See page 161.

Wound Infection

Despite your best efforts, a wound may become infected. The most common bacteria that cause wound infection are *Staphylococcus aureus* and *Streptococcus pyogenes*. The common signs of an infection include redness and

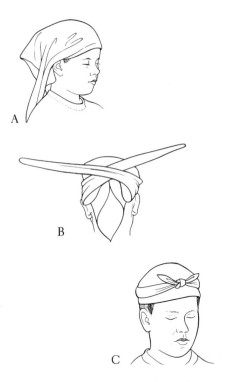

Figure 150. Head bandage. (A) Drape a triangular bandage just over the eyes. (B) Create a hem and cross behind the head, tying with a half knot in order to (C) fashion a square knot in the front. Tuck the tail that remains behind the head into the half knot.

swelling surrounding the wound, pus or cloudy discharge (pink, green, or cream colored), a foul odor (this is variable), fever, increased wound tenderness, red streaking that travels to the trunk from the wound, fever, and swollen regional lymph nodes (see figure 112).

If a wound is infected, its edges should be spread apart to allow the drainage of any pus. To do this, you need to remove some or all fastening bandages (such as butterfly bandages). The wound should then be irrigated copiously and dressed with a dry, absorbent, sterile bandage without bringing the wound edges tightly together. Begin to apply warm, moist compresses, using disinfected water, to the wound at least four times a day; also begin the victim on an antibiotic (dicloxacillin, cephalexin, or erythromycin). For a cat bite, use penicillin or tetracycline. For a wound incurred in ocean, river, or lake water, administer ciprofloxacin or trimethoprim-sulfamethoxazole as an additional antibiotic.

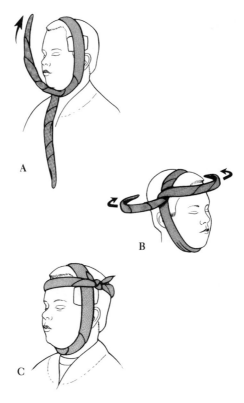

Figure 151. Securing a bandage to the side of the head. (A) Lay a cravat over the wound. (B) Cross the cravat and (C) tie it off behind the ear.

If a wound infection is advancing, the victim should be brought rapidly to a physician. If you see gas bubbles in a wound, if it is draining foul reddish gray fluid, and/or if there is a feeling of "Rice Krispies" (crepitus) in the skin surrounding a wound, it may be the onset of gangrene. This is a life-threatening infection and requires immediate advanced surgical attention.

Abscess (Boil)

See page 212.

Scalp Laceration (Cut on the Head)

See page 57.

Fishhook Removal

See page 421.

Splinter Removal

See page 422.

Blisters

See page 217.

MUSCULOSKELETAL INJURIES

Overuse Syndromes

Whenever a muscle is overused—that is, exercised past its state of conditioning—there is actual destruction of the muscle tissue and generation of lactic acid. Given a reasonable rest period, the products of metabolism are carried away in the circulation and the muscle tissue regenerates to a healthy, sometimes even stronger, condition. However, if the exercise has been vigorous and unrelenting, the participant may suffer from a variety of aches and pains that are generally categorized as overuse syndromes.

Muscle Fatigue

Simple fatigue, with depletion of energy stores within the muscle, is manifested as weakness, pain on exertion, soreness to the touch, and cramping. In many cases, this is compounded by dehydration, deficiencies of electrolytes (usually sodium and/or potassium), lack of sufficient caloric intake, or a specific injury. The sufferer has been informed by his body that it is time to rest. Sufficient time should be allowed to remove waste products, restore energy sources, correct dehydration, and regenerate muscle tissue. The victim should avoid vigorous physical activity for 12 to 24 hours, and should eat and drink amply. Pharmaceutical muscle relaxants are of little value, and pain medication is generally not necessary. Massage of the involved muscle groups is relaxing, although it probably does not hasten recovery.

Shin Splints

Shin splints is the term used to describe a painful disorder generated by excessive walking, running, or hiking. The sufferer has irritated the thin membrane that connects his two lower leg bones along the longitudinal axes where the membrane attaches to the bones. With every footstep, there is further irritation of the membrane, so that it can become impossible to walk rapidly. The victim should attempt to curtail running or vigorous walking activity, and may benefit from the administration of aspirin or a nonsteroidal anti-inflammatory drug (such as ibuprofen or naproxen). A shoe that is well cushioned (particularly its ball and heel) is very important for prevention and recovery. More complex orthotics may be required.

Plantar Fasciitis

Plantar fasciitis is inflammation of the fascia (tough connective sheath tissue) that encloses the muscles and tendons that traverse the bottom of the foot. It is a syndrome of overuse, caused by excessive walking or running, particularly associated with repetitive impact upon the bottom of a foot that is improperly cushioned or without appropriate arch support. Symptoms include pain in the bottom of the foot (ball, arch, and/or heel), worsened by weight bearing. It occurs commonly in athletes and long-distance hikers, particularly if they wear poorly fitting shoes or boots.

Treatment consists of rest, elevation of the foot with cold (ice packs) applied to the tender areas at the end of the hiking day, wearing orthotics, and administration of an oral nonsteroidal anti-inflammatory drug, such as ibuprofen. Worn at night, a splint that holds the foot in neutral position—thus keeping the plantar fascia slightly stretched—may help.

If the victim must continue to walk on the painful foot, it can be taped to provide arch support; this can do much to reduce pain. It is accomplished as follows: Apply a thin layer of benzoin or spray tape adhesive onto the bottom of the foot. Fix an anchor strip of ¾" (1.9 cm) adhesive tape in a U shape around the heel from just under the malleoli (prominences of the ankle) up to just behind the level of the "knuckles" of the

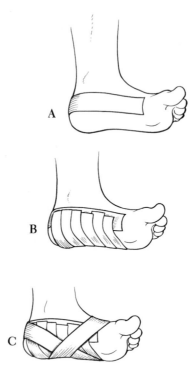

Figure 152. Taping for arch support. (A) Fix an anchor strip under the heel. (B) Attach strips across the bottom of the foot. (C) Lock the crosspieces.

toes (figure 152A). Next, lay fairly tight cross-strips of ½" (1.3 cm) tape across the bottom of the foot, with their ends torn to lay on the anchor strip (figure 152B). This creates a "sling" of tape under the foot for support. Finally, apply another U-shaped piece of tape around the heel that crosses under the center of the arch and locks down the crosspieces (figure 152C).

Torn Muscle

A torn muscle ("pulled" muscle) is recognized as sudden pain in a muscle group associated with a particular vigorous exertion, such as sprinting or lifting a heavy object. Depending on the severity of the injury, there may be associated bruising, swelling, loss of mobility, and/or weakness. For instance, a small tear in the deltoid muscle of the shoulder may cause minor discomfort upon lifting the arm over the head, while a complete separation of the quadriceps group in the anterior thigh will cause inability to straighten the leg at the knee, extreme local pain, blue discoloration of the knee, and a defect in the shape of the muscles above the knee that is easily felt and seen.

In general, a minor muscle injury can be distinguished from a bone injury by evaluating active and passive range of motion. Active range of motion is the range of normal activity the victim can manage without rescuer assistance; this will be painful with both muscle and bone injuries. Passive motion is movement of a body part performed only with the aid of the rescuer; no effort is provided by the victim, who should attempt to relax the muscle completely. If there is no pain on passive (assisted) motion, but there is pain present on active motion, then the injury is most likely muscular, because an injured bone will hurt no matter how it is moved. If there is pain on passive motion, with or without pain on active motion, suspect a bone injury.

Minor muscle injuries should be treated in the first 24 hours with immobilization, the application of cold (insulated ice packs or chemical cold packs, for example; do not apply ice directly to the skin) for 30 to 45 minutes every 2 to 3 hours, and elevation. After 48 to 72 hours, the application of heat (warm water or a heating pad, *not* ointments) and gentle movement should be started. If a significant injury is suspected (for example, complete tear of the biceps muscle or quadriceps muscle group), the injury should be immobilized as for a fracture (see page 61) and the victim transported to a physician.

The best way to prevent a pulled muscle is to stretch and warm up adequately. This allows the local blood flow to increase and minimizes the risk for small tears that can cause spasm, which in turn leads to decreased flexibility.

Sprains and Strains

Sprains and strains are injuries to ligaments (which attach one bone to another) and tendons (which attach muscle to bone) that are incurred by twisting, direct blunt trauma, or overexertion. Symptoms include pain, swelling and/or deformity, decreased range of motion secondary to pain, and bruising. The treatment is the same as for a suspected fracture. The injured part should be elevated, immobilized (see page 61), and treated with cold applications for the first 24 to 48 hours ("RICE": rest, ice, compression, and elevation). After 72 hours, heat may be applied. It is important to prevent reinjury (ankles are notorious) by proper wrapping or the application of a splint. Because the injured joint is immediately weakened, it should not be relied upon for great exertion.

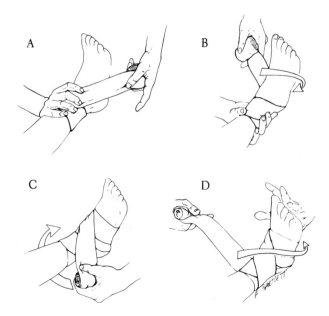

Figure 153. Wrapping the ankle with a figure-of-eight bandage. (A) Start above the ankle and (B) wrap down under the foot. (C) Cross back and forth over the top of the foot and (D) continue in a figure-of-eight pattern to secure the ankle.

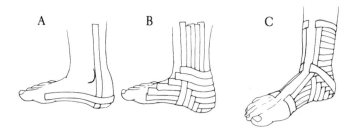

Figure 154. Taping a sprained ankle. (A) Strips of adhesive tape are placed perpendicular to each other to (B) lock the ankle with a tight weave. (C) The tape edges are covered to prevent peeling.

The most common sprain is of an ankle. If the injury is minor (no chance of a fracture) and/or if the victim needs to put weight on the ankle in order to seek help, the ankle may be wrapped snugly with an elastic wrap in a figure-of-eight method (figure 153) or taped in a criss-cross weave (figure 154). During the wrapping or taping, have the victim

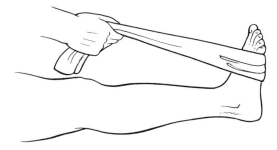

Figure 155. Pulling up on the toes to attain proper ankle position for wrapping.

point his toes and ankle upward by passing a slender rope or strap around the ball of the foot and pulling toward the body (figure 155). This allows the ankle to be strapped with the foot perpendicular to the leg and the ankle ligaments in the shortened position in which they best heal. A splint can be fashioned from a SAM Splint (see figures 78 and 79) to provide additional support. If the sprain is severe, splint the ankle as for a fracture. An Aircast Air-Stirrup ankle brace is excellent for in-shoe support.

The Achilles tendon, which runs from the heel into the lower calf, may become irritated or inflamed due to recurrent impact or repetitive stretching, particularly if the heel is not well padded. An inflamed Achilles tendon that is painful should be protected against further irritation by limiting vigorous exercise and using a heel cup or extra padding underneath the heel in order to reduce stretch forces upon the tendon.

Knee sprain is discussed on page 94.

Arthritis

Arthritis is irritation and inflammation of a joint that can be caused by overuse, infection, or various diseases (such as gout, caused by deposition of uric acid crystals). Symptoms include pain in the joint with motion, swelling (fluid collection), redness, and warmth. If there is an infection within the joint, the condition can rapidly become serious. Generally, people with such infections have high fever, shaking chills, weakness, a recent infection elsewhere in the body, or recent direct injury (often penetrating through the skin) to the joint. Differentiating between an arthritic and an infected joint is often impossible until a physician inserts a needle to see if bacterium-laden fluid or pus is present within the joint, and to

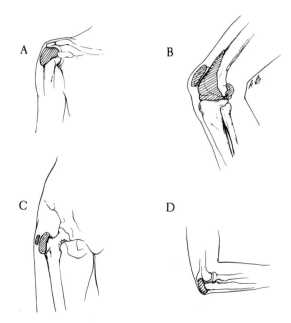

Figure 156. Bursitis affects the lubricating sacs (bursae) near the (A) shoulder, (B) knee, (C) hip, and (D) elbow.

obtain fluid for a culture. If infection is a possibility, the victim should be started on dicloxacillin, erythromycin, or cephalexin immediately.

If there is little chance of infection and you know the joint problem is due to overuse, have the victim take aspirin or a nonsteroidal anti-inflammatory drug, such as ibuprofen or naproxen. Rest the affected joint, keep it elevated if it is swollen, and adjust goals for the trip accordingly.

Bursitis

Bursitis is irritation and inflammation of the lubricating sac (bursa) that allows muscles to move freely around a joint. Common areas of irritation include the sac in front of the kneecap (irritated by prolonged kneeling), behind the elbow (irritated by a fall), in the shoulder (irritated by arm swinging), and on the outside of the hip (irritated by walking, hiking, or falling) (figure 156). Evaluation and treatment are the same as for arthritis.

Thrombophlebitis

Thrombophlebitis is inflammation in a vein associated with the development of a blood clot. This occurs in conditions of injury to the veins (cuts, bruises), or after periods of prolonged rest in a single position (sitting on a plane, cramped in a cave); it may also be associated with other risk factors (pregnancy, tobacco use, cancer, varicose veins). A blood clot irritates the lining of the vein and causes local redness, swelling, warmth, and pain. If the clot enlarges, an entire limb length can become affected. If the clot is in a deep vein, it may break off and travel to the lungs, where it causes a serious condition known as pulmonary embolism (see page 41).

It is easy to confuse the presentation of thrombophlebitis with that of an infection. If you suspect the former, have the victim elevate the limb and apply hot packs or soaks for 60 minutes every 3 hours. Seek immediate medical attention. If you are more than 24 hours from help and not absolutely certain whether you are treating infection or inflammation, administer an antibiotic (dicloxacillin, erythromycin, or cephalexin).

Back Pain

The most common back injury is muscle strain. Symptoms include muscle pain and spasm adjacent to the vertebrae. If these occur in the lumbar (lower-back) region, treatment consists of maximum rest while lying supine on a firm supporting surface. The knees may be drawn up on a pillow or rolled blanket. All possible lifting and forward bending should be discontinued. The victim should take aspirin or a nonsteroidal anti-inflammatory drug to control inflammation, and additional pain medicine as necessary. Gentle massage and alternating applications of ice packs and heat are often soothing.

If one of the cushioning intervertebral (between the vertebrae) disks has been injured (see figure 157), additional symptoms may be noted, which include numbness and/or tingling of parts of the leg (indicating impingement of the disk upon a nerve root arising from the spinal cord), shooting pains through the buttocks and posterior leg (indicating irritation of the sciatic nerve [sciatica]), leg weakness, foot drop, constipation, or difficulty with urination. The acute treatment is the same as for muscular back strain.

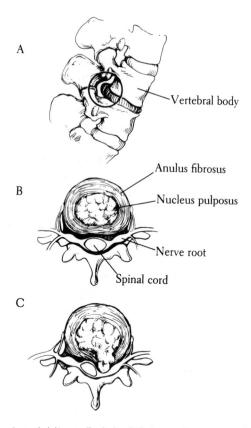

A

Vertebral body

Anulus fibrosus

B

Nucleus pulposus

Nerve root

Spinal cord

C

Figure 157. Herniated (slipped) disk. (A) Posterior protrusion of the disk into the spinal (cord) canal. (B) Cross section of the normal disk. (C) Protruding disk impinges on the spinal cord nerve root.

DISORDERS OF THE KIDNEYS AND BLADDER

Bladder Infection

Bladder infections occur frequently in females, because the shorter female urethra does not protect the bladder from bacteria as efficiently as does the male organ. A person with a bladder infection complains of discomfort (sharp pain, cramping, or burning) upon urination, frequent urination, difficulty initiating urination, lower abdominal cramping, and sometimes bloody urine, which may be as severe as small clots. Similar symptoms may be suffered by males who harbor infections in the prostate gland.

Treatment involves the administration of an antibiotic and increased oral fluid intake. Because many antibiotics are well concentrated in the urine, there are a number of acceptable treatment regimens. For the sake of simplicity, the female victim may be treated with trimethoprim-sulfamethoxazole (Bactrim or Septra) in one double-strength tablet twice a day for 3 days, or two double-strength tablets in one dose; ciprofloxacin 250 mg twice a day for 3 days, or 500 mg in one dose; ofloxacin 200 mg twice a day for 3 days, or 400 mg in one dose; nitrofurantoin monohydrate/macrocrystals (Macrobid) 100 mg capsule twice a day for 7 days with meals; or fosfomycin tromethamine (Monurol) 3 g in a single dose. If the symptoms do not completely resolve, or they recur within a few days of therapy, use the same or a different drug (in the lower dose) for 10 days.

Chlamydia are bacterium-like "germs" that are increasingly the cause of reproductive tract infections in women and genitourinary tract infections in men. Because the penicillins (such as ampicillin) are not effective against *Chlamydia,* any male with a bladder or prostate infection should be treated with tetracycline (500 mg four times a day), doxycycline (100 mg twice a day), or trimethoprim-sulfamethoxazole (one double-strength tablet twice a day) for 10 days, or with azithromycin 1 g in a single dose. Any male who develops a bladder or prostate infection should be seen by a physician when he returns from his journey.

The incidence of bladder infections in older women may be decreased by a daily 8 oz (237 ml) glass of cranberry juice. It takes several weeks of juice drinking before this effect begins to occur.

Kidney Infection

Kidney infection is considerably more serious than bladder infection. Symptoms may include all of those for bladder infection, as well as flank or lower-back pain, severe abdominal pain, fever, chills, nausea and vomiting, weakness, and cloudy urine with or without a foul odor. The pain is characterized as aching, and may become exquisite if you punch the victim gently just under the ribs adjacent to the spine on the affected side.

The field treatment is just the same as for bladder infection, except that the chosen antibiotic must be at a higher dose and continued for at least 14 days. Begin the victim on trimethoprim-sulfamethoxazole (one double-strength tablet twice a day), ciprofloxacin (500 mg twice a day), ofloxacin (400 mg twice a day), or cefadroxil (500 mg twice a day). By definition, the victim is more ill and may require hospitalization for an intravenous antibiotic(s). Therefore, anyone who is suspected to have a kidney infection should be evacuated immediately.

Kidney Stone

See page 121.

Blood in the Urine

Blood in the urine is caused by bladder or kidney infection, the passage of a stone(s), blunt or penetrating injury to the flank (kidney region), bleeding disorder, or tumor of the genitourinary tract. After heavy exertion or high fever, a person may break down a small amount of muscle tissue and release myoglobin (an oxygen-carrying protein found in muscle) into the bloodstream. In cases of burns, severe injury, or certain infections, red blood cells can be destroyed and will release their oxygen-containing protein (hemoglobin) into the bloodstream. Hemoglobin and myoglobin are filtered through the kidneys and may be concentrated in the urine, giving it a pink to reddish brown hue. If the urine is not made dilute (by drinking large amounts of fluid to increase its volume), the concentration of these pigments in the kidney can clog the filtration system and cause sudden kidney failure. Although after vigorous exercise some individuals may normally pass a small amount of reddish urine, anyone who develops darkened urine after fever or exertion should be placed at maximum rest, cooled to a normal body temperature (see page 283), encouraged to drink as much fluid as possible, and rapidly transported to a medical facility. If you are more than 24 hours away from a doctor, the urine rapidly clears with rest and increased fluids, and the victim appears in good health, the journey may continue.

Urine can also be discolored by the ingestion of chemical agents, such as urinary tract anesthetics (blue-green or orange), beets (pink-red), or bile pigments (brown, seen with hepatitis).

Acute Urinary Retention

There are rare occasions when a person cannot urinate and the bladder becomes distended with urine. This is seen more often in males than females, because a common cause is obstruction of the urethra where it passes through the male prostate gland. If the gland is enlarged (benign prostatic hypertrophy, or BPH), which occurs in elder males almost exclusively, then the passageway for urine can be narrowed to the point where it becomes obstructed. Early symptoms, which develop as the passage narrows, are difficulty initiating a stream, a weak stream, dribbling (leakage of urine), and urinating small amounts. On occasion, it may become painful to urinate. If the obstruction becomes complete, it causes urine to collect in the bladder, which becomes painfully distended and can be felt as a hard mass in the lower abdomen. Unless the obstruction can be relieved, this is an emergency. The usual treatment is to pass a small tube (catheter) through the penis directly into the bladder. This can be difficult and should only be attempted by someone trained in the technique. It is a good idea for someone properly trained to carry a urinary catheter(s) and lubricant on any expedition that will include elder males as participants.

If a male has an enlarged prostate, drugs that are anticholinergic (such as certain antispasmodics) or that contain atropine and its derivatives can precipitate acute urinary retention. For instance, an elder male with BPH on a diving expedition who takes anti-motion-sickness medication may suffer urinary retention as a side effect of the medication. A new medication that relieves the symptoms of BPH in some men is tamsulosin (Flomax), which can create its own side effects of dizziness and low blood pressure upon arising, similar to what is seen with dehydration. Therefore, it is important for people using this medication to stay well hydrated and avoid situations in which a dizzy spell or fainting might create a serious injury.

MALE GENITAL PROBLEMS

Painful Testicle

If a male complains of a painful testicle, examine both testicles. Look for discoloration or swelling. If a testicle has been injured by a blow, provide support with an improvised jockstrap and apply ice packs. If a testicle becomes acutely painful, particularly in an adolescent, and appears swollen and/or discolored, usually without a penile discharge, it may be twisted, or torsed. Since this usually happens if the testicle rotates inward (toward the midline) (see figure 158), gently see if you can rotate it outward within the scrotum. If this causes a dramatic relief of pain, you may have saved the testicle. If you believe an unresolved torsion is present, this is an emergency and the victim should be rushed to a physician.

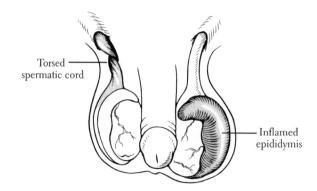

Figure 158. Rotation of the right testicle in a torsion; an inflamed epididymis of the left testicle.

If a testicle is swollen and the victim complains of pain or burning on urination, he may suffer from an infection or inflammation of the epididymis, which is part of the sperm-collection pathway (figure 158). This should be treated with doxycycline, tetracycline, or trimethoprim-sulfamethoxazole for 7 days.

Penile Discharge

If a male complains of a discharge from his penis, particularly if it follows sexual intercourse by a few days and is yellow or greenish in color, you must suspect gonorrhea. In this case, it is safest to treat the victim for both gonorrhea and a chlamydial infection. If more than 24 hours will pass before a doctor can be reached, start the victim on tetracycline 500 mg four times a day or doxycycline 100 mg two times a day for 10 days (to treat *Chlamydia*). Azithromycin 1 g in a single dose is also effective against chlamydial infection. To treat the gonorrhea, administer cefixime 400 mg orally as a single dose. Alternative single-dose therapies for gonorrhea are cefpodoxime 200 mg, cefuroxime 1000 mg, ciprofloxacin 500 mg, ofloxacin 400 mg, azithromycin 2 g, and norfloxacin 800 mg. To treat gonorrhea and chlamydial infection at the same time (the two germs often "travel" together), you can use the one-dose azithromycin therapy. Remember, syphilis may also have been transmitted, so the victim should be tested upon return to civilization.

If there has been no sexual intercourse and a penile discharge develops, particularly if it is white or clear, treat with doxycyline or azithromycin.

In this day and age, no person should engage in casual unprotected sexual intercourse. A man should wear a latex (not lambskin) condom that has been stored in a cool, dry place. The package should show no evidence of leakage. The spermicide nonoxynol-9 (condom lubricant or vaginal foam) offers additional protection against viruses.

PSYCHIATRIC EMERGENCIES

The wilderness experience can be quite stressful, and a member of the party may behave in an unusual fashion. This may be directly related to the events at hand or reflect an underlying psychiatric disorder. It is imperative that someone recognize warning signs early and evacuate anyone who cannot retain mental stability, to avoid placing the impaired individual and his traveling companions at risk for injury.

Anxiety

Anxiety is the most common psychiatric symptom, and may range from appropriate and adaptive minor doubts about success to a full-blown panic reaction. Minor anxiety is expressed as general discomfort about a situation. The excessive worrier may become timid and withdrawn, and may lose his enthusiasm for participation. His anxiety may be clothed in criticism of plans or refusal to cooperate. It is important that every member of the expedition voice fears and objections at the outset, so as not to be caught in a panic when crossing treacherous terrain or performing rescues.

The treatment is reassurance and support. Frequently, practice sessions that build up to a completed effort will relieve anxiety and improve the performance of the group. In no case should anyone be made to feel ashamed of his fears. Rather, the leader should seek to help the victim conquer them.

Approach what problems you can directly. Most people do much better if fear is identified and managed than if it is never confronted.

Panic

Panic is anxiety in the extreme. The victim loses all judgment and becomes consumed with efforts at escape and self-preservation. Panic renders the victim unable to make reasonable decisions and immediately places him and all around him at risk for injury. The rescuer must assume a strong authoritative posture with the panic victim, assuring him in no uncertain terms that the situation is under control and the panic behavior is detrimental. Depending on the situation, this can be done with verbal explanations, convincing arguments, or demonstrations of safety. If the victim places other individuals at immediate risk for injury, he should be subdued, with force if necessary.

Those who use cocaine, smoke marijuana or phencyclidine (PCP, angel dust), or ingest LSD are prone to panic reactions under conditions of stress. The management of these reactions is little different from that previously outlined; the exception is the risk of violent behavior from anyone under the influence of cocaine or PCP. If a person appears to be under the influence of psychotropic drugs, do your best to keep him from hurting anyone, but be careful not to become injured yourself in the process.

Hyperventilation

One manifestation of anxiety that verges on panic is the hyperventilation syndrome, in which the victim, overcome by his fears, begins to breathe at an inappropriately rapid rate—40 to 100 times per minute. This causes the level of carbon dioxide in his blood to fall precipitously and to render the blood alkaline (from its normal neutral state). The symptoms are dizziness; fainting spells; numbness and tingling in the hands, feet, and around the mouth; muscle spasm in the hands and wrists; and, occasionally, seizures. If you are certain that the victim is hyperventilating because of anxiety (that is, there is no reason to suspect a collapsed lung, pneumonia, or other medical problem), place a paper bag or similar device over his mouth and nose for about 5 minutes. The victim breathes in and out of this bag (encourage "slowly and deeply"), and rebreathes his own expired carbon dioxide, allowing normalization of the level in the bloodstream and correction of the symptoms. At the same time, reassure the victim that he will be all right. After the episode, make an attempt to identify the cause of the anxiety.

Depression

Depression occurs in the outdoor setting in response to situations that are perceived as hopeless. Some victims who are injured, lose their way, or are weakened by starvation and exposure may lose the will to continue. They become listless, fatigued out of proportion to their physical condition, uninterested, inattentive, without appetite, sleepy, and tearful. Clearly, the rescuer must encourage all party members to maintain their survival instincts, to continue to help others and to help themselves. In a cold environment, it is important to remember that hypothermia (see page 269) is a significant cause of apathy and should be corrected, if possible. An individual with chronic depression may go on a vacation trip with the enthusiastic expectation that his psychiatric disease will be alleviated or that his most recent depression has lifted. The sudden realization that such expectations are not fulfilled may put that person at risk for severe mood depression. Do not be afraid to inquire about a past history of psychiatric illness.

Reaction to an Injury or Illness

People's reactions to stress differ; they may become irrational, angry, apathetic, confused, or withdrawn following an accident or harsh environmental exposure. The most common reaction, given the presence of a strong leader, is to become dependent. It is crucial for the rescuer to bolster the victim's self-confidence and self-esteem at every opportunity, for it may take extraordinary physical and mental effort to survive a catastrophe in the wilderness.

Try to individualize your approach to each person. To best understand the changing needs of victims and families, try to maintain regular dialogue intended solely for the purpose of psychological support. Stay with the victim as much as possible. Use frequent touch and reassurances to relay your sense of concern and offer comfort. As best possible, involve the victim in his treatment and rescue, so that his thoughts are attuned to survival rather than to fear or grief.

When you are under stress, do your best to be supportive to others with less emotional control. Anger is rarely successful and commonly worsens an already difficult situation.

Equally important, the rescuer must constantly be alert for true medical problems that masquerade as psychological disorders. The uninterested victim may be hypothermic, the belligerent climber hyperthermic, the intoxicated hiker hypoglycemic, or the irritable child stricken with acute mountain sickness.

PART FOUR

Disorders Related to Specific Environments

INJURIES AND ILLNESSES DUE TO COLD

Hypothermia (Lowered Body Temperature)

The body generates heat through metabolic processes that can be maximized with involuntary shivering to roughly 5 times the basal level (up to 10 times with maximum exercise). However, shivering is abolished after a few hours of exposure, because of exhaustion and depletion of muscle energy supplies. When a victim loses the ability to shiver, the cooling process becomes quite rapid. Skin, surface fat, and superficial muscle layers then act as an insulating "shell" for the core of vital organs (heart, lungs, liver, kidneys, and so on). Normal skin temperature in cool weather is 90 to 93° F (32.2 to 33.9° C); this can drop to 70 to 73° F (21.1 to 22.8° C) before core cooling begins. Mild hypothermia is defined as a core (measured rectally) body temperature of less than 98.6° F (37° C) but greater than 95° F (35° C); moderate hypothermia is defined as a core body temperature of less than 95° F (35° C) but greater than 90° F (32.2° C); severe hypothermia is defined as a core body temperature of less than 90° F (32.2° C).

Heat is lost from the body to the environment by direct contact (conduction), air movement (convection), infrared energy emission (radiation), the conversion of liquid (sweat) to a gas (evaporation), and the exhalation of heated air from the lungs (respiration). It is important to note that the rate of heat loss via conduction is increased 5-fold in wet clothes and at least 25-fold in cold-water immersion. Windchill refers to the increase in the rate of heat loss (convection) that would occur when a victim is exposed to moving air (see figure 159). This chill can be compounded further if the victim is wet (conduction, convection, and evaporation).

Immersion hypothermia refers to the particular case in which a victim has become hypothermic because of sudden immersion into cold water. Again, water has a thermal conductivity approximately 25 times greater than air, and a person immersed in cold water transfers heat from his skin into the water approximately 100 times faster than into air. The actual rate of core temperature drop in a human is determined in part by these phenomenona and in part by how quickly heat is transferred from the core to the skin, skin thickness, the presence or absence of clothing, the initial core temperature, gender, fitness, water temperature, drug effects, nutritional status, and behavior in the water.

WIND SPEED (MPH)	OUTSIDE AIR TEMPERATURE (°F)															
	35	30	25	20	15	10	5	0	−5	−10	−15	−20	−25	−30	−35	−40	−45
	EQUIVALENT TEMPERATURE (°F)															
5	32	27	22	16	11	6	0	−5	−10	−15	−21	−26	−31	−36	−42	−47	−52
10	22	16	10	3	−3	−9	−15	−22	−27	−34	−40	−46	−52	−58	−64	−71	−77
15	16	9	2	−5	−11	−18	−25	−31	−38	−45	−51	−58	−65	−72	−78	−85	−92
20	12	4	−3	−10	−17	−24	−31	−39	−46	−53	−60	−67	−74	−81	−88	−95	−103
25	8	1	−7	−15	−22	−29	−36	−44	−51	−59	−66	−74	−81	−88	−96	−103	−110
30	6	−2	−10	−18	−25	−33	−41	−49	−56	−64	−71	−79	−86	−93	−101	−109	−116
35	4	−4	−12	−20	−27	−35	−43	−52	−58	−67	−74	−82	−89	−97	−105	−113	−120
40	3	−5	−13	−21	−29	−37	−45	−53	−60	−69	−76	−84	−92	−100	−107	−115	−123
45	2	−6	−14	−22	−30	−38	−46	−54	−62	−70	−78	−85	−93	−102	−109	−117	−125

Figure 159. Windchill determination. To determine windchill, find the ambient air temperature on the top line, then read down the column to the line that corresponds with the current wind speed. Example: When the air temperature is 10° F and the wind speed is 20 mph, the rate of heat loss is equivalent to -24° F under calm conditions. To convert to metric or Celsius use the following: 1 mile = 1.61 kilometers; C = 5/9 (F − 32).

A sudden plunge into cold water causes the victim to hyperventilate (see page 264), which may lead to confusion, muscle spasm, and loss of consciousness. The cold water rapidly cools muscles and the victim loses the ability to swim or tread water. Anyone pulled from cold water should be presumed to be hypothermic.

The progression of hypothermia leads to predictable physiologic responses, which roughly correspond to different body temperatures. Although not invariable, the signs and symptoms are as follows:

95 to 98.6° F (35 to 37° C). Sensation of cold; shivering; increased heart rate; urge to urinate; slight incoordination in hand movements; increased respiratory rate; increased reflexes (leg jerk when the knee is tapped); red face.

90 to 95° F (32.2 to 35° C). Increased muscular incoordination; stumbling gait; decreased or absent shivering; weakness; apathy, drowsiness, and/or confusion; slurred speech.

85 to 90° F (29.4 to 32.2° C). Loss of shivering; confusion progressing to coma; inability to walk or follow commands; paradoxical undressing (inappropriate behavior); complaints of loss of vision; decreased respiratory rate; decreased reflexes.

Below 85° F (29.4° C). Rigid muscles; decreased blood pressure, heart rate, and respirations; dilated pupils; appearance of death.

The first principle of therapy is to suspect hypothermia. Any person who is found in a cold environment should be suspected of suffering from hypothermia. The definition of "cold environment" is variable. Someone who is wet, improperly dressed, and intoxicated with alcohol can become hypothermic in 70° F weather. Do not use yourself as an indicator of warmth—you may be perfectly comfortable while your companion is lapsing into hypothermia.

Unless the victim is found frozen in a block of ice or has been recently pulled from frigid waters, the most likely clue to a hypothermic state is altered mental status. The winter hiker who gradually loses interest and lags behind the group ("Just leave me behind—I'll catch up"), who dresses inappropriately for the weather or begins to undress, or who begins to stumble and make inappropriate remarks should be immediately evaluated for low body temperature. A hypothermic individual may become anxious, repeat himself, or even become delusional. *Never leave a victim of even mild hypothermia to fend for himself.*

The second principle of therapy is to measure the victim's temperature. This should be done, if possible, with a thermometer calibrated to read below 94° F (34.4° C), which is the cutoff for most standard oral thermometers. Hypothermia thermometers with a range of 75 to 105° F (23.9 to 40.5° C) are available. Temperature ideally should be measured rectally, although this is often impractical. Oral and axillary (armpit) temperatures are unreliable in this situation, and should be used only to screen for low body temperature. That is, if they are normal, the victim will have at least a normal body temperature, but could be hotter. However, if they are low, they may grossly understate how cold the victim really is, and should be followed with a rectal measurement. Digital electronic eardrum scanners used to measure temperature may also yield a false (compared to the core) reading.

Unless the victim has suffered a full cardiopulmonary arrest, the hypothermia itself may not be harmful. Unless tissue is actually frozen, cold is in many ways protective to the brain and heart. However, if a hypothermic victim is improperly transported or rewarmed, the process may precipitate ventricular fibrillation, in which the heart does not contract, but quivers in such a fashion as to be unable to pump blood. *The burden of rescue is to transport and rewarm the victim in a way that does not precipitate ventricular fibrillation.*

The following general rules of therapy apply to all cases:

1. Handle all victims gently. Rough handling can cause the heart to fibrillate (cause a cardiac arrest).

2. If necessary, protect the airway (see page 17) and cervical spine (see page 31).

3. Prevent the victim from becoming any colder. Provide a shelter. Remove all his wet clothing and replace it with dry clothing. Don't give away all of your clothing, however, or *you* may become hypothermic. Replace wet clothing with sleeping bags, insulated pads, bubble wrap, blankets, or even newspaper.

Cover the victim's head and neck. Insulate the victim from above *and below* with blankets. Do not change blankets unless necessary to keep the victim dry. If possible, put him in a sleeping bag sandwiched between two warm rescuers. But remember that in this situation, no heat is really contributed by the bag itself. Do not count on a sleeping bag to be adequately prewarmed by a normothermic rescuer's body heat. Another technique is to blow warm air from an electric hair dryer into the bag with the victim. Hot water in bottles, *well insulated with clothing to prevent skin burns,* may be placed next to the victim in areas of high heat transfer, such as the neck, chest wall, and groin.

4. Do not attempt to warm the victim by vigorous exercise, rubbing the arms and legs, or immersing in warm water. This is "rough handling" and can cause the heart to fibrillate if the victim is severely hypothermic.

5. Seek assistance as soon as possible.

Mild Hypothermia (Core Temperature Above 95° F, or 35° C)

The victim of mild hypothermia is awake, can answer questions intelligently, and complains of feeling cold. He may or may not be shivering.

Prevent the victim from becoming any colder. Get him out of the wind and into a shelter. If necessary, build a fire or ignite a stove for added warmth. Gently remove wet items of clothing and replace them with dry garments. If no dry replacements are available, the clothed victim should be covered with a waterproof tarp or poncho to prevent evaporative heat loss. Cover the head, neck, hands, and feet. Insulate the victim above and below with blankets. If the victim is coherent and can swallow without difficulty, encourage the ingestion of warm sweetened fluids. Avoid heavily caffeinated beverages. If a dry sleeping bag is available, one or more rescuers should climb in with the victim and share body heat. Do not apply commercial heat packs, hot-water-filled canteens, or hot rocks directly to the skin; they must be wrapped in blankets or towels to avoid serious burns.

Moderate Hypothermia (Core Temperature 90 to 95° F, or 32.2 to 35° C)

The victim of moderate hypothermia has become apathetic and mildly confused, wishes to be left behind, and is uncooperative. Speech is often slurred, and logic is on the wane. The victim rapidly becomes uncoordinated and clumsy, often stumbling. He has ceased to shiver, and shows signs of muscle stiffness. Unless you have a thermometer to measure this victim's temperature, you must assume that he is severely hypothermic or will soon become so. Follow the directions for mild hypothermia, with the added cautions that it is best not to allow this victim to walk about until he is fully alert; in addition, do not give him fluids to drink until he becomes wide awake and understands what is going on.

Severe Hypothermia (Core Temperature Less than 90° F, or 32.2° C)

Depending on the body temperature, a victim who appears to be asleep may be in a complete coma. Below 65° F (18.3° C), humans become poikilothermic like a snake, and take on the temperature of the environment.

Examine the victim carefully and gently for signs of life. Listen closely near the nose and mouth and examine chest movement for spontaneous breathing. Feel at the groin (femoral artery) and neck (carotid artery) for a weak and/or slow pulse (see page 26).

If the victim shows any signs of life (movement, pulse, respirations), do not initiate the chest compressions of CPR. If the victim is breathing regularly, even at a subnormal rate, then his heart is beating. Because hypothermia is protective, the victim does not require a "normal" heart rate, respiratory rate, and blood pressure. Pumping on the chest unnecessarily is "rough handling," and may induce ventricular fibrillation.

If the victim is breathing at a rate of less than 6 to 7 breaths per minute, you should begin mouth-to-mouth breathing (see page 24) to achieve an overall rate of 12 to 13 breaths per minute.

If help is on the way (within 2 hours) and there are no signs of life whatsoever, or if you are in doubt (of whether the victim is hypothermic, for instance), you should begin standard CPR (see page 28). If possible, continue CPR until the victim reaches the hospital. Rescue breathing should take priority over chest compressions, particularly in the victim of cold-water immersion. There have been documented cases of "miraculous" recoveries from complete cardiopulmonary arrest associated with environmental hypothermia after prolonged resuscitation, presumably because of the protective effect of the cold. Remember, "no one is dead until he is warm and dead." However, all of these victims were ultimately resurrected in the hospital, after they had been fully rewarmed.

A victim of severe hypothermia cannot be rewarmed in the field. If a hypothermic victim suffers what you determine to be a cardiac arrest in the wilderness, transport should be the first priority. If enough rescuers are present to allow CPR and simultaneous transport, then do both. If you are the only person present, do not bother with CPR, because you will not be able to resuscitate the victim until he is rewarmed. Your only hope is that the victim is in a cold-protected state ("metabolic icebox") and that you can extricate him (as gently as possible!) to sophisticated medical attention.

In any case of severe hypothermia, transport should be undertaken as soon as possible. Take care to cover the victim with dry blankets and to handle him as gently as possible. Rapid rewarming or restoration of circulation will release cold acid-laden blood from the limbs back to the core organs, which may cause a profound deterioration of the victim.

Preparing a Hypothermic Victim for Transport

1. Keep the victim dry. Replace all wet clothing. Lay the victim on a sleeping bag and then cover him with a layer of blankets. Cover everything with a plastic sheet.
2. Keep the victim horizontal. Do not allow massage of the extremities. Do not allow the victim to exert himself.
3. Splint and bandage all injuries as appropriate.
4. Limit rewarming to methods that prevent further heat loss. Place insulated hot-water bottles in the victim's armpits and groin. Keep his head and neck covered.

A Special Note about the Victim of Cold-Water Drowning

If a victim is pulled from icy waters and appears to be clinically dead (fixed dilated pupils, no respirations, no detectable pulse), perform CPR until a qualified medical person is available to intervene or you become exhausted. Because of the physiology of cold-water immersion, the victim may be sufficiently protected to survive the event.

Prevention of Hypothermia

1. Carry adequate food and thermal wear, such as Thermax, Capilene, and/or polypropylene ("polypro") or wool undergarments. Anticipate the worst possible weather conditions. Dress in layers so that you can adjust clothing for overcooling, overheating, perspiration, and external moisture. Use a foundation layer to wick moisture from the body to

outer layers. Add an insulation layer to provide incremental warmth. For shirts, use wool, Capilene, or polypropylene. Consider a turtleneck or neck gaiter. For pants, wear wool or pile, with a fly. Carry windproof and waterproof outer garments, mittens or gloves (with glove liners), socks, and a hat. In very cold weather, up to 70% of generated heat may be lost by radiation from an uncovered head. Boots should be large enough to accommodate a pair of polypropylene socks plus at least one pair of heavy wool socks without cramping the toes. Stay dry. Carry a properly rated (for the cold) sleeping bag stuffed with Hollofil II, Quallofil, or down.

2. Do not exhaust yourself in cold weather. Avoid perspiring. Do not sit down in the snow or on the ice without insulation beneath you.

3. Seek shelter in times of extreme cold and high winds. Don't sit on cold rocks or metal. Insulate yourself from the ground with a pad, backpack, log, or tree limb.

4. Do not become dehydrated. In the cold, dehydration is caused by evaporation from the respiratory tree, increased urination, and inadequate fluid intake. Drink at least 3 to 4 quarts (liters) of fluid daily. During extreme exercise, drink more—5 to 6 quarts per day. Ingesting snow is an inefficient way to replace water, because it worsens hypothermia. Do not skip meals. Do not consume alcoholic beverages in cold weather. They cause an initial sensation of warmth because of dilation of superficial skin blood vessels, but this same effect contributes markedly to heat loss.

At night, fill a canteen or Nalgene water container with at least 1 quart (liter) of water, and sleep with it to keep it from freezing.

Frostbite

Frostbite is an injury caused by the actual freezing of tissues. Factors that predispose a person to frostbite include poor circulation (caused by previous cold injuries, tobacco use, alcohol ingestion, diseases of the blood vessels, constricting garments, poorly fitting boots, old age) and extremes of cold exposure. Windchill contributes markedly to frostbite risk. For instance, at an air temperature of 20° F (–6° C), a 45 mph (73 km per hour) wind causes the same rate of heat loss as a 2 mph (3.2 km per hour) breeze at an air temperature of –22° F (approximately –30° C). Furthermore, since a human in motion creates his own wind (while riding a snowmobile, for example), the risk for frostbite for such a person increases.

During exposure, once the temperature of a hand or foot drops to 59° F (15° C), the blood vessels maximally constrict and minimal blood flow occurs. As the limb temperature declines to 50° F (10° C), there may be brief periods of blood vessel dilation, alternated with constriction, as the body attempts to provide some protection from the cold. This is known as the "hunting response" and is seen more commonly in the Inuit (Eskimos) and those of Nordic descent. Below 50° F (10° C), the skin becomes numb and injury may go unnoticed until it is too late. Tissue freezes at or below a temperature of 24.8° F (–4° C). Once circulation is abolished, the skin temperature may drop at a rate in excess of 1° F (0.56° C) per minute.

The major immediate symptom of a frostbite injury is numbness, occasionally preceded by itching and prickly pain. The frostbitten area will appear to be white, with a yellow or bluish (grayish) waxy (sometimes mottled) tint. If the injury is superficial, as commonly occurs on the face, the skin is firm and may indent with a touch, because the underlying tissue is still soft and pliable. If the injury is deep, the skin may feel hard and actually be frozen solid. A hand or foot may feel clumsy or absent. The areas most commonly affected are the fingertips and toes (particularly in cramped footwear), followed by the earlobes, nose tip, cheeks, and other exposed skin. These parts have little heat-generating capability and no significant insulation. Male joggers have had their genitals frostbitten.

Rapid rewarming is the standard therapy. However, *do not thaw out a frostbitten body part if it cannot be kept thawed.* In other words, if you come upon a lost hiker 10 miles (16 km) back in the woods who has frostbitten toes, do not use your stove to heat water to thaw out his feet if he will then have to put his wet boots back on and hike out—refreezing his toes in the process. Frostbitten tissue is severely damaged and is prone to reinjury; refreezing causes an injury that will far exceed the initial frostbite wound. It is much better to walk out on frostbitten toes until safety is reached than to thaw and allow refreezing. Thus, if a victim needs to be transported to another site for rewarming, do not allow "slow" or partial rewarming, particularly if there is a chance that the tissue will be allowed to refreeze. Pad the affected body part, apply a protective splint, and hustle the victim to the site where the definitive thaw will take place.

Once the victim has reached a location (shelter) where refreezing will not occur, remove all constrictive jewelry and wet clothing. Replace wet clothes with dry garments. Immerse the frostbitten part in water heated to 102 to 108° F (39 to 42.2° C). Do not induce a burn injury by using hotter water. You can estimate 108° F water by considering it to be water in which normal skin can be submerged for a prolonged period with minimal discomfort. Heated tap water is too hot. Never use a numb frostbitten finger or toe to test water temperature. It is best to use your own hand or the victim's uninjured hand to test the temperature. Circulate the water to allow thawing to proceed as rapidly as possible. When adding more hot water, take the body part out, add the water, test the temperature, and then reimmerse the part. It is best to use a container in which the body part can be immersed without touching the sides; for instance, a 20-quart (-liter) pot will accommodate a foot. If the skin is frozen to mittens or metal, use heated water to remove them. *Never rewarm the skin by vigorous rubbing or by using the heat of a campfire, camp stove, or car exhaust,* because you most certainly will damage the tissues.

If the victim is hypothermic, attend first to the hypothermia. Thawing should not be undertaken until the core body temperature has reached 95° F (35° C) (see page 272).

Thawing of the skin usually requires 30 to 45 minutes. It is complete when the skin is soft and pliable, and color (usually red; rarely, bluish) and sensation have returned. Allowing the limb to move in the circulating water is fine, but massage may be harmful. Moderate to extreme burning pain may occur during the last 5 to 10 minutes of rewarming.

Thawed frostbite may be present in a number of stages, much like a burn injury. These are recognized as:

First degree. Numbness, redness, and swelling; no tissue loss.
Second degree. Superficial blistering, with clear (yellowish) or milky fluid in the blisters, surrounded by redness and swelling.
Third degree. Deep blistering, with purple blood-containing fluid in the blisters.
Fourth degree. Extremely deep involvement (including bone); induces mummification.

Blisters appear 6 to 24 hours after rapid rewarming. Leave these blisters intact. After thawing the skin, protect it with fluffy, sterile bandages (aloe vera lotion, gel, or cream should be applied, if available). Pad gently between the digits with sterile cotton or wool pads, held in place by a loose, rolled bandage. Transport the victim to a medical facility. Administer ibuprofen 400 mg or aspirin 325 mg twice a day. If frostbite involves the feet, try to minimize walking. Do not allow tobacco use or the drinking of alcohol. Keep the victim well hydrated with warm beverages.

After the thaw, if the victim is days away from hospital care, manage the wound as follows:

1. If you don't have sufficient sterile bandages to redress the wounds at least once a day until you reach a hospital, allow blisters to remain intact. Apply topical aloe vera gel or lotion twice a day. Cover with sterile gauze.

2. If white or clear blisters begin to leak, trim them away and apply antiseptic ointment (mupirocin or bacitracin) or cream (mupirocin). Cover with a sterile dressing (see page 242), taking particular care to pad with cotton or gauze between fingers and toes.

3. If at all possible, keep purple or bloody blisters intact, because they provide a covering that keeps the underlying damaged tissue from drying out. Apply topical aloe vera gel or lotion twice a day. Cover with sterile gauze.

4. Elevate the affected part.

5. Apply a protective splint (see page 65) if necessary to surround the bulky cushion dressing.

6. For the first 72 hours after the injury, administer dicloxacillin, cephalexin, or erythromycin.

7. If the skin blackens and begins to harden, apply topical mupirocin or bacitracin ointment, or mupirocin cream, daily to the margin where the dying skin meets the normal skin.

Throbbing pain may begin a few days after rewarming and continue for up to a few weeks. After the pain subsides, it is not unusual for the victim to notice a residual tingling sensation. If there is no tissue loss, the duration of abnormal sensation may be only a month; with extensive tissue loss, it can exceed 6 months. Intermittent burning pain or electric-current-like sensations may be present.

Tissue that has been destroyed by frostbite will usually harden and turn black in the second week after rewarming, forming a "shell" over the viable tissue underneath. If the destruction is extensive, the affected area will wither and shrivel beneath the blackness, and self-amputate over 3 to 6 months. If the victim cannot seek medical care in that interval, the wound should be kept clean and dry, and signs of infection (see page 247) treated appropriately with antibiotics.

The corneas can be frostbitten if people (such as snowmobilers) force their eyes open in situations of high windchill. Symptoms include blurred vision, aversion to light, swollen eyelids, and excessive tearing. The treatment is the same as for a corneal abrasion (see page 161).

Prevention of Frostbite

1. Dress to maintain body warmth. Wear adequate properly fitting clothing, particularly boots that can accommodate a pair of polypropylene socks and at least one pair of wool socks without cramping the toes or wrinkling the socks. Take care to cover the hands, feet, and face

(particularly the nose and ears). Wear mittens in preference to gloves, to decrease the surface area available for heat loss from the fingers. Carry pocket, hand, and/or foot warmers and use them properly. Choices include fuel-burning warmers or chemical (such as Grabber hand warmer) packs, reusable sodium acetate thermal packs, or air-activated, single-use hand and pocket warmers.

2. Keep clothing dry. Avoid perspiring during extremely cold weather.

3. Do not touch bare metal with bare skin. Remember that certain liquids (such as gasoline) become colder than frozen water before they freeze, and can cause frostbite. Cover all metal handles with cloth, tape, or leather. For brief periods of exposure when dexterity is required, wear silk or rayon gloves.

4. Do not maintain one position in the cold for a prolonged period of time. Avoid cramped quarters.

5. Wear a sunscreen with a cream or grease base to prevent windburn.

6. Stay well hydrated. Eat enough food to maximize body-heat production. Avoid becoming fatigued.

7. Do not overwash exposed skin in freezing weather. The natural oils are a barrier to cold injury. Shave sparingly or not at all for cosmetic reasons. If skin becomes exceedingly dry, apply a thin layer of petrolatum-based ointment.

8. Do not drink alcohol or use tobacco products.

9. Keep fingernails and toenails properly trimmed.

10. Do not climb during extreme weather conditions.

Frostnip

Frostnip is reversible ice-crystal formation that occurs on the surface of the skin. It is distinct from frostbite in that actual freezing of the tissues does not occur. However, because the symptoms (numbness, frosted appearance) may resemble those of frostbite, it should be taken as a serious warning that the skin is not adequately protected.

Immersion Foot (Trench Foot)

Immersion, or "trench," foot (affecting lower limbs) is caused by prolonged (hours to days) exposure to cold water or to conditions of persistent cold (32 to 50° F, or 0 to 10° C) and high humidity, without actual freezing of tissues. Early symptoms include itching, tingling, and burning pain. The skin looks red immediately after exposure, then becomes mottled or pale with a gray-blue tint within a few hours to days. At the same time, skin numbness, swelling, and muscle cramps develop. After 2 to 7 days, the skin once again appears red, with accompanying tingling, swelling, blisters, oozing, and occasional gangrene.

If you suspect immersion foot, carefully cleanse and dry the limb, and rewarm it in an environment where it can be kept warm. With the exception of rewarming, treat the injury as a combination of frostbite and a burn wound, using daily dressing changes, topical antiseptic ointments, and antibiotics if necessary to treat any infection. If left unattended, it can lead to prolonged disability.

Prevention of immersion foot involves keeping the feet dry and warm. Change socks as often as necessary to accomplish this, and attempt to promote circulation. Avoid constrictive or nonventilated (rubber) footwear. Wear properly fitting boots.

Chilblain (Pernio)

Chilblain is less severe than immersion foot. It mostly afflicts women, who develop patches of redness or blue discoloration, nodules, and, rarely, blisters or ulcerations on the lower legs, toes, hands, and ears. The skin changes appear approximately 12 hours after cold exposure, and are accompanied by itching and burning or tingling sensations.

Treatment involves rewarming the affected skin, keeping it washed and dried, and covering it with dry, soft, and sterile bandages. Affected limbs should be elevated to minimize swelling. After rewarming, tender blue skin nodules may develop and persist for up to 2 weeks. Once healing has occurred, the skin may remain darkened.

Women with a past history of pernio or history of Raynaud's syndrome (constriction of small blood vessels, leading to painful hands and feet that become pale or blue upon exposure to cold) seem to be more prone to an episode. A topical lanolin-based lotion or emollient (hydrating) cream may be helpful in prevention.

Hives Induced by Exposure to Cold

See page 210.

Snow Blindness

See page 166.

INJURIES AND ILLNESSES DUE TO HEAT

Burn Injuries

See page 98.

Heat Illness (Hyperthermia)

The human core temperature is maintained at 98.6° F (37° C), with little variation from individual to individual. Heat is generated by all of the metabolic processes that contribute to life, from the blink of an eyelid to the completion of a marathon, and must be shed constantly to avoid a condition of overheating. The resting person generates enough heat (60 to 80 kilocalories per hour) to raise body temperature by 1.8° F (1° C) per hour. A person exposed to the sun can absorb 150 kilocalories of energy an hour. Vigorous exercise can increase endogenous heat production 10-fold. As outlined in the section on hypothermia (see page 269), heat is lost to the environment through conduction, convection, radiation, and evaporation. In the normal situation, the skin is the largest heat-wasting organ, and radiates approximately 65% of the daily heat loss. The skin is also largely responsible for evaporation (of sweat). Extreme humidity impedes evaporation and greatly diminishes human temperature control. The National Weather Service heat index (see figure 160) roughly correlates air temperature and relative humidity to derive an "apparent temperature." To summarize these recommendations:

APPARENT TEMPERATURE RANGE	DANGERS/PRECAUTIONS AT THIS RANGE
80–90° F 27–32° C	Exercise can be difficult; enforce rest and hydration
90–105° F 32–41° C	Heat cramps and exhaustion; be extremely cautious
105–130° F 41–54° C	Anticipate heat exhaustion; strictly limit activities
130° F and above 54° C and above	Setting for heat stroke; seek cool shelter

	AIR TEMPERATURE (°F)										
	70	75	80	85	90	95	100	105	110	115	120
RELATIVE HUMIDITY (%)	APPARENT TEMPERATURE (°F)										
0	64	69	73	78	83	87	91	95	99	103	107
10	65	70	75	80	85	90	95	100	105	111	116
20	66	72	77	82	87	93	99	105	112	120	130
30	67	73	78	84	90	96	104	113	123	135	148
40	68	74	79	86	93	101	110	122	137	151	
50	69	75	81	88	96	107	120	135	150		
60	70	76	82	90	100	114	132	149			
70	70	77	85	93	106	124	144				
80	71	78	86	97	113	136	157				
90	71	79	88	102	122	150	170				
100	72	80	91	108	133	166					

Figure 160. Heat index. Humidity contributes greatly to the accumulation of heat; when both are excessive, human temperature control is diminished.

When maximally effective, the complete evaporation of 1 quart (liter) of sweat from the skin removes 600 kilocalories of heat (equivalent to the total heat produced with strenuous exercise in 1 hour). Sweat that drips from the skin without evaporating does not contribute to the cooling process, but may contribute to dehydration. World-class distance runners who are acclimated to the heat can sweat in excess of 3½ quarts per hour. Since the maximum rate of gastric emptying (a surrogate for fluid absorption) is only 1.2 quarts per hour, it is easy to see how a person can become dehydrated. Thus, a person should be able to tolerate a 1 quart per hour sweat rate and manage rehydration with oral fluids.

When heat-control mechanisms are overloaded, the body responds unfavorably. As opposed to hypothermia, in which moderate cooling may offer a protective effect, the syndromes of true hyperthermia (in which core body temperature is measurably elevated) can rapidly become life threatening as the heat destroys the vital organs and dismembers chemical systems essential to life. Fever in and of itself can set off a vicious cycle, because raising the body temperature by 1° C (1.8° F) can increase metabolism by approximately 13%, which hastens the generation of more heat. Dehydration may by itself raise body temperature. For all these reasons, it is crucial to be familiar with heat illness, and to be prepared to respond promptly and decisively.

Heat Exhaustion and Heatstroke

Heat exhaustion and heatstroke are part of the same continuum, but of differing severity. Heat exhaustion is illness caused by an elevation of body temperature that does not result in permanent damage. Heatstroke is life threatening and can permanently disable the victim.

The signs and symptoms of heat exhaustion are minor confusion, irrational behavior, a rapid weak pulse, dizziness, nausea, diarrhea, headache, and mild temperature elevation (up to 105° F, or 40.5° C). It is important to note that *sweating may be present or absent,* and that *the skin of the victim may feel cool to the touch.* It is the core temperature that is elevated and that must be measured (rectally).

The signs and symptoms of heatstroke are extreme confusion, unconsciousness, low blood pressure or shock (see page 54), seizures, increased bleeding (bruising, vomiting blood, bloody urine), diarrhea, vomiting, shortness of breath, darkened ("machine oil") urine, and major core body temperature elevation (up to 115° F, or 46.1° C, has been reported). Again, it is important to note that *sweating may be present or absent.* It is rare for someone to feel cool externally when his temperature exceeds 105° F (45° C), but it is not impossible.

The skin will usually be warm or hot to the touch when a victim suffers heat exhaustion or heatstroke, but, again, this is not absolutely constant. *Carry a rectal thermometer so you can take a temperature reading.* If no thermometer is available, and you are fairly certain that the victim is suffering from heat exhaustion or heatstroke, proceed with therapy.

The most important aspect of therapy is to *lower the temperature as quickly as possible.* The body may lose its ability to control its own temperature at 106° F (41.1° C), so from that point upward, temperature can skyrocket. Manage the airway (see page 17) and administer oxygen (see page 383) at a flow rate of 10 liters per minute by face mask. Do not give liquids by mouth unless the victim is awake and capable of purposeful swallowing. Cooled liquids do not assist the cooling process enough to risk choking the uncooperative or confused victim.

Cooling the Victim

1. Remove the victim from obvious sources of heat. Shield him from direct sunlight and remove his clothing.

2. Wet down the victim and begin to fan him vigorously. Evaporation is a very efficient method of heat removal. Use cool or tepid water; *do not sponge the victim with alcohol.* If electric fans are available, use them. Do not be concerned with shivering, so long as you continue to aggressively cool the victim.

3. Place ice packs in the armpits, behind the neck, and in the groin. There is controversy surrounding total body immersion in ice water to treat hyperthermia; one argument is that such action causes constriction of superficial blood vessels and redirection of hot blood to the core circulation, temporarily increasing core temperature. This is of no concern in a life-threatening field situation. If the only method available for cooling is immersion in a cold mountain stream, do it!

4. Recheck the temperature every 5 to 10 minutes, to avoid cooling much below 98.6° F (37° C). When you have cooled the victim to 99.5 to 100° F (37.5 to 37.8° C), taper the cooling effort. After the victim is cooled, recheck his temperature every 30 minutes for 3 to 4 hours, because there will often be a rebound temperature rise.

5. *Do not use aspirin or acetaminophen unless the victim has an infection.* These specific drugs are used to combat fever that is caused by the release of chemical compounds from infectious agents into the bloodstream. Such compounds affect the portion of the brain (hypothalamus) that serves as the body's thermostat, causing body temperature to rise. Aspirin or acetaminophen acts to block this chemical interaction in the brain, and thus eliminates the fever. If elevated body temperature is not caused by an infection, then aspirin or acetaminophen will not work—and may in fact be harmful, leading to bleeding disorders or liver inflammation, respectively.

6. If the victim is alert, begin to correct dehydration (see page 184). Be certain that the concentration of carbohydrates or sugar in the beverage does not exceed 6%, so as not to inhibit intestinal absorption. Try to get 1 to 2 quarts (liters) into the victim over the first few hours. For every pound (0.45 kg) of weight loss attributed to sweating, have the victim ingest a pint (473 ml) of fluid. This may take up to 36 hours.

Muscle Cramps

Muscle cramps in a warm environment accompany overuse (see page 250) or water and salt losses in the individual who exerts strenuously. A well-trained athlete can lose 2 to 3 quarts (liters) of sweat per hour (a potential 20 g sodium loss each day). In most cases, cramps are caused by replacement of water without adequate salt intake.

Treatment for cramps consists of gentle motion, massage, and stretching of the affected muscles, accompanied by fluid and salt replacement. This can be done by drinking water and balanced salt solutions or sports beverages prior to and during heavy exertion. One recommendation is to drink a solution that contains 3.5 g of sodium chloride and 1.5 g of potassium chloride in a quart (liter) of water. As a rough measure, ¼ to ½ tsp (1.3 to 2.5 ml) of salt in water will suffice. With proper fluid and electrolyte replacement, salt tablets (which irritate the lining of the stomach) are usually unnecessary.

Heat Swelling

In warmer climates, normal people, particularly elders, may suffer from swelling of the feet and ankles. This is noted after prolonged periods of walking or sitting and is not necessarily indicative of heart failure. Often, the swelling will disappear as a person becomes adjusted to the warm environment over several days. The swelling is painless and there is no sign of infection (redness). Body temperature is not elevated.

Treatment for heat swelling is to minimize periods of walking and to use support stockings that rise at least to midthigh. The legs should be elevated whenever possible. There is no reason to use fluid pills (diuretics). If the sufferer is short of breath or otherwise ill in association with leg swelling, he should seek the advice of a physician.

Fainting

Fainting has many causes (see page 150). Fainting due to heat exposure occurs when a person (particularly an elder) adapts by dilating blood vessels in the skin and superficial muscles in order to deliver warm blood to the surface of the body, where the excess heat energy can be delivered back to the environment. The expansion of the superficial blood vessels allows a greater-than-normal proportion of the circulating blood volume to be away from the central circulation—which supplies, among other organs, the brain. This lack of sufficient central pressure is worsened when a person is on his feet for a prolonged period of time, because gravity allows a significant blood volume to pool in his lower limbs. Combined with fatigue and mild dehydration, the diversion of blood leads to a fainting episode, because not enough blood (with oxygen and glucose) is pumped to the brain. Dehydration can also stimulate the vagus nerve, which causes the heart rate to slow ("vasovagal" episode).

A victim who has suffered a fainting episode in the heat should be examined for any head or neck injuries, as well as other possible breaks or cuts. Other causes of fainting (low blood sugar, abnormal heart rhythm, and so on) must be considered. If fainting is due to the heat, the victim will reawaken shortly, because assuming a horizontal position returns blood to the brain and solves the major problem. In general, body temperature is not elevated.

The victim of a fainting spell due to heat should be rested in a horizontal position for 15 to 30 minutes, and should not immediately assume a standing posture without first sitting for 5 minutes. Encourage him to consume a pint or two (½ to 1 liter) of cool sweetened liquid (such as Gatorade). To avoid further episodes, efforts should be made to avoid dehydration, missing meals, or standing in one position for a prolonged period. Support hose may help, as might regular leg muscle exercise. The victim should learn to recognize the warning signs of a fainting spell, which include dizziness, light-headedness, nausea, weakness, sweating, blurred vision, or seeing flashing lights. When a warning sign occurs, the victim should immediately assume a horizontal position or at least sit and lower his head to a position between his knees.

Avoiding Heat Illness

1. Avoid dehydration. Drink 1 pint (473 ml) of liquid 10 to 15 minutes before beginning vigorous exercise. Drink at least 1 pint to 1 quart (½ to 1 liter) of liquid with adequate electrolyte supplementation (see below) each hour during heavy exercise with sweating in a hot climate. *Adequate water ingested during exercise is not harmful, does not cause cramps, and will prevent a large percentage of cases of heat illness.* Encourage rest and fluid breaks. The temperature of the fluid ingested should be cool, to encourage it to empty from the stomach. It is a myth that ingesting cold fluid causes abdominal cramps, so long as the amount ingested is prudent.

A unique device for carrying water is the CamelBak Hydration system, which allows you to sip continuously from an over-the-shoulder delivery tube.

If the urine becomes darkened or scant, then fluid requirements are not being met. As a general rule, people outdoors should consume at least 3 quarts (liters) of fluid each day to replenish that lost through urination, exhaled moisture, skin evaporation, and defecation. With moderate activity, this should be increased to at least 4 to 5 quarts. Do not rely upon thirst as an absolute guide to fluid requirements. In general, merely quenching thirst does not adequately replace fluid losses in heat stress or high-altitude conditions. It is possible to sweat up to 3 quarts per hour when exercising in extremely hot and humid conditions. During heavy exertion in hot weather, consider drinking at least a quart of liquid per hour.

With a normal diet, there is no need to take salt tablets. Electrolyte requirements can be met with food salted to taste. Electrolyte- and sugar-enriched drinks, such as Gatorade, should be used when normal meals cannot be eaten or when sweating is excessive (during athletic training or military forced marching, for example). A home brew (see page 184) may be used if a Gatorade-type beverage is not available.

The normal daily diet may be safely supplemented during times of extreme sweating (greater than ½ to 1 quart, or liter, per hour) with 5 to 10 g of sodium (normal daily dietary intake is 4 to 6 g; most adults would be fine with 1 to 3 g) and 2 to 4 g potassium. Supplemental salt is advised when weight loss from sweating exceeds 5 lb (2.3 kg) in a single session, particularly early in the acclimatization period when salt losses in sweat are great. Consume 0.5 g (1/10 tsp) sodium chloride (table salt) with a pint (473 ml) of water for each pound (0.45 kg) of weight loss over 5 lb. If large quantities of electrolytes are lost and not replaced (for instance, if large quantities of water are consumed without salt), a person can become quite ill. Similarly, salt without water can be harmful. Salt tablets can be very irritating to the stomach, and should not be used unless salt-containing solutions are not available. Coffee, tea, and alcohol-containing beverages cause increased fluid loss through excessive urination (diuretic effect) and should be avoided.

2. Be watchful of the very young and very old. Their bodies do not regulate body temperature well and can rapidly become too hot or too cold. Do not bundle up infants in warm weather.

3. Stay in shape. Obesity, lack of conditioning, insufficient rest, and ingestion of alcohol and/or illicit drugs all contribute to an increased risk for heat illness.

4. Condition yourself for the environment. Gradual increased exposure to work in a hot environment for a minimum of an hour a day for 10 days will allow you to acclimatize. More time spent in the heat hastens the process. Acclimatization is manifested as increased sweat volume with a decreased electrolyte concentration (more efficient sweating), greater peripheral blood vessel dilatation (more efficient heat loss), lowered heart rate, decreased skin and rectal temperatures during exercise, increased water and salt conservation by the kidneys, and enhanced metabolism of energy supplies. Eat potassium-rich vegetables and fruits, such as broccoli and bananas.

5. Wear clothing appropriate for the environment. Dress in layers so that

you can add or shed clothing as necessary. Clothing should be light-weight and absorbent. Wear a loose-fitting broad-brimmed hat. Do not wear plastic or rubber sweat suits in the heat.

6. Towel off your face and scalp frequently, because 50% of sweating occurs from these areas. Remove headgear when possible in order to allow evaporation from the head.

7. Keep out of the sun on a hot day. Resting on hot ground increases heat stress; the sun can heat the ground by more than 40° F (22.2° C) above the air temperature. If you must lie on the ground, dig a shallow (a few inches, or cm) trench to get down to a cooler surface.

8. Avoid taking drugs that inhibit the sweating process (such as atropine, antispasmodics, anti-motion-sickness), diminish cardiac output (beta blockers), disrupt certain features of physiologic activity (antidepressants, antihistamines), increase muscle activity (hallucinogens, cocaine), or pro-mote dehydration (diuretics).

WILDLAND FIRES

The wilderness adventurer or casual hiker in a forest or timbered park may find himself face to face with a wildland fire. This section will discuss high-risk situations, survival techniques, and medical considerations. Review the sections on burns (see page 98), lightning injuries (see page 350), heat ill-ness (see page 281), and inhalation injuries (see page 103) as well.

High-Risk Situations

The risk for a wildland fire is increased under certain environmental con-ditions. Pay heed to posted warnings of fire hazard, and do not venture into the woods unprepared to escape. Be particularly cautious when:

1. There are drought conditions. Low humidity, higher air temperatures, and gusty winds create dry fuel for a fire.

2. You are in an area rich with abundant fuel, such as dead grass, pine needles, shrubs, fallen trees, and the like.

3. You travel through gullies, canyons, along steep slopes, or other regions where wind and fuel are ideal for rapid advance of an estab-lished fire.

4. Fires have occurred recently in the vicinity.

Standard Fire Encounter Principles

1. Have advance knowledge of weather conditions prior to undertaking an expedition. Do not travel in hazardous regions in times of high fire risk. Local ranger stations are the best source of information. *Never plan an extended journey without leaving an itinerary with the proper authorities.*

2. At every campsite, take a few moments to prepare a plan for an evacuation, with at least two escape routes.

3. If a fire is in the area, pay attention to it. If there is any chance that it can involve your party, *get out early.*

4. If you see smoke or fire at a distance, post a lookout to watch for any changes that might indicate increased danger.

5. In all situations, stay calm and act with authority. Give orders concisely and be sure that they are understood.

6. Do not attempt to fight the fire. Your first responsibility is to evacuate all potential victims and provide necessary first aid. Leave fire fighting to professionals.

7. Do not sleep near a wildland fire. If the wind and fire direction change, you may be overcome with smoke and unable to escape.

What to Do When Caught in a Wildland Fire

1. Try not to panic. This is difficult, but if anything will save your life, it will be a clear head.

2. Don't move downhill toward a fire, because fires have a tendency to run uphill.

3. Unless the path of escape is clear, don't start running. Conserve your strength, and seek the flank of the fire. Continually observe changes in speed and direction of the fire and smoke to choose travel away from fire hazards. Be alert, keep calm, and avoid injury from rolling or falling debris.

4. Enter a burned area, particularly one with little fuel (grass or low shrubs). Although there is a chance that the area might burn again, you are better off here than in an area of fresh fuel. If you have to cross the fire line, cover your skin as well as possible, take a couple of deep breaths, and dash through the lowest flames (less than 3', or 92 cm, deep and where you can see through them). If smoke is dense, crawl along the ground for better air and visibility.

5. Try to avoid breathing smoke. Hold a moistened cloth over your mouth. If the air is very hot, use a dry cloth (dry heat is less damaging to the lungs than is steam). If you have a choice of clothing, cover your skin with closed-toe shoes, a long-sleeved cotton or wool shirt, cotton or wool pants, a hat, and gloves.

6. Seek refuge from the radiant heat. Take shelter in a trench, in a pond, behind rocks, or in a stream, vehicle, or building. Do not climb into elevated water tanks, wells, caves, or any other place where you might be trapped or quickly use up the available oxygen.

7. If all else fails and you cannot escape the advancing flames, lie face-down on the ground and cover your exposed skin as best possible. This is better than standing or kneeling.

8. If you are near a vehicle, and there is no route for escape, it is better to stay in the vehicle than to run from the fire. Try to position the vehicle in an area of little natural vegetation. Avoid driving through dense smoke. Turn off the headlights and ignition. Roll up the windows, close the air vents, and shield yourself from the radiant heat by covering up with floor mats or hiding under the dash. Stay in the vehicle as long as possible (it is rare for a gasoline tank to explode, and it takes a minute or two for the vehicle to catch on fire). Do not be overly alarmed if the vehicle rocks, or if smoke and sparks enter the vehicle. When the fire passes, cover your nose and mouth with a moistened cloth to avoid inhaling fumes from burning plastics and paint. Use urine if no other liquid is available.

9. If you are in a building and a fire is approaching, attach hoses to external water fixtures to achieve as much water spray coverage as possible. Place lawn sprinklers on the roof or use the hoses to soak down the roof. Put a ladder outside that will reach the roof. Locate and position buckets, rakes, axes, and shovels. Soak down shrubs and combustible foliage within 20' (6 m) of the building. If you have time, also do the following:

- Close windows, vents, doors, and blinds. Remove combustible drapes and window dressings.
- Turn off the gas at the meter. Turn off all pilot lights (heater, range, oven, and so on). Turn off any propane tanks.
- Open the fireplace damper and close the fireplace screens.
- Turn on a light in each room (for visibility if smoke accumulates).
- Move flammable furniture away from windows and sliding glass doors.
- Move flammable patio furniture indoors or far away from the building.
- Keep all of your pets in one room.
- If you have a car or truck, back it into the garage or park it in an open space facing the direction of escape. Shut the doors and roll up the windows. Leave the key in the ignition. Close the garage

door(s) and windows, but leave them unlocked. Disconnect any automatic garage door opener.

How to Report a Fire

If you suspect a wildland fire, *immediately* report it to local fire protection authorities. You should be prepared to give your name and location, the location of the fire, a description of the fire (flames, color, smoke), and a list of any people in the area, with their most exact locations.

Medical Considerations

The three most common medical problems in a wildland fire situation are burns (see page 98), smoke inhalation (see page 103), and dehydration (see page 184), followed by heat illness (see page 281) and poison ivy or oak exposure (see page 205). Anyone exposed to the constant and intense heat of a forest fire should consume at least a pint to a quart (½ to 1 liter) of fluid per hour.

Carbon Monoxide Poisoning

In general, there is not a shortage of oxygen in the region of an outdoor fire, so long as there is adequate ventilation. However, in an enclosed space, oxygen may be rapidly depleted as toxic gases and smoke accumulate. This can occur when people cook inside a tent or snow cave. The most commonly inhaled toxin is carbon monoxide, which is the odorless and colorless product of incomplete combustion. Carbon monoxide binds to hemoglobin (the oxygen-carrying pigment in red blood cells) with 100 times the affinity of oxygen. Thus, a human victim suffers from markedly diminished delivery of oxygen to all organ systems. Symptoms of carbon monoxide intoxication include:

Mild (10% level measured in the blood). Decreased exercise tolerance, decreased ability to concentrate, headache, nausea.

Moderate (20% level). Severe headache, vomiting, poor coordination, decreased vision, decreased hearing, shortness of breath.

Severe (30% level). Confusion, lethargy.

Catastrophic (40 to 60%). Fainting, unconsciousness, gasping respirations, seizures, shock, death.

If a person is suspected to have inhaled any toxic gas, he should be moved to fresh air as soon as possible, and have oxygen (see page 383) administered at a flow rate of 5 to 10 liters per minute by face mask. Anyone overcome with smoke inhalation should be rapidly transported to a hospital. Be prepared to manage the airway (see page 17). The definitive treatment for severe carbon monoxide poisoning is treatment with oxygen in a hyperbaric chamber. If a person suffers from carbon monoxide poisoning and is allowed to breathe normal air, it takes 4 to 5 hours for half of the carbon monoxide in his system to be eliminated. This elimination time ("half life") is decreased to 45 to 60 minutes if he breathes 100% oxygen through a face mask, however, and can be decreased to 15 to 20 minutes if oxygen is breathed under 3 atmospheres of pressure in a hyperbaric chamber.

ALTITUDE-RELATED PROBLEMS

Altitudes of 8,000 to 14,000' (2,438 to 4,267 m) are attained regularly by skiers, hikers, and climbers in the continental United States. Outside the U.S., mountain climbers may reach altitudes of up to 29,028' (8,856 m) (Mount Everest).

Most difficulties at high altitude are a direct result of the lowered concentration of oxygen in the atmosphere. Although the percentage of oxygen in the air is relatively constant at about 20%, the absolute amount of oxygen decreases with the declining barometric pressure. Thus, at 18,000' (5,487 m) there is half the oxygen that is available at sea level. A person transported suddenly to this altitude without time to acclimatize or without the provision of supplemental oxygen would probably lose consciousness; sudden transport to the summit of Mount Everest (where the amount of inspired oxygen is one-third that at sea level) would cause rapid collapse and death.

Habitation at high altitude causes a generalized decreased tolerance for exercise and physical stress. To a certain extent, humans can adapt to high altitude and become more efficient in the oxygen-poor environment. The prevention of altitude-related disorders is best accomplished by gradual acclimatization to the lowered oxygen content of atmospheric air. In this process, you increase the rate and depth of your breathing; this removes more carbon dioxide from your body. This, along with changes that occur in kidney function, cause your blood to become more alkaline, which allows it to take up and deliver more oxygen to your tissues. Resting heart rate gradually increases. Over time, red blood cell production is increased, and your heart and skeletal muscles become more efficient.

Prevention of Altitude-Related Disorders

Acclimatization requires gradual exposure to altitude, with a rate of ascent not to exceed 1,500' (457 m) per day at altitudes above 8,000' (2,438 m). Rest days at a constant altitude are essential at heights above 10,000' (3,048 m). Acclimatization is achieved by adhering to a schedule of ascent:

For any climb above 8,000' (2,438 m), spend an initial 2 to 4 days at 5,000 to 7,000' (1,524 to 2,134 m). The first day should be a rest day. If anyone shows signs of altitude-related illness, spend additional time at this altitude.

For any climb above 13,000' (3,962 m), all members of the party should add 2 to 4 days for acclimatization at 10,000 to 12,000' (3,048 to 3,658 m). Subsequent climbing should not exceed 1,500' (457 m) per day. Scattered rest days are advised, along with an extra night for acclimatization with any ascent of 2,000' (609 m) or more. The party should sleep at the lowest altitude that does not interfere with the purpose of the expedition.

In addition, the drug acetazolamide (Diamox) has proven to be useful in stimulating breathing, diminishing the sleep disorder associated with acute mountain sickness (see page 296), facilitating the body's normal adjustment to high altitude, and thus improving nocturnal oxygenation. It is administered in a dose of 125 mg twice a day beginning 24 hours before ascent, and continued for a period of 1 to 2 days; within this period, the initial physiological acclimatization process should become operative. It may also be given as a 500 mg sustained-action capsule every 24 hours. Acetazolamide should be used if an ascent will be unavoidably rapid.

Children who have previously suffered from acute mountain sickness may benefit from acetazolamide, which should be administered in a dose of 5 mg per kg (2.2 lb) of body weight per day, in two divided doses, up to 125 mg per day. Diamox has a diuretic (increased urination) effect, so that it is extremely important to drink sufficient fluids to prevent dehydration. Fluid losses are generally greater at high altitude, so do not rely upon thirst as a gauge of adequate fluid intake. Drink enough to keep the urine clear and light colored. *Diamox is no substitute for proper acclimatization!*

When you're traveling at high altitudes, avoid the use of alcohol, stay warm, keep out of the wind, avoid exhaustion, and eat regularly to avoid weight loss. A diet relatively high in carbohydrates is preferable to one high in fat and protein.

Since oxygen is transported in red blood cells, it is advisable to avoid being anemic at high altitude. Iron-deficiency anemia is common in women, related to menstrual bleeding. If this is recognized, it should be corrected under the supervision of a physician with the administration of ferrous sulfate 300 mg per day; note that a side effect is constipation.

In addition to the effects of less oxygen available at high altitude, mountaineers are subjected to other environmental hazards. Temperature decreases with altitude by an average of 11.7° F (6.5° C) per 3,280' (1,000 m). Ultraviolet light penetration increases approximately 4 to 6% per 984' (300 m) gain in altitude. Sunlight reflecting off glaciers absent a cooling wind can transfer intense radiant heat. The dry air predisposes to dehydration.

High-Altitude Pulmonary Edema

Pulmonary edema is excess fluid in the lungs, either in the lung tissue itself or in the space normally used for gas exchange (oxygen for carbon dioxide). Fluid in the lungs renders them unable to perform their normal task, and thus the victim cannot get enough oxygen.

High-altitude pulmonary edema (HAPE) usually occurs in an unacclimatized individual—typically a male—who rapidly ascends to an altitude that exceeds 8,000' (2,438 m), particularly if heavy exertion is involved. Prior traditional physical conditioning is not a factor; many cases involve young, previously healthy individuals. If the victim exercises above 8,000' but sleeps at a lower altitude (such as 6,000', or 1,829 m), his risk for developing HAPE is much less.

Symptoms begin 1 to 3 days after arrival at high altitude. They include shortness of breath, cough, weakness, easy fatigue (especially when walking uphill), and difficulty sleeping. Signs of acute mountain sickness (AMS, see page 296) are often present. As greater amounts of fluid accumulate in the lungs, the victim develops drowsiness, severe shortness of breath, and rapid heart rate; his initial dry and gentle ("soft") cough produces white phlegm and then blood (pink, frothy sputum—a late sign); he exhibits confusion and cyanosis (bluish discoloration of the skin, particularly noticeable in the nail beds and lips). If you place an ear to the victim's chest, you may hear crackling or gurgling noises. The symptoms worsen at night. Rapidly, the victim becomes extremely agitated, disoriented, and sweaty; he is in obvious extreme respiratory distress. Confusion, collapse, and coma follow. The victim may show a fever of up to 101.3° F (38.5° C).

As soon as the earliest signs of HAPE are present, the victim should be evacuated (carried, if necessary) to a lower altitude at which there were previously no symptoms. Such warning signs include rapid heart rate (greater than 90 to 100 beats per minute at rest), weakness, shortness of breath, cough, difficulty walking, inability to keep up, and poor judgment. Maximum rest is advised. The definitive treatments are descent and the administration of oxygen; if it is available, oxygen at a flow rate of 5 to 10 liters per minute should be administered by face mask (see page 383). Improvement is rarely noted until oxygen is administered or descent of at least 1,000 to 2,000' (304 to 608 m) is accomplished.

In no case should a victim be left to descend by himself. Always have a healthy person accompany him. If the victim must be carried down, he should be kept in a sitting position, if possible. Keep him warm, as well.

The administration of fluid pills (diuretics) is controversial and should be done only under strict medical supervision, as should the administration of morphine.

Some aid stations in high-altitude regions are equipped with an inflatable pressure bag (such as a Gamow bag) large enough to enclose a human. This is used to simulate conditions at lower altitude and may be used to treat moderate or severe high-altitude illness. The cylinder-shaped Gamow container is a small, portable hyperbaric chamber that can be pressurized with a foot pump to 2 lb (0.9 kg) per square inch, which simulates a descent of approximately 5,248' (1,600 m); the exact equivalent depends upon the altitude at which the bag is deployed. In addition, oxygen from a tank can be administered to the victim by face mask (see page 383) within the bag.

A drug that physicians are using successfully to treat HAPE is nifedipine, which lowers obstructive pressure in the pulmonary arterial circulation (which carries deoxygenated blood from the heart through the lungs). The first dose is 10 mg chewed, then swallowed. This is followed by 10 mg every 4 to 6 hours, or 30 mg extended-release preparation (Adalat CC) every 12 hours. Since this drug is also used to treat high blood pressure, a side effect can be low blood pressure and dizziness, particularly if the victim is dehydrated. These particular side effects seem to be minimal when the extended-release preparation is used. Nifedipine has also been used successfully to prevent HAPE in subjects with a history of repeated episodes, but is not yet recommended for prevention in the general population.

Once a victim has been judged to suffer from any degree of HAPE, he should no longer be a candidate for high-altitude travel until cleared by a physician. Such a precaution does not include routine jet airplane transportation.

High-Altitude Cerebral Edema

High-altitude cerebral edema (HACE) is the medical term for a disorder (theoretically linked to brain swelling) that involves an alteration of mental status seen at high altitude, related to diminished atmospheric oxygen. Symptoms include difficulty walking (inability to walk a straight line, staggering, or frank inability to walk), headache (often throbbing), confusion, difficulty in speaking, drowsiness, vomiting, and, in severe cases, blindness, unconsciousness, paralysis, and/or coma. A victim may suffer from HACE and HAPE at the same time. Other symptoms may include hallucinations, paralysis of an arm and/or leg, and seizures. Victims are often gray or pale in appearance. Imbalance or the inability to walk heel to toe in a straight line is a very worrisome sign and should prompt immediate action to treat the victim.

The treatment for HACE is immediate descent to an altitude below one at which the victim previously had no symptoms, and the administration of oxygen at a flow rate of 5 to 10 liters per minute by face mask or nasal cannula (tube) (see page 383). If the victim becomes severely ill, he should be brought (carried, if necessary, and preferably in the sitting position) to a lower altitude (below 5,000', or 1,524 m). In addition, administration of the steroid drug dexamethasone (Decadron) 8 mg first dose, then 4 mg every 6 hours until descent is accomplished, may be helpful. The pediatric dose of Decadron is 0.5 mg per kg (2.2 lb) of body weight for the first dose, followed by 0.1 mg per kg every 6 hours. Again, *never leave a potentially seriously ill person to fend for himself.* A victim of HACE or HAPE can deteriorate rapidly, and most will need to be transported down the mountain. As with HAPE, a Gamow bag can be used for treatment. Because the early symptoms of acute mountain sickness (see below) and HACE are similar, pay close attention to the condition of ill members of your climbing party.

Acute Mountain Sickness

Acute mountain sickness (AMS) is the most common altitude-related disorder. It affects those who ascend to altitudes above 8,200' (2,500 m) from below 4,922' (1,500 m) and are unable to keep pace with acclimatization. A person who is partially acclimatized may be stricken if he ascends rapidly to a higher altitude, overexerts, or uses sleep medication (which can be a respiratory depressant). Symptoms, which may be quite subtle in the beginning, include headache, insomnia, fatigue, loss of appetite, nausea, dizziness, drowsiness, weakness, and apathy. Some people have described the suffering associated with AMS as similar to a hangover. Children are prone to nausea and vomiting as a manifestation of AMS. The lips and fingernails may have a blue discoloration (cyanosis) if HAPE is present.

The most common and disabling symptom of AMS is headache that typically occurs on the second or third day at high altitude and may be complicated by difficulty in walking (particularly if HAPE is present) and impaired memory. The headache is mild to severe, throbbing, in both temples or the back of the head, worse during the night and upon awakening, and worsened by straining or bending over. Mild symptoms of HACE accompany AMS; they include decreased appetite, mood swings, and lack of interest in activity. Some victims complain of a deep inner chill.

One hallmark of AMS, known as periodic breathing, is an alteration of the normal sleeping pattern. Sleep is fitful, with periods of wakefulness or disturbing dreams. The pattern of breathing becomes irregular, such that the sleeper has periods of rapid breathing (very deep breaths) alternated with periods of no breathing. The latter can be quite startling to the casual observer—intervals of 10 seconds may pass without a breath. Acetazolamide, 125 mg at bedtime, diminishes periodic breathing, improves oxygenation, and is safe to use as a sleeping aid. Insomnia from other causes may respond to short-acting drugs for sleep, such as triazolam (Halcion) 0.125 mg, zolpidem (Ambien) 5 mg, or temazepam (Restoril) 15 mg, but these medications are potentially dangerous in a person who is suffering incipient AMS because he may suffer respiratory depression, which leads to decreased oxygenation. Also, sleep medication may mask the symptoms of HACE.

Treatment for AMS includes rest, adequate fluid intake to avoid dehydration, and mild pain medicine for the headache. The victim should be led to a lower altitude, preferably at least 1,640' (500 m) below that where symptoms began. However, many victims of AMS will adjust to the current altitude in 3 to 4 days, and therefore may remain at a stable altitude if symptoms are mild. *In no case should a person attempt to climb to (or, particularly, sleep at) a higher altitude until the symptoms of AMS have completely subsided.* With mild AMS, acetazolamide (Diamox) can be administered in a dose of 125 to 250 mg by mouth every 8 to 12 hours until symptoms diminish. The dose in children is 5 mg per kg (2.2 lb) of body weight per day, in two divided doses, up to 250 mg per day.

Prochlorperazine (Compazine) 10 mg by mouth or 25 mg by suppository can be given for nausea and vomiting, with the added benefit that it may stimulate the beneficial ventilatory (breathing) response that is triggered by a low oxygen content in the blood (associated with altitude and called the "hypoxic ventilatory response"). The dose in children older than 2 years of age is 0.4 mg per kg (2.2 lb) of body weight per day, by mouth or by oral suppository, in three or four divided doses. Promethazine (Phenergan) is fine as an alternative for adults.

If an oxygen cylinder is available (see page 383), low flow (0.5 to 1 liter per minute) oxygen by nasal cannula (tube) or face mask is particularly effective if used for sleep. This alone may be adequate to halt the progression of mild AMS and allow a victim to acclimatize without descent to a lower altitude. However, if this approach is taken, the victim should not be left alone until all symptoms of AMS have resolved. The victim who spends a few hours in a Gamow bag will probably notice diminution of symptoms.

If AMS is severe and HACE seems to be developing (the victim is vomiting, cannot walk a straight line, and is becoming confused), administer dexamethasone as previously recommended for HACE. AMS can progress to HACE with coma in 24 hours.

Minor Disorders of High Altitude

Fluid Retention

Swelling of the face, hands, and feet may occur after 4 to 10 days at increased altitude. Women are more commonly affected than are men, and they note puffiness of the hands, feet, eyelids, and face, particularly in the morning after a night's sleep or just prior to a menstrual period. Ten or more lb (4.5 kg) can be gained in fluid retention. The swelling persists for 1 to 3 days after return to lower altitude, then spontaneously disappears (increased urination is noted at this time). The disorder is a nuisance, but of no real medical hazard. Salt intake should be controlled so as not to be excessive. Avoid fluid pills (diuretics), which promote dehydration and rarely reduce the swelling to any significant degree. A person who retains fluid at high altitude should be examined for signs and symptoms of HACE and HAPE.

High-Altitude Flatus Expulsion (HAFE)

HAFE is the spontaneous and unwelcome passage of increased quantities of rectal gas noted at high altitude. It may become an embarrassment but is of no true medical concern. Avoid foods such as chili and beans that are known to induce flatulence at low altitudes, and show consideration for other members of the party in sleeping arrangements. If stricken, a traveler may benefit from chewable tablets or simethicone (Mylicon 80 mg) or simethicone 80 mg with activated charcoal 250 mg (Flatulex tablets) once or twice a day. Charcoal Plus is another simethicone-activated charcoal preparation.

Altitude Throat

Altitude throat is a sore throat caused by nasal congestion and mouth breathing during exertion at high altitudes. Because the air is dry and cold, the protective mucous coating of the throat is dried out and the throat becomes extremely irritated, with redness and pain. In general, this can be distinguished from a bacterial or viral infection (see page 173) by the absence of fever, swollen lymph glands in the neck, or systemic symptoms (fatigue, muscle aches, sweats, and the like). Prevention is difficult and treatment is only mildly satisfying. The victim should keep his throat moist by sipping liquids and sucking on throat lozenges or hard candies (Life Savers, for instance). As soon as convenient, nighttime breathing of warm humidified air should be instituted. Avoid anesthetic gargles, since they will mask the signs of a true infection.

High-Altitude Bronchitis

Most bronchitis has an infectious cause (see page 181). High-altitude bronchitis is more likely to be caused by relative hyperventilation of cold, dry air. This causes the secretions in the respiratory passages to thicken. The resulting airway irritation causes a persistent cough, which can cause coughing fits sufficiently severe to lead to rib fractures. Treatment consists of humidification of inspired air, which can be accomplished transiently by cautiously breathing steam, and over the longer term by breathing through a porous scarf or balaclava that allows retention of moisture and heat.

Snow Blindness

See page 166.

SNAKEBITE

Poisonous Snakes

Two types of poisonous snakes are indigenous to the United States: pit vipers (rattlesnake, cottonmouth [water moccasin], copperhead) and coral snakes. Their distributions are as follows:

Northeast. Cottonmouth, copperhead, timber rattlesnake.
Southeast. Cottonmouth, copperhead, eastern diamondback rattlesnake, pygmy rattlesnake, eastern coral snake.
Central. Cottonmouth, copperhead, massasauga rattlesnake, timber rattlesnake, prairie rattlesnake.
Southwest. Cottonmouth, copperhead, pygmy rattlesnake, massasauga rattlesnake, northern black-tailed rattlesnake, prairie rattlesnake, sidewinder, Mojave rattlesnake, western diamondback rattlesnake, red diamondback rattlesnake, Texas coral snake, Sonoran coral snake.
Pacific Coast. Northern Pacific rattlesnake, southern Pacific rattlesnake, Great Basin rattlesnake, western diamondback rattlesnake, red diamondback rattlesnake, sidewinder, Mojave rattlesnake.

In the United States, 98% of venomous bites are from pit vipers. In addition, many "nonvenomous" species, such as colubrid (rear-fanged) snakes (including the red-neck keelback), are capable of producing venomous bites. There are no indigenous venomous snakes in Hawaii or Alaska.

Pit vipers are typified by rattlesnakes, which have a characteristic triangular head, vertical elliptical pupils ("cat's eyes"), two elongated and hinged fangs in the front part of the jaw, heat- (infrared-) sensing facial pits on the sides of the head midway between and below the level of the eyes and the nostrils, a single row of scales on the underbelly leading to the tail (not seen in nonpoisonous snakes), and rattles on the tail (figure 161). The snake's age is not determined by the number of rattles, since molting may occur up to four times a year. Because fangs are replaced every 6 to 10 weeks in the adult rattlesnake, bites may demonstrate from one to four large puncture marks. An adult pit viper can strike at a speed of 8' (2.4 m) per second. The rattlesnake may strike without a preliminary warning rattle.

Coral snakes are characterized by their color pattern, with red, black, and yellow or white bands encircling the body (see figure 162). A general

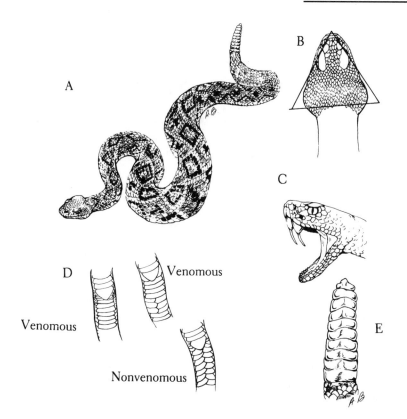

Figure 161. Rattlesnake. (A) Typical rattlesnake appearance, with features of identification that include (B) triangular head, (C) hinged fangs, (D) single row of underbelly scales leading up to the anal plate, and (E) a rattle on the tail.

rule is "red on yellow—kill a fellow [venomous]; red on black—venom lack [nonvenomous]." The fangs are very short and fixed; the snakes have round pupils, and they bite with a chewing, rather than striking, action.

Signs of Envenomation

Most snakebites do not result in envenomation, because either the snake does not release venom, the skin is not penetrated, or the venom is not potent. Therefore, it is important to recognize the signs of envenomation, in order to avoid needless worry, evacuation, and improper therapy.

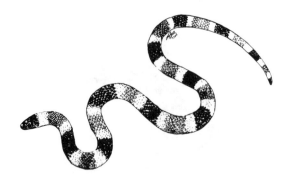

Figure 162. Coral snake.

The most common signs of envenomation are:

Pit Vipers

1. One or more fang marks. Most snakebites (venomous and nonvenomous) will demonstrate rows of markings from the teeth. In the case of venomous snakes, there will be one to four larger distinct markings from the elongated fangs that inoculate the victim with venom (figure 163). Venomous snakebite wounds tend to bleed more freely than bites from animals and insects.

2. Burning pain at the site of the bite. *This may not be present with the bite of the Mojave rattlesnake.*

3. Swelling at the site of the bite. This usually begins within 5 to 10 minutes of envenomation and may become quite severe. *This may not be present with the bite of the Mojave rattlesnake.*

4. Numbness and tingling of the lips, face, fingers, toes, and scalp 30 to 60 minutes after the bite. This can also be present if the victim hyperventilates with fear and excitement (see page 264). If a victim of a snakebite has immediate symptoms, these are likely to be due to hyperventilation.

5. Twitching of the mouth, face, neck, eye, and bitten extremity muscles 30 to 90 minutes after the bite.

6. Rubbery or metallic taste in the mouth 30 to 90 minutes after the bite.

7. Sweating, weakness, nausea, vomiting, and fainting 1 to 2 hours after the bite. Additional symptoms include chest tightness, rapid breathing rate (20 to 25 breaths per minute), rapid heart rate (125 to 175 beats per minute), palpitations, headache, chills, and confusion.

8. Bruising at the site of the bite. This usually begins within 2 to 3 hours. Large blood blisters may develop within 6 to 10 hours.

9. Difficulty breathing, increased bleeding (bruising, bloody urine,

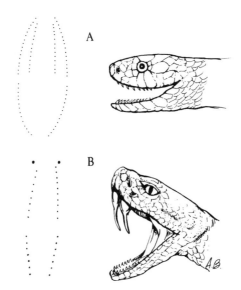

Figure 163. Snakebite patterns. (A) Nonvenomous snake. (B) Venomous snake.

bloody bowel movements, vomiting blood), and collapse 6 to 12 hours after the bite.

Coral Snakes

1. Burning pain at the site of the bite may be present or absent. There is generally very little local swelling or bruising, and certainly much less than that seen with the bite of a pit viper.
2. Numbness and/or weakness of a bitten arm or leg within 90 minutes.
3. Twitching, nervousness, drowsiness, giddiness, increased salivation and drooling in 1 to 3 hours. Vomiting may occur.
4. Slurred speech, double vision, difficulty talking and swallowing, and impaired breathing within 5 to 10 hours.
5. Death from heart and lung failure.

Treatment of Snakebite

If a person is bitten by a snake that could be poisonous, act swiftly. *The definitive treatment for serious snake venom poisoning is the administration of antivenin (sometimes called "antivenom"). The most important aspect of therapy is to get the victim to an appropriate medical facility as quickly as possible.*

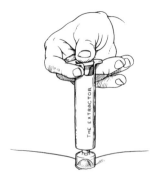

Figure 164. Application of the Extractor to a snakebite wound.

1. Don't panic. Most bites, even by venomous snakes, do not result in medically significant envenomations. Reassure the victim and keep him from acting in an energy-consuming, purposeless fashion. If the victim has been envenomed, increased physical activity may increase his illness by hastening the spread of venom. If the victim is hyperventilating from fear, manage according to the instructions on page 264.

2. Retreat out of the striking range of the snake, which should be considered to be the snake's body length (for pit vipers, it is approximately half the body length). A rattlesnake can strike at a speed of 8' (2.4 m) per second.

3. Locate the snake. If possible, identify the species. If you cannot do this with confidence (which is really only important for the Mojave rattlesnake and coral snake), kill the animal with a blow on the neck from a long, heavy stick. Collect the snake and bring it along for proper identification. Doing this may be extremely important in estimating the amount of antivenin necessary; however, never delay transport of the victim in order to capture a snake. Take care to carry the dead animal in a container that will not allow the head of the snake to bite another victim (the jaws can bite in a reflex action for 20 to 60 minutes after death). If you are not sure how to collect the snake, it is best just to get away from it, to avoid creating an additional victim.

4. Apply the Extractor suction device according to the manufacturer's instructions (figure 164). This removes venom without the need for a skin incision.

5. Splint the bitten body part, to avoid unnecessary motion. Allow room for swelling within the splint. Maintain the bitten arm or leg at a level below the heart. Remove any jewelry that could become an inadvertent tourniquet.

6. Transport the victim to the nearest hospital.

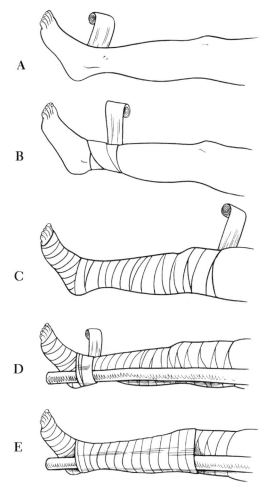

Figure 165. The pressure immobilization technique. (A) Begin to wrap the limb directly over the bite site with an elastic bandage. (B) Continue wrapping up the limb. (C) Wrapped limb. (D) Begin to apply a splint. (E) Wrapped and splinted limb.

7. *Do not apply ice directly to the wound or immerse the part in ice water.* An ice pack placed over the wound is of no proven value. Application of extreme cold can cause an injury similar to frostbite.

8. If the victim is more than 2 hours from medical attention, and the bite is on an arm or leg, use the pressure immobilization technique (figure 165): Place a 2" x 2" (5 cm) cloth pad (¼", or 0.6 cm, thick) over the bite and apply an elastic wrap firmly around the involved limb directly over the padded bite site with a margin of at least 4 to 6" (10 to 15 cm) on either side of the wound, taking care to check for adequate circulation in the fingers and toes (normal feeling and color). An alternative method is to simply wrap the entire limb at the described tightness with an elastic bandage. The wrap is meant to impede absorption of venom into the general circulation by containing it within the compressed tissue and microscopic blood and lymphatic vessels near the limb surface. You should then splint the limb to prevent motion. If the bite is on a hand or arm, also apply a sling.

An alternative to the pressure immobilization technique is a constriction band (not a tourniquet) wrapped a few inches closer to the heart than the bite marks on the bitten limb. This should be applied tightly enough to only occlude the superficial veins and lymph passages. The band may be advanced periodically to stay ahead of the swelling. It is of questionable usefulness if 30 minutes have intervened between the time of the bite and the application of the constriction band (or pressure immobilization technique).

9. The only indications for incision and suction are if all four of the following conditions are present: The bite is from a rattlesnake, the victim is more than 1 hour from medical care, the Extractor cannot be applied, and the procedure can be performed within 5 minutes of the bite. The incisions should be made *only by a person experienced in the procedure* with a razor blade or sharp knife directly over the fang marks, in a parallel fashion (not crisscross), ⅛" to ¼" (0.3 to 0.6 cm) long and ⅛" to ¼" deep (just through the skin). The purpose is to enlarge the fang marks and facilitate suction. Apply suction for 30 minutes with the rubber device from a snakebite kit—use your mouth only as a last resort. *The impression of most snakebite experts is that incision and suction are of little value and probably should be abandoned.* It appears that little venom can actually be removed from the bite site unless a perfectly placed incision is made immediately after the bite and followed by superb suction. Furthermore, mouth contact with a crisscross incision invariably creates a nasty infection that leaves a noticeable scar; there is also the risk of transmission of blood-borne disease.

10. "Snakebite medicine" (whiskey) is of no value and may actually be harmful if it increases circulation to the skin.

11. There is not yet scientific evidence that electrical shocks applied to snakebites are of any value. To the contrary, there are experiments that refute this concept.

12. The bite wound should be washed vigorously with soap and water, and the victim treated with dicloxacillin, erythromycin, or cephalexin.

Watch for an allergic reaction (see page 58) caused by the snakebite. Once the victim is in the hospital, the severity of envenomation will be ascertained, and the victim treated with antivenin if necessary. Such therapy must be carried out under the supervision of a physician, because serious allergic reactions to presently available antivenins are common.

Avoidance of Poisonous Snakes

1. Avoid the known habitats of poisonous snakes, such as rocky ledges and woodpiles.

2. Do not reach into areas that you cannot visually examine first. Walk on clearly marked trails, and use a walking stick to move suspicious objects. Do not reach blindly behind rocks.

3. Wear adequate protective clothing, particularly boots to cover your feet and lower legs.

4. Never hike alone in snake territory. Carry the Extractor, an elastic wrap, and a SAM Splint (see page 66).

5. Avoid hiking at night in snake territory. Carry a flashlight and walking stick.

6. Do not handle snakes unless you know what you are doing. Remember that you can be bitten and envenomed by seemingly dead or nonvenomous snakes.

Nonpoisonous Snakes

Many snakes (for example, the gopher snake and king snake) are nonvenomous and do not create serious medical problems with a bite. However, identifying a snake from the bite puncture wounds is often extremely difficult for the amateur. Unless the snake can be positively identified as a nonvenomous species, the victim should be considered to have been bitten by a poisonous snake and managed appropriately. The snake should be captured for identification (see page 304). If the snake is known to be nonvenomous, the wound should be washed vigorously with soap and water, and the victim treated with dicloxacillin, erythromycin, or cephalexin.

Gila Monster and Mexican Beaded Lizard

The Gila monster (*Heloderma suspectum*) (see figure 166) and Mexican beaded lizard (*H. horridum*), which can grow to 14" (35 cm) long, are found in the Great Sonoran Desert area of southern Arizona and northwestern

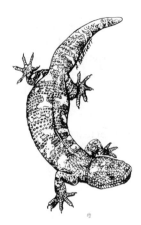

Figure 166. Gila monster.

Mexico. They possess grooved teeth and venom glands. Most envenomations occur when an animal bites and holds on, or when a tooth is shed into
the bite wound. If the Gila monster holds on, the grip may need to be loos-
ened by mechanical means or incision of the jaw muscles.

Symptoms of an envenomation include burning pain at the site of the
bite, swelling of the bite wound, red or blue discoloration, nausea and
vomiting, weakness, anxiety, rapid heart rate, and sweating. Low blood
pressure is the most serious complication. Intense pain from the bite may
last for 3 to 5 hours, and then subside after 8 hours.

The wound should be washed vigorously and all pieces of teeth removed.
The victim should have his arm or leg splinted and should be transported to
a hospital. Severe reactions are unusual; most victims recover uneventfully.
Be prepared to treat the victim for shock (see page 54). Do not administer
alcohol, stimulants, or narcotic pain medicines. Do not apply ice directly to
the wound or immerse a bitten limb in ice water.

If it will be more than 24 hours before you can reach medical care,
administer an antibiotic (cephalexin, eythromycin, or amoxicillin-
clavulanate).

HAZARDOUS AQUATIC LIFE

In general, anyone who gets an infection following a wound acquired in
an aquatic environment should be treated with an antibiotic to cover

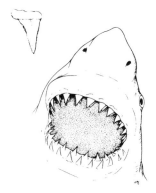

Figure 167. Jaws of the great white shark, with advancing rows of razor-sharp ripsaw teeth.

Staphylococcus and *Streptococcus* species (use dicloxacillin, erythromycin, or cephalexin), and a second antibiotic to cover *Vibrio* species (use ciprofloxacin, trimethoprim-sulfamethoxazole, or doxycycline). An infection from *Vibrio* bacteria is more likely in deep puncture wounds, if there is a retained spine (such as from a stingray), and in people who suffer from an impaired immune system (diabetes, AIDS, cancer, chronic liver disease, alcoholism, chronic corticosteroid therapy).

Sharks

The jaws of the shark contain rows of razor-sharp teeth, which can bite down with extreme force (figure 167). The result is a wound with loss of tissue that bleeds freely and can lead rapidly to shock (see page 54).

The basic management of a major bleeding wound is described on page 48. Even if a shark bite appears minor, the wound should be washed out and bandaged, and the victim taken to a doctor. Often, the wound will contain pieces of shark teeth, seaweed, or sand debris, which must be removed in order to avoid a nasty infection. Like other animal bites, shark bites should not be sewn or taped tightly shut, in order to allow drainage. This helps prevent serious infection. The victim should be started on an antibiotic to oppose *Vibrio* bacteria (ciprofloxacin, trimethoprim-sulfamethoxazole, or doxycycline).

The skin of many sharks is rough like sandpaper, and can cause a bad scrape. If this occurs, it should be managed like a second-degree burn (see page 100).

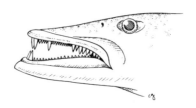

Figure 168. Barracuda, with large caninelike teeth.

Shark Avoidance

1. Avoid shark-infested waters, particularly at dusk and after dark. Do not dive in known shark feeding grounds.
2. Swim in groups. Sharks tend to attack single swimmers.
3. When diving, avoid deep drop-offs, murky water, or areas near sewage outlets.
4. Do not tether captured (speared, for example) fish to your body.
5. Do not corner or provoke sharks.
6. If a shark appears, leave the water with slow, purposeful movements. *Do not panic or splash.* If a shark approaches you while you are diving in deep water, attempt to position yourself so that you are protected from the rear. If a shark moves in, attempt to strike a firm blow to the snout.
7. If you are stranded at sea and a rescue helicopter arrives to extract you from the water, exit the water at the earliest opportunity.

Barracudas

Barracudas may bite victims and create nasty wounds with their long caninelike teeth (figure 168). These wounds are managed like shark bites (see above). Because barracudas seem to be attracted to shiny objects, the swimmer, boater, or diver is advised to not wear bright metallic objects, particularly not a barette in the hair nor anklets dangled upon a leg near the surface from a boat or dock.

Moray Eels

Although they look quite ferocious, moray eels (figure 169) seldom attack humans, unless provoked. They have muscular jaws equipped with sharp fanglike teeth, which can inflict a vicious bite. A moray tends to bite and hold on; in some instances, it is necessary to break the eel's jaws to get it to release.

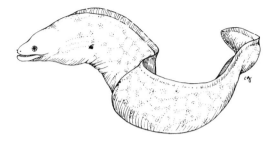

Figure 169. Moray eel.

A moray bite should be managed like a shark bite (see page 309). Even if the bite is very small, it should be examined by a physician, to be sure that all tooth fragments have been removed. If the bite is more than superficial and on the hand, on the foot, or near a joint, the victim should be started on an antibiotic (ciprofloxacin, trimethoprim-sulfamethoxazole, or doxycycline) to oppose *Vibrio* bacteria. Avoid sewing or otherwise tightly closing a large moray bite unless absolutely necessary.

Sponges

Sponges handled directly from the ocean can cause two types of skin reaction. The first is an allergic type similar to that caused by poison oak (see page 205), with the difference that the reaction generally occurs within an hour after the sponge is handled. The skin becomes red, with burning, itching, and occasional blistering. The second type of reaction is caused by small spicules of silica from the sponges that are broken off and embedded in the outermost layers of the skin. This causes irritation, redness, and swelling. When large skin areas are involved, the victim may complain of fever, chills, fatigue, dizziness, nausea, and muscle cramps.

Because it is difficult to tell precisely which type of skin reaction has occurred, if a person develops a rash after handling a sponge, undertake the following therapy:

1. Soak the affected skin with white vinegar (5% acetic acid) for 15 minutes. This may be done by wetting a gauze pad or cloth with vinegar and laying it on the skin.
2. Dry the skin, then apply the sticky side of adhesive tape to the skin and peel it off. This will remove most sponge spicules that are present. An

alternative is to apply a thin layer of rubber cement or a commercial facial peel, let it dry and adhere to the skin, then peel it off.

3. Repeat the vinegar soak for 15 minutes or apply rubbing (isopropyl 40%) alcohol for 1 minute.

4. Dry the skin, then apply hydrocortisone lotion (0.5 to 1%) thinly twice a day until the irritation is gone. Do not use topical steroids before decontaminating with vinegar; this might worsen the reaction.

5. If the rash worsens (blistering, increasing redness or pain, swollen lymph glands), this may indicate an infection, and the victim should be started on an antibiotic to oppose *Vibrio* bacteria (ciprofloxacin, trimethoprim-sulfamethoxazole, or doxycycline). If the rash is persistent but there is no sign of infection, a 7-day course of oral prednisone in a tapering dose (for a 150 lb, or 68 kg, person, begin with 70 mg and decrease by 10 mg per day) may be helpful. Corticosteroids should always be taken with the understanding that a rare side effect is serious deterioration of the head ("ball" of the ball-and-socket joint) of the femur, the long bone of the thigh.

Jellyfish

Jellyfish is the term commonly used to describe an enormous number of marine animals that are capable of inflicting a painful, and occasionally life-threatening, sting. These include fire coral, hydroids, jellyfish (including sea wasps), and anemones. The stings occur when the victim comes into contact with the creature's tentacles or other appendages, which may carry millions of microscopic stinging cysts, each cyst equipped with a toxin-laden microscopic stinger. Depending on the species, size, geographic location, time of year, and other natural factors, stings can range in severity from mild burning and skin redness to excruciating pain and severe blistering with generalized illness (nausea, vomiting, shortness of breath, muscle spasms, low blood pressure, and so on). Broken-off tentacles that are fragmented in the surf or washed up on the beach can retain their toxicity for months and should not be handled, even if they appear to be dried out and withered.

The dreaded box jellyfish *(Chironex fleckeri)* (figure 170) of northern Australia and the Indo-Pacific contains one of the most potent animal venoms known. A sting from one of these creatures can induce death in minutes from cessation of breathing, abnormal heart rhythms, and profound low blood pressure (shock).

Be prepared to treat an allergic reaction following a jellyfish sting! (See page 58.)

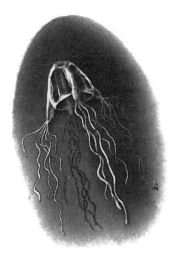

Figure 170. Indo-Pacific box jellyfish (sometimes called sea wasp).

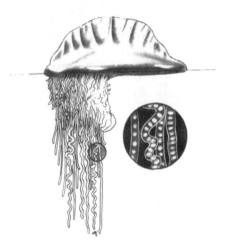

Figure 171. Portuguese man-of-war ("bluebottle"), with a close-up of sting-ing cells located on the tentacles.

The following therapy is recommended for all unidentified jellyfish and other creatures with stinging cells, including box jellyfish, Portuguese man-of-war ("bluebottle") (figure 171), Irukandji, fire coral (see figure 172), stinging hydroid, sea nettle, and sea anemone (see figure 173):

1. If the sting is felt to be from the box jellyfish *(Chironex fleckeri)*, immedi-ately flood the wound with vinegar (5% acetic acid). Keep the victim as still as possible. Continually apply the vinegar until the victim can be

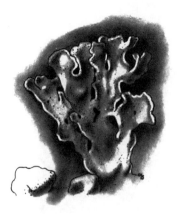

Figure 172. Fire coral.

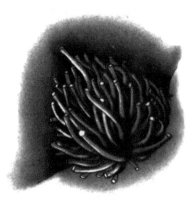

Figure 173. Sea anemone.

brought to medical attention. If you are out at sea or on an isolated beach, allow the vinegar to soak the tentacles or stung skin for 10 minutes before you attempt to remove adherent tentacles or further treat the wound. In Australia, surf lifesavers (lifeguards) may carry antivenin, which is given as an intramuscular injection at the first-aid scene. After decontamination with vinegar, consider application of the pressure immobilization technique (see page 305) until antivenin can be administered and the victim delivered to a hospital.

2. For all other stings, if a topical decontaminant (vinegar or isopropyl [rubbing] alcohol) is available, pour it liberally over the skin or apply a soaked compress. (Some authorities advise against the use of alcohol on the theoretical grounds that it has not been proven beyond a doubt to help. However, many clinical observations support its use. Since not

all jellyfish are identical, it is extremely helpful to know ahead of time what works for the stingers in your specific geographic location.) Vinegar may not work as well to treat sea bather's eruption (see page 208); a better agent may be a solution of papain (such as unseasoned meat tenderizer).

Until the decontaminant is available, you can rinse the skin with seawater. Do not rinse the skin gently with fresh water or apply ice directly to the skin. A brisk freshwater stream (forceful shower) may have sufficient force to physically remove the microscopic stinging cells, but nonforceful application is more likely to cause the cells to fire, increasing the envenomation. A nonmoist ice or cold pack may be useful to diminish pain, but take care to wipe away any surface moisture (condensation) prior to the application.

3. Apply soaks of vinegar or rubbing alcohol for 30 minutes or until pain is relieved. Baking soda powder or paste is recommended to detoxify the sting of certain sea nettles, such as the Chesapeake Bay sea nettle. If these decontaminants are not available, apply soaks of dilute (quarter-strength) household ammonia. A paste made from unseasoned meat tenderizer (do not exceed 15 minutes of application time, particularly not upon the sensitive skin of small children) or papaya fruit may be helpful. These contain papain, which may also be quite useful to alleviate the sting from the thimble jellyfish that cause sea bather's eruption (see page 208). Papain solution is available via a saturated abrasive pad in the product Wipe-Out! (see page 209). Do not apply any organic solvent, such as kerosene, turpentine, or gasoline.

4. After decontamination, apply a lather of shaving cream or soap and shave the affected area with a razor. In a pinch, you can use a paste of sand or mud in seawater and a clamshell.

5. Reapply the vinegar or rubbing alcohol soak for 15 minutes.

6. Apply a thin coating of hydrocortisone lotion (0.5 to 1%) twice a day. Anesthetic ointment (such as lidocaine hydrochloride 2.5% or a benzocaine-containing spray) may provide short-term pain relief.

7. If the victim has a large area involved (an entire arm or leg, face, or genitals), is very young or very old, or shows signs of generalized illness (nausea, vomiting, weakness, shortness of breath, chest pain, and the like), seek help from a doctor. If a child has placed tentacle fragments in his mouth, have him swish and spit whatever potable liquid is available. If there is already swelling in the mouth (muffled voice, difficulty swallowing, enlarged tongue and lips), do not give anything by mouth, protect the airway (see page 17), and rapidly transport the victim to a hospital.

To prevent jellyfish stings, an ocean bather or diver should wear, at a minimum, a synthetic nylon-rubber (Lycra [DuPont]) dive skin.

Coral and Barnacle Cuts

Cuts and scrapes from sharp-edged coral and barnacles tend to fester and become infected wounds. Treatment for these cuts is as follows:

1. Scrub the cut vigorously with soap and water, then flush the wound with large amounts of water.

2. Flush the wound with a half-strength solution of hydrogen peroxide in water. Rinse again with water.

3. Apply a thin layer of bacitracin or mupirocin ointment, or mupirocin cream, and cover with a dry, sterile, nonadherent dressing. If no ointment or dressing is available, the wound can be left open. Thereafter, it should be cleaned and redressed twice a day.

If the wound develops a pus-laden crust, you can use wet-to-dry dressing changes to remove the upper nonhealing layer in order to expose healthy, healing tissue. This is done by putting a dry, sterile gauze pad over the wound (without any underlying ointment), soaking the gauze pad with saline or a dilute antiseptic solution (such as 1 to 5% povidone iodine in disinfected water), allowing the liquid to dry, and then "brutally" ripping the bandage off the wound. The dead and dying tissue adheres to the gauze and is lifted free. The pink (hopefully), slightly bleeding tissue underneath should be healthy and healing. Dressings are changed once or twice a day. Use wet-to-dry dressings for a few days, or until they become nonadherent. At that point, switch back to the treatment in the above paragraph.

4. If the wound shows signs of infection (extreme redness, pus, swollen lymph glands), start the victim on an antibiotic to oppose *Vibrio* bacteria (ciprofloxacin, trimethoprim-sulfamethoxazole, or doxycycline).

Coral poisoning occurs if coral cuts are extensive or the cuts are from a particularly toxic species. The symptoms include a coral cut that heals poorly or continues to drain pus or cloudy fluid, swelling around the cut, swollen lymph glands, fever, chills, and fatigue. An antibiotic (see step 4, directly above) should be started, and the victim seen by a physician, who may elect to treat the victim for a week or two with a corticosteroid.

Sea Urchins

Some sea urchins are covered with sharp venom-filled spines (figure 174) that can easily penetrate and break off into the skin, or with small pincer-like appendages (figure 175) that grasp the victim and inoculate him with

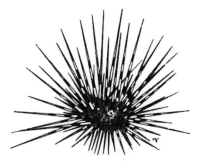

Figure 174. Spiny sea urchin.

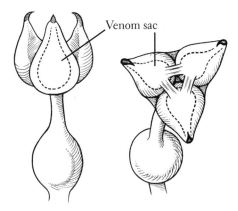

Venom sac

Figure 175. Sea urchin pincer with embedded venom sac.

venom from a sac within the pincer. Sea urchin punctures or stings are painful wounds, most often of the hands or feet. If a person receives many wounds simultaneously, the reaction may be so severe as to cause difficulty in breathing, weakness, and collapse. The treatment for sea urchin wounds is as follows:

1. Immerse the wound in nonscalding hot water to tolerance (110 to 113° F, or 43.3 to 45° C). This frequently provides pain relief. Administer appropriate pain medicine.
2. Carefully remove any readily visible spines. Do not dig around in the skin to fish them out—this risks crushing the spines and making them more difficult to remove. Do not intentionally crush the spines. Purple or black markings in the skin immediately after a sea urchin encounter do not necessarily indicate the presence of a retained spine fragment. Such discoloration is more likely dye leached from the surface of a

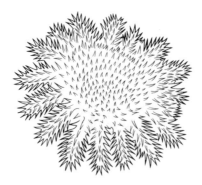

Figure 176. Crown of thorns starfish.

spine, commonly from a black urchin (*Diadema* spp.). The dye will be absorbed over 24 to 48 hours, and the discoloration will disappear. If there are still black markings after 48 to 72 hours, then a spine fragment is likely present.

3. If the sting is caused by a species with pincer organs, use hot-water immersion (step 1, page 317), then apply shaving cream or a soap paste and shave the area.

4. Seek the care of a physician if you feel spines have been retained in the hand or foot, or near a joint. They may need to be removed surgically, to minimize infection, inflammation, and damage to nerves or important blood vessels.

5. If the wound shows signs of infection (extreme redness, pus, swollen regional lymph glands) or a spine has penetrated deeply into a joint, the victim should be started on an antibiotic to oppose *Vibrio* bacteria (ciprofloxacin, trimethoprim-sulfamethoxazole, or doxycycline).

6. If a spine puncture in the palm of the hand results in a persistent swollen finger without any sign of infection (fever, redness, swollen lymph glands in the elbow or armpit), then it may become necessary to treat a 150 lb, or 68 kg, victim with a 7-day course of oral prednisone in a tapering dose (begin with 70 mg and decrease by 10 mg per day). Corticosteroids should always be taken with the understanding that a rare side effect is serious deterioration of the head ("ball" of the ball-and-socket joint) of the femur, the long bone of the thigh.

Starfish

The crown of thorns starfish (*Acanthaster planci*) is a particularly venomous starfish found in tropical oceans worldwide (figure 176). It carries sharp and rigid spines that may grow to 3" (7.5 cm) in length. The cutting edges

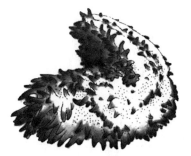

Figure 177. Sea cucumber.

easily penetrate a diver's glove and cause a painful puncture wound with copious bleeding and slight swelling. Multiple puncture wounds may lead to vomiting, swollen lymph glands, and brief muscle paralysis.

The treatment is similar to that for a sea urchin puncture (see page 316). Immerse the wound in nonscalding hot water to tolerance (110 to 113° F or 43.3 to 45° C) for 30 to 90 minutes. This frequently provides pain relief. Administer appropriate pain medicine. Carefully remove any readily visible spines. If there is a question of a retained spine or fragment, seek the assistance of a physician.

Other starfish, such as the rose star, can cause a skin rash. This may be treated with topical calamine lotion with 1% menthol or topical hydrocortisone 1% lotion.

Sea Cucumbers

Sea cucumbers (figure 177) are sausage-shaped creatures that produce a liquid called holothurin, which is a contact irritant to the skin and eyes. Because some sea cucumbers dine on jellyfish, they may excrete jellyfish stinging cells and venom as well. Therefore, anyone who sustains a skin irritation from handling a sea cucumber may benefit from the treatment for jellyfish stings described beginning on page 312. If the eyes are involved, they should be irrigated with at least a quart (liter) of water, and immediate medical attention should be sought. If the victim is out at sea, treat the eye injury as a corneal abrasion (see page 161).

Bristleworms

Bristleworms are small, segmented marine worms covered with chitinous bristles arranged in soft rows around the body (see figure 178). When a

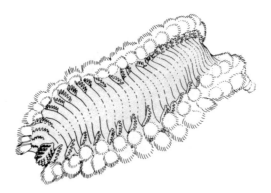

Figure 178. Bristleworm.

worm is stimulated, its body contracts and the bristles are erected. Easily detached, they penetrate skin like cactus spines and are difficult to remove. Some marine worms are also able to inflict painful bites.

The bite or sting of a marine worm may induce intense inflammation typified by burning sensation with a raised, red, and itchy rash, most frequently on the hands and fingers. Untreated, the pain is generally self-limited over the course of a few hours, but the redness and itching may last for 2 to 3 days. With multiple punctures, there may be marked swelling.

Remove all large visible bristles with tweezers. Then gently dry the skin, taking care to avoid breaking or embedding the spines farther into it. Apply a layer of adhesive tape, rubber cement, or a facial peel to remove the residual smaller spines. Then apply acetic acid 5% (vinegar), rubbing (isopropyl) alcohol 40%, dilute ammonia, or a paste of unseasoned meat tenderizer for 10 to 15 minutes. If the residual inflammation is significant, the victim may benefit from the administration of topical hydrocortisone 1% lotion.

Cone Shells (Snails)

Cone shells are beautiful, yet potentially lethal, cone-shaped mollusks that carry a highly developed venom apparatus, consisting of a rapid-acting poison that is injected by means of a dartlike, barbed tooth (figure 179). The venom causes a mild sting (puncture wound) that initially is characterized by bee-sting-like pain or, rarely, numbness and blanching. This is rapidly followed by numbness and tingling at the wound site, around the mouth and lips, and then all over the body. If the envenomation is severe,

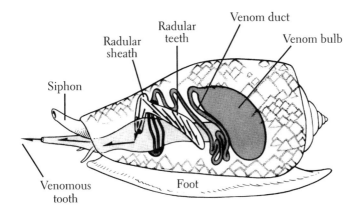

Figure 179. Cone snail, with a depiction of its venom apparatus.

the victim is afflicted with muscle paralysis, blurred vision, and breathing failure. A sting can be fatal.

There is no antivenin for a cone shell envenomation. While many first-aid remedies (such as hot-water immersion, surgical excision of the sting site, and injection of a local anesthetic) have been recommended, the one that makes the most sense is the pressure immobilization technique (see page 305) to contain the venom until the victim can be brought to advanced medical attention. Be prepared to offer the victim assistance for breathing (see page 24).

Stingrays

A stingray does its damage by lashing upward in self-defense with a muscular tail-like appendage, which carries up to four sharp, swordlike stings (see figure 180). The stings are supplied with venom, so that the injury created is both a deep puncture or laceration and an envenomation. The pain from a stingray wound can be excruciating and accompanied by bleeding, weakness, vomiting, headache, fainting, shortness of breath, paralysis, collapse, and, occasionally, death. Most wounds involve the feet and legs, because unwary waders and swimmers tread upon the creatures hidden in the sand. If a person is struck by a stingray, immediately do the following:

1. Rinse the wound with whatever clean water is available. Immediately immerse the wound in nonscalding hot water to tolerance (110 to

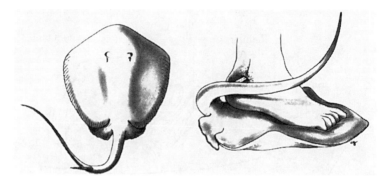

Figure 180. Stingray. The ray thrusts upward in self-defense with venom-laden spine(s) into the foot of an unwary victim.

113° F, or 43.3 to 45° C). This may provide some pain relief. Generally, it is necessary to soak the wound for 30 to 90 minutes. Gently extract any obvious piece of stinger.
2. Scrub the wound with soap and water. Do not try to sew or tape it closed; doing so could promote a serious infection.
3. Apply a dressing and seek medical help. If more than 12 hours will pass before a doctor can be reached, start the victim on an antibiotic (ciprofloxacin, trimethoprim-sulfamethoxazole, or doxycycline) to oppose *Vibrio* bacteria.
4. Administer appropriate pain medication.

Avoidance of Stingray Injuries

1. Always shuffle your feet when wading in stingray waters.
2. Always inspect the bottom before resting a limb in the sand.
3. Never handle a stingray unless you know what you are doing or the stingrays are definitively domesticated (such as at "Stingray City" off Grand Cayman Island in the British West Indies).

Catfish

Catfish sting their victims with dorsal and pectoral fin spines, which are charged with venom. When a fish is handled, the spines are extended and "locked" into position. The wound can be exceedingly painful, resembling the sting of a stingray. The treatment is the same as that for a stingray

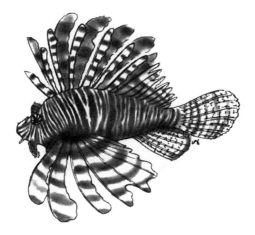

Figure 181. Lionfish (zebrafish).

wound. Soaking the wound in nonscalding hot water to tolerance (110 to 113° F, or 43.3 to 45° C) may provide dramatic relief of pain.

Tiny South American catfish of the genus *Vandellia* are known as "urethra fish" in English. They can swim up the human urethra or other urogenital openings and lodge within the victim, where they extend short spines on their gill covers. This can be extremely painful. Nonsurgical treatment is the ingestion of megadose (1 to 2 g per day) ascorbic acid (Vitamin C); when excreted in the urine, this slowly softens the spines and allows the fish to be excreted as well. Surgical removal is generally required because the victim cannot tolerate the discomfort caused by a retained urethra fish.

Scorpionfish

Scorpionfish include zebrafish (lionfish, turkeyfish) (figure 181), scorpionfish, and stonefish. They possess dorsal, anal, and pelvic spines that transport venom from venom glands into puncture wounds. Common reactions include redness or blanching, swelling, and blistering (lionfish). The injuries can be extremely painful and occasionally life threatening. The treatment is the same as that for a stingray wound. Soaking the wound in nonscalding hot water to tolerance (110 to 113° F, or 43.3 to 45° C) may provide dramatic relief of pain from a lionfish sting, is less likely to be curative for a scorpionfish sting, and may have little effect on the pain from a stonefish sting, but it should be undertaken nonetheless, because

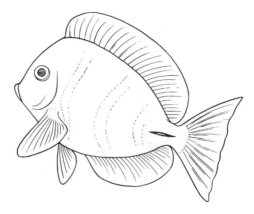

Figure 182. Surgeonfish.

the heat may destroy some of the harmful proteins contained in the venom. If the victim appears intoxicated or is weak, vomiting, short of breath, or unconscious, seek immediate advanced medical aid. Scorpionfish stings frequently require weeks or months to heal, and therefore require the attention of a physician. There is an antivenin available to physicians to help manage the sting of the dreaded stonefish.

Surgeonfish

Surgeonfish are tropical reef fish that carry one or more retractable jackknifelike skin appendages on either side of the tail (figure 182). When a fish is threatened, the appendage(s) is extended, where it serves as a blade to inflict a cut (figure 183). The appendage may carry venom, which contributes to the pain.

Treatment is to soak the wound in nonscalding hot water to tolerance (110 to 113° F, or 43.3 to 45° C) for 30 to 90 minutes or until the pain is relieved, then scrub vigorously to remove all foreign material. Watch closely for the development of an infection.

Octopuses

Octopus bites are rare. A nonvenomous octopus bite causes a local irritation that does not require any special therapy, other than wound cleansing and observation for infection. However, a bite from the Indo-Pacific blue-ringed or spotted octopus inoculates the victim with a substance extremely

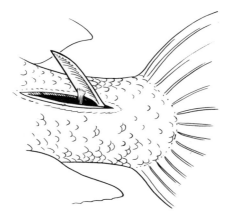

Figure 183. Surgeonfish tail, with blade extended.

similar to tetrodotoxin, one of the most potent poisons (also found in pufferfish—see page 327) found in nature.

Most victims are bitten on the hand or arm as they handle the creature or "give it a ride." The bite consists of one or two small puncture wounds, and may go unnoticed. Otherwise, there is a small amount of discomfort, described as a minor ache, slight stinging, or pulsating sensation. Occasionally, the site is initially numb, followed in 5 to 10 minutes by discomfort that may spread to involve the entire limb. By far the most common local reaction is the absence of symptoms, a small spot of blood, or a tiny blanched area.

More serious symptoms develop within 15 minutes of the bite, and include numbness of the mouth and face, followed by blurred vision, difficulty speaking, incoordination, weakness, vomiting, muscle paralysis, and breathing failure. The victim may collapse quickly and die from inability to breathe.

First aid is the pressure immobilization technique (see page 305). Be prepared to provide artificial respiration (see page 24) until the victim can be brought to advanced medical attention. If oxygen (see page 383) is available, it should be administered by face mask at a flow rate of 10 liters per minute.

Sea Snakes

Sea snakes are the most abundant reptiles on earth, though they are found only in the Pacific and Indian Oceans. They can attain a length of 9' (2.7 m)

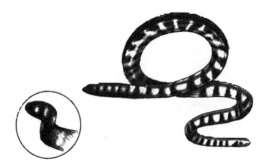

Figure 184. Sea snake, with paddle-shaped tail.

and are equipped with a paddlelike tail that allows them to swim forward and backward with considerable speed and agility (figure 184).

A sea snake can bite a victim with two to four fangs. The venom is extremely toxic, and causes paralysis, destruction of red blood cells, and widespread muscle damage.

The diagnosis of sea snake envenomation is determined as follows:

1. Unless you are handling a snake (commonly, fishermen emptying nets), you must be in the water to be bitten by a sea snake. The animals cannot move easily on land and do not survive very long there. However, you must be cautious when exploring regions of tidal variation, particularly in mangrove vegetation or near inlets where snakes breed.
2. Sea snake bites rarely cause much pain at the bite site.
3. Fang marks. These are like pinholes and may number from 1 to 4 (rarely, up to 20).
4. If symptoms do not occur within 6 to 8 hours of the bite, then significant poisoning has not occurred. The symptoms include weakness, paralysis, lockjaw, drooping eyelids, difficulty speaking, and vomiting. Later, the victim will develop darkened urine and difficulty breathing.

If a person is bitten by a sea snake, seek *immediate* medical attention, and immediately implement the pressure immobilization technique (see page 305). The definitive therapy is similar to that for a land snakebite— namely, administration in a hospital of the proper antivenin.

Skin Rashes Caused by Aquatic Plants (Seaweed Dermatitis) or Creatures (Sea Bather's Eruption, Swimmer's Itch)

See page 207.

Poisonings from Seafood

Scombroid Poisoning

Scombroid poisoning is caused by improper preservation (inadequate refrigeration or drying) of fish in the family Scombridae, which includes tuna, mackerel, bonito, skipjacks, and wahoo. Nonscombroid fish that can also cause this syndrome include mahi-mahi (dolphinfish), anchovies, sardines, and Australian ocean salmon. Most of these fish are dark fleshed. When they are not preserved properly, bacteria break down chemicals in the flesh to produce the chemical histamine, which causes an allergic-type reaction in the victim. Although the fish may have a peppery or metallic taste and "dull" appearance, they may also have normal color, flavor, and appearance.

Minutes after eating the fish, the victim becomes flushed, with itching, nausea and sometimes vomiting, diarrhea, low-grade fever, abdominal pain, and the development of hives (see page 210). Occasionally, a victim will become weak and short of breath, sometimes with wheezing. The reaction is similar to that seen with monosodium glutamate (MSG) sensitivity ("Chinese food syndrome"). Treatment is the same as for an allergic reaction (see page 58). If the victim does not improve with diphenhydramine (Benadryl), he may benefit from cimetidine (Tagamet) 300 mg by mouth. Administer the chosen antihistamine every 6 to 8 hours until symptoms resolve—generally, within 12 to 24 hours.

Puffer Poisoning

Certain puffers (blowfish, globefish, swellfish, porcupinefish [see figure 185], and so on) contain tetrodotoxin, one of the most potent poisons in nature. These fish are prepared as a delicacy (fugu) in Japan by specially trained and licensed chefs. The toxin is found in the entire fish, with greatest concentration in the liver, intestines, reproductive organs, and skin. After the victim has eaten the fish, symptoms can occur as quickly as 10 minutes later or be delayed by a few hours. These include numbness and tingling around the mouth, light-headedness, drooling, sweating, vomiting, diarrhea, abdominal pain, weakness, difficulty walking, paralysis, difficulty breathing, and collapse. Many victims die.

If someone is suffering from puffer poisoning, immediately transport him to a hospital. Pay attention to his ability to breathe, and assist his breathing if necessary (see page 24). Unfortunately, there is no antidote, and the victim will need sophisticated medical management until he

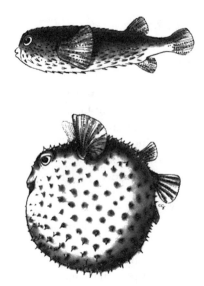

Figure 185. Porcupine (puffer) fish.

metabolizes the toxin. Eating puffers, unless they are prepared by the most skilled chefs, is dietary Russian roulette.

Ciguatera Fish Poisoning

Ciguatera fish poisoning involves a large number of tropical and semi-tropical bottom-feeding fish that dine on plants or smaller fish that have accumulated toxins from microscopic dinoflagellates, such as *Gambierdiscus toxicus.* Therefore, the larger the fish, the greater the toxicity. The ciguatoxin-carrying fish most commonly ingested include the barracuda, jack, grouper, and snapper. Symptoms, which usually begin 15 to 30 minutes after the victim eats the contaminated fish, include abdominal pain, nausea, vomiting, diarrhea, tongue and throat numbness, tooth pain, difficulty walking, blurred vision, skin rash, itching, tearing of the eyes, weakness, twitching muscles, incoordination, difficulty sleeping, and occasional difficulty in breathing. A classic sign of ciguatera intoxication is the reversal of hot and cold sensation (hot liquids seem cold and vice versa), which may reflect general hypersensitivity to temperature. Unfortunately, the symptoms persist in varying severity for weeks to months. Victims can become severely ill, with heart problems, low blood pressure, deficiencies of the central and peripheral nervous systems, and generalized collapse.

Treatment is for the most part supportive, although certain drugs are beginning to prove useful for aspects of the syndrome. An example is intravenous mannitol for abnormal nervous system behavior or abnormal heart rhythms. These therapies must be undertaken by a physician. Prochlorperazine may be useful for vomiting; hydroxyzine or cool showers may be useful for itching. There are chemical tests to determine the presence of ciguatoxins in fish and in the bloodstream of humans, but there is not yet a specific antidote. Anyone who displays symptoms of ciguatera fish poisoning should be seen promptly by a physician.

During recovery from ciguatera poisoning, the victim should exclude the following from his diet: fish, fish sauces, shellfish, shellfish sauces, alcoholic beverages, nuts, and nut oils.

Paralytic Shellfish Poisoning

Paralytic shellfish poisoning is caused by eating shellfish that contain concentrated toxins produced originally by certain planktons and protozoans in the ocean. These same microorganisms are responsible for the "red" (blue, brown, white, black, and so on) tides that occur in warm summer months. The shellfish (such as California mussels, which are quarantined each year from May through October) dine upon the microorganisms and concentrate the poison in their digestive organs and muscle tissues. Generally, crabs, shrimp, and abalone are safe to eat.

Minutes after eating contaminated shellfish, the victim complains of numbness and tingling inside and around his mouth, and of his tongue and gums. He soon becomes light headed, weak, and incoherent, and begins to suffer from drooling, difficulty swallowing, incoordination, headache, thirst, diarrhea, abdominal pain, blurred vision, sweating, and rapid heartbeat. Even if a victim becomes paralyzed, he may continue to be aware of what is happening, unless he does not receive enough oxygen to the brain (because he stops breathing).

The victim of paralytic shellfish poisoning should be brought immediately to a hospital. If he is having trouble breathing, be prepared to assist him (see page 24).

Hallucinatory Fish Poisoning

Certain reef fish of the tropical Pacific and Indian Oceans carry heat-stable toxins in their head parts, brain, and spinal cords, and (to a lesser degree) in their muscles, or flesh. Typical species include surgeonfish, goatfish, mullets, sergeants major, damselfish, and rudderfish. The toxicity of the fish can vary with the season.

Symptoms occur within 90 minutes of ingestion, and include dizziness, numbness and tingling around the mouth and lips, sweating, weakness, incoordination, auditory and visual hallucinations, nightmares, shortness of breath, brief paralysis, and sore throat. People do not die from this affliction. Treatment is supportive. The victim should be observed closely to see that he does not injure himself by exercising bad judgment.

Anisakiasis

Anisakiasis is caused by penetration of the nematode *Anisakis simplex* worm larvae through the lining of the stomach. This occurs when someone eats raw or undercooked fish, such as sushi. The most common carriers, which serve as intermediate hosts via sea mammals, are mackerel, Pacific herring and cod, coho salmon, hake, anchovies, squid, silvergray and yellowtail rockfish, bocaccio, and, in rare cases, tuna.

Symptoms begin within 1 hour of eating the fish, and include severe pain in the upper abdomen, nausea, and vomiting. The victim may appear quite ill. Occasionally, he may present with the symptoms of an allergic reaction.

If the worm(s) is not removed by a physician, who must do this physically through an endoscope passed through the esophagus into the stomach, it dies within a few days. However, implantation can initiate an abscess. Some worms don't implant, but are coughed up, vomited up, or passed in the stool. If a worm crawls into the esophagus or throat, an unusual tingling feeling can develop.

A worm that passes through the stomach and implants in the intestine (up to 7 days after ingestion) causes abdominal pain, nausea, vomiting, diarrhea, and fever. It may penetrate completely through the bowel. Often an operation is performed for suspected appendicitis or intestinal cancer, only to discover the true cause of the victim's symptoms.

Unfortunately, there is no drug or purgative treatment that will eliminate the parasite once it has been ingested. It is either passed in the stool by the victim spontaneously or has to be physically removed, which can be as complicated as surgically removing a section of intestine.

To prevent this problem, any fish should be cooked to a temperature above 140° F (60° C) or frozen for 24 hours to −4° F (−20° C) before it is eaten. Smoking, marinating, pickling, brining, and salting may not kill the worms. A fish should be gutted as soon as possible after it is caught to prevent migration of the worms from its internal organs into its muscle tissue.

An allergic reaction may still occur from eating properly preserved or cooked, but parasitized, fish.

INSECT AND ARTHROPOD BITES

Bees, Spiders, Scorpions, and Other Small Biters

Bees, Wasps, Hornets, and Ants

This group of insects includes honeybees, bumblebees, wasps, hornets, and yellow jackets; each possesses a stinger, which is used to introduce venom into the victim. Most stings occur on the head, neck, arms, and legs.

"Killer bees" (an unfortunate misnomer) are an Africanized race of honeybees created by interbreeding of the African honeybee (brought for experiments into Brazil) with common European honeybees. The hazard from these bees is that they tend to be more irritable, swarm more readily, defend their hives more aggressively, and impose mass attacks upon humans. The venom of an Africanized bee is not of greater volume or potency than that of a European honeybee. However, the personality of the Africanized bees is such that they may pursue a victim for up to ⅔ mile (1 km), and may recruit other attacking bees by the hundreds or thousands.

The sting mechanism for a honeybee is composed of a doubly barbed stinger attached to a venom sac that pumps venom into the victim. When the bee attempts to escape after a sting, the stinger and sac are left behind and continue to operate (this kills the bee). Thus, the honeybee can sting only once, whereas a wasp, with a smooth stinger that does not become entrapped, can sting multiple times, as can yellow jackets, hornets, and bumblebees.

Pain from a bee, wasp, or hornet sting is immediate, with rapid swelling, redness, warmth, and itching at the site of the sting. Blisters may occur. Sometimes the victim will become nauseated, vomit, and/or suffer abdominal cramping and diarrhea. If the person is allergic to the insect venom, a dangerous reaction may follow rapidly (within minutes, but occasionally delayed by up to 2 hours). This consists of hives, shortness of breath, difficulty breathing, swelling of the tongue, weakness, vomiting, low blood pressure, and collapse. People have swallowed bees (undetected in beverage bottles) and sustained stings of the esophagus, which are enormously painful.

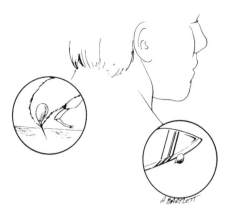

Figure 186. Honeybee sting. Because the venom sac is still attached to the stinger, both should be scraped or pulled free from the skin as soon as possible.

A severe allergic reaction may follow the sting(s) of a fire (red) ant, because it marches along the victim and leaves a trail of small, painful blisters. Harvester ants generally produce less severe reactions. A day or two after the ant bite, the fluid in the blister turns cloudy or white, and a small sterile pustule develops. This may continue to be painful and itch for a week or more.

Treatment for Insect Sting

1. Be prepared to deal with a severe allergic reaction (see page 58). If the victim develops hives, shortness of breath, and profound weakness, and appears to be deteriorating, *immediately* administer epinephrine. This is injected subcutaneously (see page 419) in a dose of 0.3 to 0.5 ml for adults and 0.01 ml per kg (2.2 lb) of body weight for children, not to exceed 0.3 ml. Epinephrine is available in allergy kits (see page 437) with instructions for use. *Anyone known to have insect allergies who travels in the wilderness should carry epinephrine.* Take particular care to handle preloaded syringes carefully, to avoid inadvertent injection into a finger. When administering an injection, *never* share needles between people.

2. Administer diphenhydramine (Benadryl) by mouth, 50 to 100 mg for an adult and 1 mg per kg (2.2 lb) of body weight for a child. This antihistamine drug may by used by itself for a milder allergic reaction.

3. Stingers or pieces of stingers left in the skin should be scraped off with a knife or other sharp (straight) edge (figure 186), if one is readily available. Because the honeybee venom sac is still attached to the stinger, if you squeeze the sac, you may inject more venom into the wound, worsening the reaction, although this has never been proven. So, it is better to flick or pull a stinger and venom sac out of the skin of the victim using a tweezer or your fingers than to waste precious time searching for a straight-edged object. An alternative is to apply the Extractor device (see figure 164), if it is available immediately after the sting has occurred.

4. Apply ice packs to the site of the sting.

5. Apply a paste made from unseasoned papain-containing meat tenderizer (such as Adolph's unseasoned meat tenderizer) and water directly to the wound for no more than 15 minutes. A paste of baking soda is of no value. Do not apply mud. If the victim is allergic to meat tenderizer, a 20% aluminum-salt-containing preparation (including many household antiperspirants) may be effective. The commercial product After Bite (Tender Corporation, Littleton, New Hampshire), a mixture of ammonium hydroxide and mink oil, is moderately effective for relief of pain and itching following insect bites, but will not abort an allergic reaction. Stingeze liquid (Wisconsin Pharmacal, Jackson, Wisconsin) is a mixture of camphor, phenol, benzocaine, and diphenhydramine. This is a good agent to control itching and mild pain following any insect bite. Itch Balm Plus (Sawyer Products, Safety Harbor, Florida) is a similar mixture of hydrocortisone, diphenhydramine, and tetracaine.

6. If a person stung by an insect develops more than a mild local reaction, transport him to a hospital.

Avoidance of Stinging Insects

1. Store garbage, particularly fruit, at a distance from the campsite.

2. Remove *(carefully)* beehives and wasp nests from children's play areas.

3. Wear light-colored clothing. Dark-colored clothing is attractive to insects and may evoke a defensive (sting or bite) response. Keep shirt sleeves closed and tuck pants into boots. Wear light-colored socks.

4. Avoid wearing sweet fragrances that make you smell like a flower.

5. Do not anger bees or wasps. If confronted by a swarm, cover your face and move rapidly from the area. Do not poke sticks or throw rocks into bee holes.

6. Avoid rapid or jerky movements near bees. Do not swat at them.

Spiders

Although over 20,000 different species of spiders live in the United States, only a few pose any real hazard to humans. The troublemakers

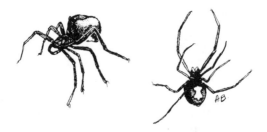

Figure 187. Female black widow spider with typical hourglass marking on the underside of the abdomen.

are those that bite and introduce venom from venom glands into the wound. The nature of the reaction depends on the type and quantity of venom.

Black Widow Spider

In the United States, the female black widow spider (*Latrodectus mactans*) is about ⅝" (15 mm) in body length, black or brown, and with a characteristic red (or orange or yellow) hourglass marking on the underside of the abdomen (figure 187). The top side of the spider is shiny and features a fat abdomen that resembles a large black grape. The longest legs are directed toward the front. This species and other *Latrodectus* species are found scattered in rural regions, in barns, within harvested crops, and around outdoor stone walls. Some are arboreal.

The bite of the black widow spider is rarely very painful (usually more like a pinprick) and often causes little swelling or redness, although there can be a warm and reddened area around the bite. If much venom has been deposited, the victim develops a typical reaction well within an hour. Symptoms include muscle cramps, particularly of the abdomen and back; muscle pain; muscle twitching; numbness and tingling of the palms of the hands and bottoms of the feet; headache; droopy eyelids; facial swelling; drooling; sweating; restlessness and anxiety; vomiting; chest muscle spasms, causing difficulty in breathing; fever; and high blood pressure. A man may develop a persistent penile erection (priapism). A small child may cry persistently. A pregnant woman may develop uterine contractions and premature labor.

Untreated, most people recover without help over the course of 8 hours to 2 days. However, very small children and elderly victims may suffer greatly, with possible death.

Treatment for a Black Widow Spider Bite

1. Apply ice packs to the bite.

2. *Immediately* transport the victim to a medical facility.

3. Once the victim is in the hospital, the doctor will have a number of therapies to use, which include intravenous calcium solutions and muscle relaxant medicines for muscle spasm; antihypertensive drugs for elevated blood pressure; pain medicine; and, in very severe cases, antivenin to the venom of the black widow spider.

4. If you will be unable to reach a hospital within a few hours and the victim is suffering *severe* muscle spasms, you may administer an oral dose of diazepam (Valium), if you happen to be carrying it. The starting dose for an adult who does not regularly take the drug is 5 mg, which can be augmented in 2.5 mg increments every 30 minutes up to a total dose of 10 mg, so long as the victim remains alert and is capable of normal, purposeful swallowing. The starting dose for a child age 2 to 5 years is 0.5 mg; for a child age 6 to 12 years the starting dose is 2 mg. Total dose for a child should not exceed 5 mg; *never* leave a sedated child unattended.

Brown Recluse Spider

At least five species of recluse spiders are found in the United States. The brown recluse spider (*Loxosceles reclusa*) is the best known and found most commonly in the South and southern Midwest. However, interstate commerce has created new habitats in many other parts of the country for the brown recluse and related species. The spider is brown, with an average body length of just under ½" (10 mm). A characteristic dark violin-shaped marking ("fiddleback") is found on the top of the upper section of the body (see figure 188). The brown recluse spider is found in dark, sheltered areas, such as under porches, in woodpiles, and in crates of fruit. It is most active at night. It commonly bites when it is trapped, but is not otherwise aggressive toward humans.

The bite of the brown recluse spider may cause very little pain at first, or a sharp sting may be felt. The stinging subsides over 6 to 8 hours, and is replaced by aching and itching. Within 1 to 5 hours, a painful red or purplish blister sometimes appears, surrounded by a bull's-eye of whitish blue (pale) discoloration, with occasional slight swelling. The red margin may spread into an irregular fried-egg pattern, with gravitational influence, such that the original blister remains near the uppermost part of the lesion. The victim may develop chills, fever, weakness, and a generalized red skin rash. Severe allergic reactions

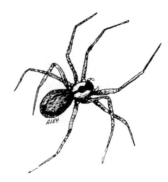

Figure 188. Brown recluse spider with typical violin-shaped marking on the top side of the cephalothorax.

within 30 minutes of the bite occur infrequently. Over 5 to 7 days, the venom causes a violet discoloration and breakdown of the surrounding tissue, leading to an open ulcer that may take months to heal. If the reaction has been severe, the tissue in the center of the wound becomes destroyed, blackens, and dies.

A rare reaction is "systemic loxoscelism," in which the venom binds to red blood cells and induces severe symptoms within 24 to 72 hours. These include a flulike presentation with fever, chills, headache, fatigue, weakness, nausea, vomiting, muscle and joint aches, blood in the urine, yellow skin discoloration (jaundice), kidney failure, and even shock, seizures, and coma. This is more common in children and requires intensive medical therapy.

Treatment for a Brown Recluse Spider Bite

Because the bite of the brown recluse spider typically causes severe tissue destruction, the victim should see a physician, who will prescribe medicine or another therapy as soon as possible. In the meantime, apply cold packs to the wound for as long as is practical and administer an antibiotic (erythromycin or cephalexin). Do not apply a heating pad or hot packs. Depending upon the severity of the reaction, the doctor will either advise medicines or surgical excision of the bite. Dapsone, a drug used to inhibit certain cells that are part of the inflammatory response, has been used effectively. Hyperbaric oxygen therapy is recommended by some clinicians.

Until you receive other advice, treat the wound with a thin layer of mupirocin or bacitracin ointment, or mupirocin cream, underneath daily dressing changes.

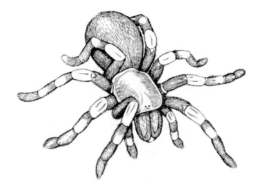

Figure 189. Tarantula.

Other Spiders

Other spiders that may produce painful bites and a small amount of local tissue breakdown include the tarantula, wolf spider, jumping spider, yellow sac spider, orb weaver, and hobo spider *(Tegenaria agrestis)*. The bites should be treated with ice packs, pain medicine, and standard wound care.

Some tarantulas (figure 189) carry hairs that can irritate the skin, eyes, and mucous membranes of humans. When the spider is threatened, it rubs its hind legs over its abdomen and flicks thousands of hairs at its foe. These hairs can penetrate human skin and cause swollen bumps, which can itch for weeks. Treatment is with an oral antihistamine and topical medication such as Stingeze liquid or Itch Balm Plus (see page 333).

The hobo spider may cause a reaction similar to, but less severe than, a brown recluse spider. The bite wound should be treated accordingly; see previous page.

Scorpions

Scorpions are found in deserts and warm tropical climates, hidden under stones, fences, and garbage. In the United States, the most dangerous species is the nocturnal bark scorpion *Centruroides exilicauda,* which is found almost exclusively in the southwestern states and can be up to 2" (5 cm) long. This yellowish brown (straw-colored), solid or striped species is distinguished from other scorpions by its slender body and a small tubercle (telson) at the base of its stinger (see figure 190). The sting is inflicted with the last segment of the tail, and it is immediately exquisitely

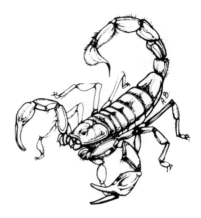

Figure 190. Scorpion.

painful; the pain is made much worse by tapping on the site of the injury. Other symptoms include excitement, increased salivation, sweating, numbness and tingling around the mouth, nausea, double vision, nervousness, muscle twitching and spasms, rapid breathing, shortness of breath, high blood pressure, seizures, paralysis, and collapse. A child under the age of 2 is at particular risk for a severe reaction. Stings by nonlethal scorpion species are similar to bee stings.

If someone is stung by a scorpion, immediately apply an ice pack to the wound and immobilize the affected body part. Seek immediate care, particularly for stings of *C. exilicauda*. In Arizona and New Mexico, antivenin is available to physicians for treatment.

To prevent scorpion stings, be careful when handling deadwood and working in piles of leaves. Clothing, shoes, bedrolls, and sleeping bags should be shaken out and inspected before use. *C. exilicauda* is fluorescent under an ultraviolet light (Wood's lamp or "black light") and can be spotted glowing green at night in this manner.

Mosquitoes

Female mosquitoes bite humans in quest of a blood meal, in order to lay eggs. Because they breed in water, they are most frequently found in marshy, wetland, or wooded areas. Although many tend to swarm at dusk, different species feed at different times. The insects are attracted to host odors (long-range), exhaled carbon dioxide (midrange), and heat and moisture (short-range). During a bite, mosquito saliva is injected into the victim. This liquid contains the substances that cause the classic reaction—

a small white or red bump that itches, then disappears. Those who have been sensitized because of previous bites can have delayed (12 to 48 hours) reactions, which include intense swelling and itching. In addition, mosquitoes transmit diseases such as malaria (see page 131) and various types of encephalitis. To date, mosquitoes in Alaska have not been found to transmit any diseases.

Therapy for mosquito bites is limited to cool compresses and skin hygiene to prevent infections. If someone is bitten intensely and suffers a severe delayed allergic reaction, he may benefit from a course of prednisone similar to that used to treat poison oak (see page 205). Oral antihistamines, such as cetirizine hydrochloride, given prior to mosquito exposure, may lessen the reaction to mosquito bites in highly sensitized persons.

Insect repellents are discussed on pages 347 and 453.

Biting Flies

A midge (also called a gnat or no-see-um) is a small biting fly that creates a painful red bump that seems out of proportion to the insect's size. After your immune system has become sensitized to these bites, your reactions seem to become worse with repeated assaults, and you may develop blisters or small sores.

Blackflies, buffalo gnats, turkey gnats, and green-headed flies create larger punctures that may bleed. The immediate pain, swelling (welt), and redness are usually intense and persistent. The sores may last for weeks, and be accompanied by weakness and fever when there are multiple bites. Swollen lymph glands may occur, particularly in children. Horsefly, deerfly, mango fly, breeze fly, and sand fly bites are generally less noxious, but may on occasion be severe.

Treatment is symptomatic and similar to that applied under step 5 for the local reaction to an insect sting (see page 333), with the exception that the application of meat tenderizer has never been suggested to be of benefit for a fly bite.

Fleas

Fleas are parasitic on mammals and birds. The wingless body enables the critters to run and jump with ease. They live on blood. They are more active in warmer climates, and are commonly associated with domestic animals. A flea bite usually is a small dark red or purplish dot surrounded by a circular area of lighter redness and swelling. Itching is common. Those who have been sensitized may develop blisters or ulcers. Flea bites may appear in unpatterned clusters, most commonly on the legs, ankles, and feet.

Treatment is symptomatic and similar to that applied under step 5 for the local reaction to an insect sting (see page 333), with the exception that the application of meat tenderizer has never been suggested to be of benefit for a flea bite.

The female *Tunga penetrans* flea (burrowing flea, chigo, sand flea, jigger) causes tungiasis in Central and South America and in Africa. The impregnated female flea burrows into a human's skin until only the flea's posterior end remains external. The insect sucks blood, becomes larger, and appears as a firm, itchy nodule the size of a small pea, which has a dark spot in the center (the hind end of the flea). The most common sites of infestation are the feet, buttocks, or perineum of humans who don't wear shoes or who squat into dusty soil. The burrowed flea can be killed with topical ether; it must then be surgically removed, or severe infection can develop.

Chiggers

Chiggers (red bugs, harvest mites) are an enormous nuisance, particularly in the southeastern United States. The adult mites lay their eggs on vegetation (such as grass). The newly hatched larvae attach themselves to a human and inflict the bites; each is terribly itchy, and marked initially with a small red dot that becomes a red welt over the next 24 hours. Bites may number in the hundreds. Blisters, weeping, and severe swelling may appear. The feet and ankles are most commonly affected. The lesions resolve over 2 weeks, but not without flare-ups of intense itching and discomfort.

Treatment is symptomatic and similar to that applied under step 5 for the local reaction to an insect sting (see page 333). One percent phenol in calamine may be helpful. Home remedies for chigger bites are common, and include application of dabs of clear nail polish or meat tenderizer. None is of proven scientific benefit. If a person is bitten intensely and suffers a severe reaction, he may benefit from a course of prednisone similar to that used to treat poison oak (see page 205).

Centipedes and Millipedes

Centipedes bite their victims with their fangs, not with their feet or rear-end appendages. *Scolopendra* species bites have been reported to cause burning pain, swelling, redness, and swollen lymph glands. More severe

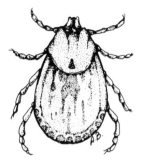

Figure 191. Tick.

reactions are rare. Treatment is symptomatic and similar to that applied under step 5 for the local reaction to an insect sting (see page 333), with the exception that the application of meat tenderizer has never been suggested to be of benefit for a centipede bite.

Millipedes do not bite their human victims; instead, they eject secretions that can cause skin irritation. In tropical regions, this has been reported to begin with brown skin staining, followed by a burning sensation with blisters. Millipede secretions that enter the eye may cause severe irritation similar to a corneal abrasion (see page 161). There is no specific treatment, other than to irrigate the affected area promptly and thoroughly with disinfected water or saline solution, then treat as a burn (see page 98) or, if the eye is injured, as a corneal abrasion (see page 161).

Ticks

Ticks (figure 191) are ubiquitous in wooded regions and fields, and readily attach to the skin of victims, most commonly in the scalp, armpits, groin, and other cozy (for a tick) areas. They like shade and moist skin, and may wander for a while in search of a comfortable spot. Once in place, they hang on with their mouthparts and feed on the victim's blood. The tick is the intermediate host for the vectors of many diseases, such as Rocky Mountain spotted fever (see page 138), Colorado tick fever (see page 139), relapsing fever (see page 135), ehrlichiosis (see page 141), babesiosis (see page 142), and Lyme disease (see page 139).

A tick bite can cause a local reaction that ranges from the common small, itchy nodule to an extensive ulcer. With large or multiple bites, the victim may suffer fever, chills, and fatigue in the absence of infection.

Normally, the bite wounds resolve over a week or two. A persistent lump may be a collection of reactive (to tick saliva) tissue that requires surgical excision.

Tick Paralysis

If a person (particularly a young girl with long hair) is traveling in or has just returned from tick country and begins to complain of fatigue and weakness, you may have discovered a case of tick paralysis.

The disorder is most common in spring and summer when ticks are feeding. Certain female ticks attach to the skin and slowly (over several days) release a neurotoxin that causes profound lethargy and muscle weakness in the victim. At first he may be irritable and restless, and complain of numbness and tingling in his hands and feet. Over the next day or two, the victim becomes weak, with an ascending (beginning in the feet and advancing toward the head) paralysis, which can become total. Just a portion of the face can be paralyzed if a tick is lodged behind the ear.

Search the skin (particularly the hair-covered areas) thoroughly for ticks and remove them properly (see below). Improvement is usually noted within hours, while complete recovery occurs in 24 to 48 hours after removal of the tick. However, if the tick isn't removed, the victim can die.

Tick Avoidance

When traveling in forests and fields, it is a good idea to inspect the body thoroughly (particularly the hairline, groin, underarms, navel, scalp, and other hair-covered areas) for ticks each day. Don't forget to brush ticks out of the fur of all dogs and pack animals.

Wear proper clothing to prevent tick attachment. Keep shirts tucked into pants and trouser cuffs tucked into socks. Light-colored clothing displays ticks. The deer tick, which transmits the infectious agent of Lyme disease, is extremely small, particularly in juvenile stages. The best repellent is permethrin (Permanone) applied to clothing, not to skin (see page 347), but DEET is also effective.

Tick Removal

The proper way to remove a tick is to grasp it close to its mouthparts with tweezers or with the fingernails and pull it straight out with a slow and

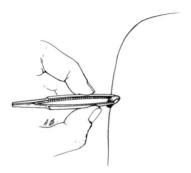

Figure 192. Removing a tick with tweezers.

steady motion (figure 192). Another excellent way to remove a tick is with a grooved or V-shaped device designed to slide between the tick and the skin to trap the tick and allow it to be pulled from the skin. Do not twist the tick. If you must remove it with your fingers, use tissue paper or cloth to prevent skin contact with infectious tick fluids. Do not touch the tick with a hot object (such as an extinguished match head) or cover it with mineral oil, alcohol, kerosene, camp stove fuel, or Vaseline; these remedies might cause the tick to struggle and regurgitate infectious fluid into the bite site. Viscous lidocaine 2% applied to a tick for 5 minutes will cause it to detach its grip, but it is not known if the tick regurgitates. If a tick head is buried in the skin, you can apply permethrin (Permanone insect repellent), using a cotton swab, to the upper and lower body surfaces of the tick. After 10 to 15 minutes, the tick will relax and you will be able to pull it free. After the tick is removed, carefully inspect the skin for remaining head parts, and gently scrape them away.

Caterpillars

The puss caterpillar, *Megalopyge opercularis* (see figure 193), is found in the southern United States. The gypsy moth caterpillar, *Lymantria dispar* (see figure 194), and the flannel moth caterpillar, *M. cirpata,* are found in the northeastern U.S. The numerous bristles that cover the bodies of these species cause skin irritation when the caterpillar is directly touched, or when there is contact with detached bristles deposited on outdoor bedding or hung clothes. Shortly after exposure, the victim suffers a rash with redness, itching, burning discomfort, and hives. Blisters are rare. If a large area of skin is involved, the victim can become nauseated and weak, and can suffer from high fever. If the small bristle hairs are inhaled, shortness

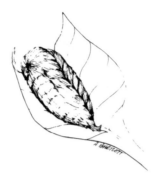

Figure 193. Puss caterpillar.

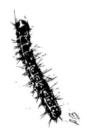

Figure 194. Gypsy moth caterpillar.

of breath or asthmalike (see page 39) symptoms may follow. If the eyes come into contact with these hairs, symptoms include redness, itching, tearing, and swollen eyelids. Handling particularly venomous species can cause intense pain, headache, fever, vomiting, and swollen lymph glands.

Treatment of the skin consists of applying adhesive tape (duct tape is best) to attempt removal of the bristles, followed by an application of calamine lotion. A good alternative is to apply a commercial facial peel or thin layer of rubber cement, allow it to dry, and then peel it off; the bristles will be carried with it. Management of an allergic reaction similar to that from poison oak is described on page 205. If the redness and swelling are prominent, the victim may be treated with a nonsteroidal anti-inflammatory drug for 5 days.

Beetles

Beetles are the largest group of insects. Fortunately, no beetle has a bite or sting that can envenom a human, although some types produce toxic secretions that can be deposited on the skin.

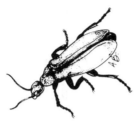

Figure 195. Blister beetle.

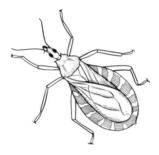

Figure 196. Triatomid "kissing bug."

Blister beetles of the *Epicauta* species (figure 195) are found throughout the eastern and southern United States. These insects are usually about ½" (1.3 cm) long and extremely agile. When they make contact with the skin, they release a chemical substance (cantharidin) that is very irritating. Initial contact is painless. Within a few hours, blisters appear, which are not particularly painful unless they are large and broken. If a blister beetle is squashed on the skin, an enormous blister follows.

The treatment is the same as for a second-degree burn (see page 100). If "beetle juice" enters the eye, the eye should be irrigated copiously and the injury managed as you would snow blindness (see page 166).

Sucking Bugs

These insects have sucking mouthparts, and are typified by the assassin bugs and their subset of triatomids ("kissing bugs," "wheel bugs," and Mexican bedbugs). Aquatic sucking bugs include the giant water bugs and "water scorpions."

Triatomids (figure 196) usually bite humans during the night on exposed body parts, and feed for up to 30 minutes. The initial bite is painless without any immediate reaction. However, the wheel bug, black corsair, or masked bedbug hunter bite may cause pain like a hornet sting.

A triatomid may continue to bite until there is a cluster or line of red, itchy bumps that may last for up to a week. If the reaction is more severe, there are large hives, swollen lymph glands, fever, and blisters. Bedbug bites often create an itchy bump with a central red spot.

Treatment is symptomatic and similar to that applied under step 5 for the local reaction to an insect sting (see page 333), with the exception that the application of meat tenderizer has never been suggested to be of benefit for a sucking bug bite.

Skin Infestation by Fly Larvae

Skin infestation by fly larvae is called myiasis, and is most commonly noted in Mexico and Central and South America, the latter two with the botfly *Dermatobia hominis.* The fly egg, which may actually be carried by another species of insect (such as the mosquito), is deposited onto human skin, where it hatches, allowing the emerging larva to burrow into the skin through the insect bite or another opening (such as a hair follicle or small scratch or nick).

The larva then develops within a dome-shaped cavity (swelling) that enlarges over 4 to 7 weeks. A central breathing pore drains clear or slightly bloody fluid. Drainage may begin within the first 2 weeks after penetration. There is often redness and itching. Movement may be felt under the skin as the larva wiggles. This may also feel like a crawling sensation or brief flash of sharp pain, because the larva has many parallel rows of bristly spines.

The mature larva will attempt to exit the skin through the breathing pore, and is noticed as a small white object "peeking" through the hole. You can force it to exit through the hole by suffocating it: Cover the breathing pore with bacon fat, a strip of meat, chewing gum, wax, fingernail polish, or a plug of grease. Usually, 12 hours of occlusion will cause the larva to exit the hole or die from asphyxiation. Moistened tobacco leaves or nicotine drops will paralyze the larva. It is unwise to make a rough incision to remove the larva, because if the creature is ruptured, it will leak substances into the wound that cause inflammation and promote infection. It is sometimes possible to simply squeeze the lesion and force extrusion of the larva, but care must be taken not to rupture the larva. If nothing is done to force the larva to leave the skin, it will do so on its own in a few weeks, but this is generally not recommended because of the pain and potential for abscess (see page 212) formation.

Other fly larvae that can invade humans and cause myiasis may "migrate," or travel under the skin, usually settling over the head or shoulders. They may emerge from the lesions or die where they are, in which case they don't need to be removed.

Wound myiasis describes the situation in which flies (including the green- or bluebottle fly, housefly, black blowfly, and flesh fly) have deposited eggs into a wound, where the larvae feed on the decaying tissue. This is seen most commonly in elderly victims with underlying chronic diseases. The "maggots" are unsightly, but do not harm the victim. Screwworms, on the other hand, which originate from outbreaks among livestock, may invade humans and cause destructive ulcers, particularly if they enter through the nose.

For wound myiasis confined to the skin, a mixture of 5% chloroform in olive oil kills the larvae, so that they can be removed manually. In the absence of this mixture, simple irrigation and mechanical removal of the larvae will suffice.

Insect Repellents

In insect-laden areas, where contact is inevitable, the traveler must wear proper clothing. Cover the head and neck with a full-brimmed hat (with or without netting) and scarf (temperature permitting). Shield the ankles and wrists. Tuck pant cuffs into socks. Light-colored clothing is less attractive than dark clothing to biting insects, and also makes it easier to spot any mosquitoes, ticks, and flies that have landed.

Nylon (particularly double layered) and sailcloth are more difficult for insects to hang on to or penetrate and are generally preferred over cotton or cloth with a loose weave. Loose-fitting clothing made with tightly woven fabric, along with a T-shirt underlayer, makes for reasonable upper-body protection. Where clothing can be pulled tight against the skin, a mosquito can bite through.

Clothing needs to be checked regularly and brushed free of insects; this is best done with the sticky side of adhesive tape.

Portable insect screens and bed nets should be deployed when necessary. The use of artificial lights, which draw insects, should be avoided.

Insect repellents applied to clothing are extremely effective and avoid skin irritation. It is a good idea to test the repellent on a small area of clothing before general application, to be certain that it will not blemish the fabric.

Chemical insect repellents are mandatory whenever you travel through mosquito, sand fly, or tick territory. Different repellents work by different mechanisms and therefore their effectiveness varies for different types of insects, but I can make some general recommendations that will be applicable in most situations.

The best repellents contain the chemicals DEET (N,N-diethyl-3-methylbenzamide), Indalone (butyl 3,4-dihydro-2,2-dimethyl-4-oxo-2H-pyran-6-carboxylate), Rutgers 612 (2-ethyl-1,3-hexanediol), and DMP (dimethyl phthalate). Di-n-propyl isocinchomeronate (R-326) has been promoted as useful against biting flies. See page 453 for brand names.

Citronella and Avon Skin-So-Soft bath oil or skin stick are far less effective (1 hour of protection versus 7 hours with 25% DEET). There is some evidence that p-methane-3,8-diol isolated from eucalyptus oil may be an effective repellent. Along with isopulegol and citronellal, it is contained in the product Mosiguard Natural. Ingesting vitamin B1 has not been proven to deter biting insects. It may decrease the skin irritation that follows an insect bite, but this would not diminish the transmission of infectious disease(s) via the bite.

To be effective, a repellent should be applied to the skin (liquid) and clothing (spray). After you swim, bathe, or perspire excessively, reapply it. In windy conditions, repellents evaporate quickly and may need to be reapplied. Children under 2 years of age should not have insect repellent applied to the skin more than once in 24 hours (it is more effective to apply it to the clothing, anyhow). If you're applying both a sunscreen and an insect repellent, apply the sunscreen first, so that it can be absorbed; wait 30 minutes, then apply the insect repellent. There are also newer sunscreen–insect repellent combinations, such as Coppertone Bug & Sun and Banana Boat Bite Block. Bug Guard contains Skin-So-Soft (mostly mineral oil) in combination with citronella, enhanced by a sunscreen.

With regard to DEET-containing products, do not use repeated applications or concentrations greater than 15% in children under the age of 6 (Skedaddle, Skintastic, and other preparations intended for use on children contain approximately 6.5 to 10% DEET). In adults, skin irritation and/or rare severe side effects may be seen following the use of concentrated (75 to 100%) products. Most authorities recommend avoidance of concentrated products, noting the effectiveness of a 50% concentration in jungle settings. A concentration not to exceed 30 to 50% for routine adult use seems reasonable. Two recommended products are Ultrathon Insect Repellent and Sawyer Gold Insect Repellent. It has been stated that a 20 to 30% concentration applied to clothing is 90% effective in preventing tick attachment. A new product that may significantly decrease absorption of DEET is Sawyer Controlled Release Deet Formula, which uses a protein that encapsulates the DEET and allows slow (sustained) release. It should be applied to skin, not clothing.

The following recommendations are offered to avoid toxicity:

1. Apply repellent sparingly, and only to exposed skin or clothing. Keep it out of the eyes.
2. Avoid high-concentration products on the skin, particularly with children.
3. Do not inhale or ingest repellents.
4. Use long-sleeved clothing and apply repellent to fabric rather than to skin.
5. Don't use repellent on children's hands, which may be rubbed in the eyes or placed in the mouth.
6. Do not reapply repellent in normal weather conditions.
7. Wash repellent off the skin after the insect bite risk has ended.

Permethrin (Permanone Tick Repellent; Duranon Tick Repellent) is a synthetic form of pyrethrin (contact insecticide) that may be applied to clothing and footwear. A single application is usually good for 1 to 2 weeks, or 20 washings. It is effective against ticks and mosquitoes. N-octyl bicycloheptene dicarboximide synergist combined with DEET (Sawyer Products' Gold; S. C. Johnson's Ticks OFF or Deep Woods OFF) is a tick repellent, also effective against biting flies and gnats, that can be applied directly to the skin.

PermaKill 4 Week Tick Killer is a 13.3% permethrin liquid concentrate that is diluted (⅓ oz, or 10 ml, in 16 oz, or 473 ml, of water) to be sprayed from a pump bottle. It can also be diluted 2 oz (59 ml) in 1½ (355 ml) cups of water to soak a bed net, shirt, and pants, which are then air-dried.

Fleas, horseflies, blackflies, sand flies, deerflies, chiggers, gnats, and other assorted nuisances may not be driven away by insect repellents. Protective netting and a lot of swatting may be your only defenses. A head net may be invaluable during times of high mosquito infestation. If you use a bed net, be certain that it is free of holes and has its edges tucked in. The net needs to be woven to a tightness of 18 threads per inch (6 to 7 per cm). Tighter mesh may hinder ventilation and create an uncomfortable environment. A net that has been dipped in an insecticide, usually permethrin, is more effective.

Electric-light traps with electrocution grids, ultrasound devices, and audible sound devices have not been shown scientifically to repel insects or to decrease the concentration of biting insects in their vicinity.

To date, plant products, with the potential future exception of an extract of eucalyptus oil, do not appear to repel insects as well as DEET. Although allspice, bay, camphor, cedar, cinnamon, citronella, geranium, lavender, nutmeg, pennyroyal, peppermint, pine, thyme, and verbena may have repellent properties, they are limited in effectiveness in comparison to DEET.

Leeches

Leeches are parasitic annelid worms that live on land or in water. They attach to human skin with a painless bite in order to extract blood through the skin. Some of them release a substance called hirudin, which is an anti-coagulant (causes increased tendency to bleed). Aquatic leeches are found in fresh water, and are considered more dangerous than those on land, because they can attach inside the mouth, throat, lungs, vagina, urethra, and other internal sites.

To remove a leech, don't pull it off—the residual sore may be larger. Instead, apply lemon juice, salt, vinegar, tobacco juice, or insect repellent. Using a lighted or recently extinguished match or glowing ember may cause a skin burn. If the detached leech sticks to your fingers, roll it between them. If a leech is attached to someone's eye, shine a flashlight close to it; it may move toward the light and away from the eye. The medical considerations for a leech bite are itching (see page 444) and secondary infection (see page 247). Insect repellents (see page 347), particularly DEET applied to clothing and skin, will discourage leech attachment. Slippery grease (such as petroleum jelly) applied to exposed skin may also help. Wear waterproof boots when wading in leech-infested water, and tuck in pant legs.

LIGHTNING STRIKE

Lightning strikes the earth at least 100 times per second during an estimated 3,000 thunderstorms per day. Fortunately, the odds of being struck by lightning are not very great. Still, 200 to 400 people per year are victims of fatal strikes in the United States. The wise traveler respects thunderstorms and seeks shelter at all times during a lightning storm.

Lightning is the direct-current electrical discharge associated with a thunderstorm; it releases an initial charge (the vast majority of which travels from ground [positive] to cloud [negative]) of approximately 30 million volts to neutralize a potential difference (within a hundredth to a ten-thousandth of a second) of 200 million to a billion volts. A lightning flash may be made up of multiple (up to 30) strokes, which causes lightning to seem to flicker. Each stroke lasts less than 500 milliseconds. The diameter of the main stroke is 2½ to 3" (6 to 8 cm); the temperature has been estimated to be anywhere from 14,432 to 90,032° F (8,000 to 50,000° C—four times as hot as the surface of the sun). Within milliseconds, the temperature falls to 3,632 to 5,432° F (2,000 to 3,000° C).

Thunder is attributed to the nearly explosive expansion of air heated and ionized by the stroke of lightning. To estimate the approximate distance in miles from your location to the lightning strike, time the difference in seconds between the flash of light and the onset of the thunder, and divide by five.

Lightning can injure a person in five ways:

1. Direct hit, which most often occurs in the open.
2. Splash, which occurs when lightning hits another object (tree, building). The current seeks the path of least resistance, and may jump to a human. Splashes may occur from person to person, or from a metal fence.
3. Contact, when a person is holding on to a conductive material that is hit or splashed by lightning.
4. Step (stride) voltage (or ground current), when lightning hits the ground or an object nearby. The current spreads like waves in a pond.
5. Blunt injury, which occurs from the victim's own muscle contractions and/or from the explosive force of the shock wave produced by the lightning strike. These can combine to cause the victim to be thrown, sometimes a considerable distance.

When lightning strikes a person directly, splashes at him from a tree or building, or is conducted along the ground, it usually largely flows around the outside of the body (flashover phenomenon), which causes a unique constellation of signs and symptoms. The victim is frequently thrown, clothes may be burned or torn ("exploded" off by the instantaneous conversion of sweat to steam), metallic objects (such as belt buckles) may be heated, and shoes removed. The victim often undergoes severe muscle contractions—sufficient to dislocate limbs. In most cases, the person struck is confused and rendered temporarily blind and/or deaf. In some cases, there are linear 1 (½ to 2", or 1.3 to 5 cm, wide, following areas of heavy sweat concentration), "feathered" (fernlike; keraunographism; Lichtenberg's flowers—cutaneous imprints from electron showers that track over the skin) (see figure 197A) or "sunburst" patterns of punctate burns over the skin (see figure 197B), loss of consciousness, ruptured eardrums, and inability to breathe. Occasionally, the victim ceases breathing and suffers a cardiac arrest. Seizures or direct brain damage may occur. Eye injuries occur in half of victims.

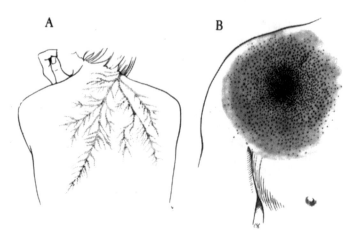

Figure 197. (A) Ferning lightning burn. (B) Punctate (starburst) lightning burn.

A victim struck by lightning may not remember the flash or thunder, or even recognize that he has been hit. The confusion, muscle aches, body tingling, and amnesia can last for days. With a more severe case, the skin may be mottled, the legs and/or arms may be paralyzed, and it may be difficult to locate a pulse in the radial (wrist) artery (see page 26), because the muscles in the wall of the artery are in spasm. First-, second-, or third-degree skin burns may be present. Broken bones are not uncommon.

If a person is found confused, burned, or collapsed in the vicinity of a thunderstorm, consider the possibility that he was struck by lightning. The victim is not "electrified" or "charged"—you will not be jolted or stunned if you touch him.

1. Maintain the airway and assist breathing (see page 24). Continue to perform artificial respiration and CPR (see page 28) until sophisticated help can be obtained. Victims of lightning strike may have paralysis of the breathing mechanism for a period of 15 to 30 minutes, and then make a remarkable recovery. A seemingly lifeless individual may be saved if you breathe for him promptly after the injury. Do not assume that dilated or nonreactive (to light—see page 30) pupils are a sign of death, because they may represent direct injury to the eye(s).

2. Assume that the victim has been thrown a considerable distance. Protect the cervical spine (see page 31).

3. Examine the victim for any other injuries and treat accordingly.

4. Transport the victim to a hospital.

5. If you are in the vicinity of a thunderstorm, seek shelter for the victim and yourself. Lightning *can* strike twice in the same place!

Lightning Avoidance

1. Know the weather patterns for your area. Don't travel in times of high thunderstorm risk. Avoid being outdoors during a thunderstorm. Carry a radio to monitor weather reports. Lightning can lash out from many miles in front of a storm cloud, in seemingly clear weather. If you calculate that a nearby lightning strike is within 3 miles (5 km) of your location, anticipate that the next strike will be in your immediate area.

2. If a storm enters your area, immediately seek shelter. Enter a hard-roofed auto or large building, if possible. Tents and convertible autos offer little or no protection from lightning. Tent poles are lightning rods. Metal sheds are dangerous because of the risk of side splashes. Indoors, stay away from windows, open doors, fireplaces, and large metal fixtures.

3. Do not carry a lightning rod, such as a fishing pole or golf club. Avoid tall objects, such as ski lifts and power lines. Avoid being near boat masts or flagpoles. Do not seek refuge near power lines or tall metal structures. If you are in a boat, try to get out of the water. If you are swimming in the water, get out. Do not stand near a metal boat. Insulate yourself from ground current by crouching on a sleeping pad, backpack, or coiled rope.

4. Move off ridges and summits. In the woods, avoid the tallest trees (stay at a distance from the tree that's at least equal to the tree's height) or hilltops. Shelter yourself in a stand of smaller trees. Avoid clearings—you become the tallest tree. Don't stay at or near the top of a peak or ridge. Avoid cave entrances. In the open, crouch down or roll into a ball.

5. Stay in your car. If it is a convertible, huddle on the ground at least 50 yards (46 m) from the vehicle.

6. If you are part of a group of people, spread the group out so that everyone isn't struck by a single discharge.

7. If your hair stands on end, you hear high-pitched or crackling noises, or see a blue halo (St. Elmo's fire) around objects, there is electrical activity near you that precedes a lightning strike. If you can't get away from the area immediately, crouch down on the balls of your feet and keep your head down. Don't touch the ground with your hands.

Tornado Avoidance

1. Watch the cloud formations in a stormy sky. If you see revolving, funnel-shaped clouds, you are in danger.

2. Take shelter immediately. The best location is an underground cave or concrete structure. Do not remain in a tent or camper.

3. If you are caught outside in open country, hunker down or lie flat in a depression, ditch, culvert, or ravine. Cover your head with your arms.

4. Do not try to outrun a tornado. There is no way to predict when it will change direction.

What to Do in an Earthquake

If you are caught in an earthquake in a wilderness setting, do the following:

1. Seek a safe location, out of the path of a rockfall, mudslide, or snow avalanche. If you can, move into a clearing away from buildings, trees, and power lines. If the ground shaking is extreme, position yourself on your hands and knees.

    If you are in a moving vehicle, drive to a clearing and stay in the vehicle until the shaking stops.

    If you are indoors, stay put until you are certain that it's safe to go outside. Move away from glass windows.

2. Eliminate any obvious fire hazards. If you are in a cabin supplied with natural gas, turn it off at the source if there is any odor or you believe there might be a leak.

3. Be prepared for aftershocks.

4. Secure a supply of drinking water. Be certain that you are prepared for a period of time without electrical power.

5. Prepare a shelter, store sufficient food, and locate equipment necessary for survival. Keep first-aid supplies and a flashlight within easy reach.

UNDERWATER DIVING ACCIDENTS AND NEAR-DROWNING

On land at sea level, the human body is constantly exposed to 14.7 lb (6.7 kg, or 1 atmosphere) of pressure due to the weight of the atmosphere (an air column 165 miles, or 266 km, high). As a human descends under water

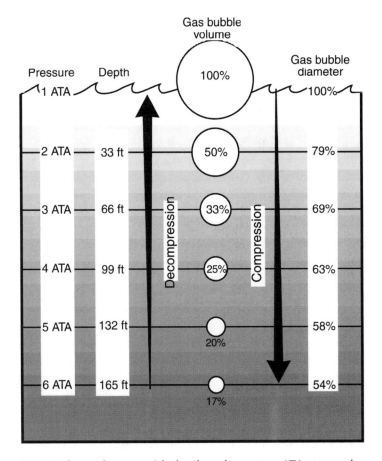

Figure 198. Volume changes with depth and pressure. ATA=atmosphere.

in the ocean, with every 33 feet (13 m) of depth an additional atmosphere of pressure is exerted. With increasing pressure (P) that occurs on descent, the volume (V) of gas in an enclosed space is diminished, as determined by Boyle's law: $P_1V_1 = P_2V_2$. Conversely, during ascent from the depths, the gas in an enclosed space expands. Under water, the greatest relative volume changes with increasing and decreasing pressure occur near the surface (figure 198).

Air Embolism

An air embolism occurs when there is a rupture in the barrier between the microscopic air space of a lung and its corresponding blood vessel, which carries oxygenated blood back to the heart (where it can be distributed to the body). In effect, bubbles of air are released into the arterial bloodstream, where they act as physical barriers to circulation, and can cause a stroke (see page 129), heart attack (see page 45), headache, and/or confusion. Typically, the victim is a scuba (self-contained underwater breathing apparatus) diver who ascends too rapidly without exhaling, thus allowing overexpansion of the lungs—and rupture of the tissue—as the external water pressure decreases with ascent. In other words, as a diver ascends from the depths, the air in his lungs (which was delivered from the scuba tank through a regulator at a pressure equal to the surrounding water pressure on the lungs, thereby allowing lung expansion) expands. If the rate of exhalation does not keep pace with the lung expansion, the increased pressure within the lungs causes air to be forced through the lung tissue, where it appears in the bloodstream in bubble form and travels directly to the heart. From the heart, the air circulates to and may occlude critical small blood vessels that supply the heart, brain, and spinal cord.

The most common symptoms are unconsciousness, confusion or disorientation, seizures, and/or chest pain immediately upon surfacing. Others include dizziness, visual blurring, abnormal personality, paralysis, and weakness. Any disorder that appears in a previously normal diver more than 10 minutes after surfacing is probably not due to air embolism.

Anyone suspected of having suffered an air embolism should be placed in a head-down position (with the body at a 15- to 30-degree tilt), turned onto his left side, be assisted with breathing if necessary (see page 24), and *immediately transported to an emergency facility.* If oxygen (see page 383) is available, it should be administered by face mask at a flow rate of 10 liters per minute. The treatment for arterial gas embolism is recompression in a hyperbaric oxygen chamber, which pressurizes the victim's environment and shrinks the bubbles. This must be accomplished as rapidly as possible to save the victim's life and to minimize disability. A portable recompression chamber manned by trained personnel may be utilized to initiate field treatment. If the victim is capable of purposeful swallowing, administer one adult aspirin by mouth.

If the air that expands on ascent does not rupture into a blood vessel and become an air embolism, it can rupture into the actual lung tissues or into the pleural space between the lung and the inside of the chest wall, and cause a collapsed lung (pneumothorax) (see page 35). In this case, oxygen administration is advised. Recompression in a hyperbaric chamber is not advised for a pneumothorax unless there are also severe symptoms associated with an air embolism.

When transporting a victim of air embolism, it is recommended that you use an aircraft that can be pressurized to 1 atmosphere (such as a Lear jet, Hercules C-130, or Cessna Citation), or keep the flight altitude (in an unpressurized aircraft) below 1,000' (305 m).

The Divers Alert Network at Duke University Medical Center (919-684-8111) provides a 24-hour hotline to assist in the management of all significant diving accidents, as well as evacuation to a facility with a hyperbaric chamber.

Decompression Sickness (the "Bends")

When a scuba diver descends in the water, nitrogen present in the compressed air he breathes is absorbed into the tissues of his body. This process is analogous to the introduction of carbon dioxide into a beverage for the purpose of carbonation. In the human case, there is a limit to the time and depth that a diver can tolerate before exceeding the amount of nitrogen he can absorb safely without a staged decompression (ascent). If this limit is exceeded, and/or if the diver ascends too rapidly, this nitrogen leaves his tissues and enters his bloodstream in the form of microscopic bubbles (like opening a bottle of soda pop).

The signs and symptoms caused by these bubbles in the body represent decompression sickness, also known as the "bends." Symptoms may begin immediately after ascent from a dive or may be delayed by a number of hours. These include joint pain, numbness and tingling of the arms and legs, difficulty walking, back pain, fatigue, weakness, inability to control the bladder or bowels (spinal cord "hit"), paralysis, headache, confusion, dizziness, nausea, vomiting, difficulty in speaking, itching, skin mottling ("marbling"), shortness of breath, cough, and collapse. A rapid, simplified neurological exam (see page 129), such as administered to a suspected stroke victim, may identify a subtle abnormality.

If you suspect someone of suffering the bends, immediately have him begin to breathe oxygen (at a flow rate of 10 liters per minute by face mask) (see page 383) and begin rapid transport to an emergency facility. Oxygen breathing should occur for at least 30 minutes. The definitive treatment is recompression in a hyperbaric chamber. *Do not put the diver back into the water to attempt in-water recompression;* this is very hazardous. If possible, have the victim lie down in a comfortable position, preferably on his side, but do not let him obstruct blood flow to a limb by resting his head on an arm or crossing his legs. A portable recompression chamber manned by trained personnel may be utilized to initiate field treatment.

Because the pressure inside a commercial jet aircraft flying at 30,000' (9,150 m) is equivalent to an unpressurized environmental altitude of 8,000' (2,440 m), a diver should not fly for 24 hours following a scuba dive. When transporting a victim of decompression sickness, it is recommended that you use an aircraft that can be pressurized to 1 atmosphere (such as a Lear jet, Hercules C-130, or Cessna Citation), or keep the flight altitude (in an unpressurized aircraft) below 1,000' (305 m).

The Divers Alert Network at Duke University Medical Center (919-684-8111) provides a 24-hour hotline to assist in the management of all significant diving accidents, as well as evacuation to a facility with a hyperbaric chamber.

Nitrogen Narcosis

When absorbed into the bloodstream in sufficient concentration, nitrogen acts as an anesthetic agent. Thus, at depths that exceed 90' (27 m), divers are at risk for euphoria, confusion, inappropriate judgment, and unconsciousness induced by nitrogen absorbed into the bloodstream from air breathed under pressure. The treatment is prompt (but cautious) ascent, to allow the absorbed levels of nitrogen to decrease. *No one should ever dive alone. Always pay attention to your dive buddy's behavior. If he acts in a strange manner, assist him to the surface.*

Ear Squeeze

As a diver descends in the water, the external water pressure on his eardrum increases rapidly. If he cannot equalize this pressure from within by forcing air into the eustachian tube (a small passageway that connects the middle ear and the throat) and into the middle ear, the eardrum stretches inward (extremely painful) and then ruptures (figure 199). This rupture allows water to rush into the middle ear, with resultant severe pain, hearing loss, vertigo (see page 154), nausea, vomiting, and disorientation. If the diver cannot make his way to the surface, he may drown. If the eardrum is injured but not ruptured, the pain is similar to that of an ear infection.

Inability to "clear" the ears (equalize pressure from within) in order to prevent inward bulging and rupture of the eardrum should keep a diver out of the water. A person with an upper respiratory tract infection (and narrowed eustachian tube) should not dive, and should avoid travel in an unpressurized aircraft.

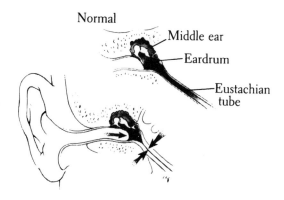

Figure 199. Middle ear squeeze. When a diver descends, air in the middle ear contracts, the eustachian tube collapses, and the eardrum bulges inward, causing pain. If the external water pressure is sufficient, the eardrum can rupture.

If a diver suddenly feels pain in his ear and is stricken with dizziness, nausea, or visual difficulty, he should remain calm and slowly ascend to the surface. The ear should be allowed to drain and dry on its own. Do not insert cotton swabs into the ear, because you may poke the eardrum and increase the damage. Do not instill any medicines into the ear, unless you are carrying Cortisporin suspension (*not* "solution"). Transport the victim to an ear specialist. Suspend all diving activities until the eardrum is healed or repaired. If dizziness is profound, administer a drug(s) for motion sickness (see page 390). The victim should be started on an antibiotic (ciprofloxacin, trimethoprim-sulfamethoxazole, or doxycycline) to oppose *Vibrio* bacteria. If one of these antibiotics is not available, use amoxicillin-clavulanate. An oral or topical nasal decongestant (such as 0.5% oxymetazoline) is useful for the first few days after the episode. Because sudden dizziness may also be due to an air embolism or the bends, the victim should be observed closely for worsening of his condition.

Sinus Squeeze

Sinus squeeze occurs if pressurized air cannot be forced into the sinuses during descent. In such a case, the air within the sinus contracts, causing the walls of the sinus to bleed, accompanied by intense, sharp pain. Symptoms include pain over the affected sinus, in the upper teeth (when the maxillary, or cheek, sinus is involved), and nosebleed. A "reverse squeeze" occurs during ascent, when air expands in the sinus without being able to escape. This is also very painful, but fortunately self-limited, because the air will be absorbed slowly into the tissues that line the sinuses.

If a sinus squeeze occurs, slowly ascend to the surface. This generally alleviates most of the pain, but it may take a while for the bleeding to stop. Because the sinus may now be blood filled, the victim is at high risk for developing sinusitis (see page 172) and should be placed on amoxicillin-clavulanate or erythromycin for 4 days, along with oral and nasal decongestants to promote drainage. If the pain is severe and persists for more than 12 hours after the initial incident, the victim may benefit from a short course of prednisone: 60 mg the first day, 40 mg the second, and 20 mg the third. This combats the inflammation, but should not be given if the victim has symptoms of a sinus infection (foul nasal discharge, fever, facial tenderness).

Tooth Squeeze

Increasing pressure during descent into the water can cause entrapped gas in the interior of a tooth or in the structures surrounding a tooth to contract. In an extreme case, this can cause a tooth to crack or implode. Conversely, air under a filling or within a cavity or abscess can expand on ascent, causing a minor (and painful) "explosion." To minimize the risk of a tooth squeeze, do not enter the water for at least 24 hours after dental treatment.

Near-Drowning

One of the most common tragic accidents, particularly of children, is near-drowning. This can occur in a variety of settings, but the problems encountered seldom vary:

1. Lack of oxygen. This occurs because the lung tissue is injured by water, and oxygen transfer into the bloodstream is inhibited. Another factor is occasional spasm of the vocal cords, which blocks the passage of air through the windpipe (most commonly seen in cold-water drowning).
2. Body chemistry abnormalities. Because of the lack of oxygen delivery to the organs and tissues of the body, there is rapid accumulation of waste products that cannot be effectively removed. This results in an

accumulation of acid and other chemicals that alter the function of the heart, brain, kidneys, liver, and so on.

3. Accompanying problems, such as hypothermia (see page 269), injuries, and serious illnesses (for example, heart attack or stroke). Sadly, alcohol figures prominently in adult boating and near-drowning accidents.

If a near-drowning incident occurs, do the following:

1. *Send someone for help.*
2. Suspect a broken neck in the appropriate circumstances. For instance, someone who has been seen to collapse in a swimming pool probably hasn't broken his neck. (If he dove into the pool, that is another story!) However, someone who tumbles into the waves off a surfboard and washes up unconscious onto the beach may well have a neck injury. Do what is necessary to aid the victim, but remember to protect his neck (see page 31).
3. Check for breathing by feeling over the mouth and nose while watching the chest rise. Open the mouth and sweep it clean with two fingers. Align the victim on the ground with his head at a level below his feet. Begin mouth-to-mouth or mouth-to-mouth-and-nose (for a child) breathing, if necessary (see page 24).
4. Check for pulses and begin chest compressions if necessary (see page 28).
5. If it is impossible to perform mouth-to-mouth breathing because the stomach is full (most victims swallow a fair amount of water in the drowning process), turn the victim on his side (with his head at a level below his feet) and perform the Heimlich maneuver (see page 22). Sweep the mouth clear and resume mouth-to-mouth breathing. The Heimlich maneuver used in this fashion is to empty the stomach, not the lungs, of water. It should not be used routinely in the rescue of near-drowning victims. However, if the victim is nonbreathing and in the water, where mouth-to-mouth breathing is difficult or impractical, a few brisk Heimlich "hugs" applied to the chest may stimulate the victim to cough and begin breathing on his own.
6. Hypothermia (see page 269) is commonly associated with near-drowning. Cover the victim above and below with blankets. Gently remove all wet clothing. Because hypothermia may be protective for the heart and brain (with regard to lack of oxygen) to a considerable degree, if the victim is cold, continue the resuscitation until trained rescuers arrive or until you are fatigued (see page 274). Remember, "no one is dead until he is warm and dead."

7. If the victim responds to your measures, he should be transported to an emergency facility. Even if he feels 100% normal, he should still be evaluated by a physician, because delayed worsening of lung function is possible. A person who is already short of breath and coughing may deteriorate quickly.

8. Administer oxygen (see page 383) at a flow rate of 10 liters per minute by face mask.

Prevention of Near-Drowning

1. Watch your children. Toddlers are at greatest risk for near-drowning.

2. Fence in all pools and swimming areas. Maintain the water level in a pool as high as possible to allow a person who reaches the edge to pull himself out.

3. Teach all children to swim.

4. Never place nonswimmers in high-risk situations: small sailboats, white-water rafts, inflatable kayaks, and the like.

5. When boating or rafting, always wear a properly rated life vest with a snug fit and a head flotation collar. In a kayak or raft traversing white-water, wear a proper helmet.

6. Do not mix alcohol and water sports.

7. Know your limits. Feats of endurance and demonstrations of bravado in dangerous rapids or surf are for idiots.

8. Be prepared for a flash flood. In times of unusually heavy rainfall, stay away from natural streambeds, arroyos, and other drainage channels. Use a map to determine your elevation and stay off low ground or the very bottom of a hill. Know where the high ground is and how to get there in a hurry. Absolutely avoid flooded areas and unnecessary stream and river crossings. Do not attempt to cross a flowing stream where the water is above your knees. Abandon a stalled vehicle in a flood area.

ANIMAL ATTACKS

Most animal attacks are from "man's best friend," the pet dog. Other animals that will attack humans, given provocation, include the cat, rat, tiger, lion, skunk, squirrel, camel, elephant, bear, alligator, crocodile, bat, wolf, rhinoceros, and hippopotamus. Although there are unique variations to the nature of the wounds created by different animals (in most part related to the size of the animal, types of teeth and claws, and risk of infection), the basic out-of-hospital management of an animal bite or mauling is the same for all creatures.

General Treatment

1. If a person is bitten or mauled by an animal, apply pressure to stop any brisk bleeding, and follow the instructions for management of bleeding and cuts (see pages 48 and 227).

2. It is important to clean the wounds well. Flush any injury that has broken the skin with at least 2 quarts (liters) of disinfected water, scrub with mild soap, and flush again. If you are carrying povidone iodine (Betadine) solution 10% (not soap or scrub); benzalkonium (Zephiran) liquid 1% antiseptic; or, in a pinch, Bactine antiseptic (benzalkonium 0.13%), rinse the wound with one of these for 1 minute (to help kill rabies virus), then rinse away the solution until there is no discoloration of the wound.

3. Do not sew or tape closed any animal bite, unless it is absolutely essential to allow rescue. If a large tear is present, the wound edges can be held together with tape and wraps (see page 229). Tight closure of a contaminated wound (all animal bites and scratches introduce bacteria into the wound) can lead to a devastating infection. Apply a thin layer of bacitracin or mupirocin ointment or mupirocin cream into the wound.

4. If the victim is more than 5 hours from a physician, administer cefuroxime axetil, dicloxacillin, amoxicillin–clavulanic acid, cefixime, cephalexin, trimethoprim-sulfamethoxazole, or ciprofloxacin. If the bite is from a cat, domestic or wild, administer an antibiotic as soon as possible. If an animal bite becomes infected, the same antibiotics are recommended, with the exception that for cat (domestic and "big" cat) bites, dicloxacillin should be given with penicillin.

Special Considerations

High-Risk Wounds

Wounds at high risk for infection include bites to the hands and feet, and all puncture wounds (see page 225). These should be rinsed copiously and never cinched shut by any method. Anyone who sustains such a wound should be given antibiotics for 4 days (see step 4 on page 363). Cat, human, and primate bites are enormously prone to infection, and require prompt attention by a physician. In a typical human bite, which occurs when a closed fist strikes an opponent's teeth, the cut extends deeply into a knuckle and inoculates the underlying tendon sheath with saliva and bacteria. As the fist is opened, the wound becomes "closed," and an infection can develop quickly. If a human bite is incurred in this manner, splint the hand in the position of function (see figure 32) and administer cefuroxime axetil, ciprofloxacin plus erythromycin, or dicloxacillin plus ampicillin for 7 days.

Rabies

Rabies virus infection occurs more frequently in wild than in domestic animals. In some foreign countries where immunization of animals is infrequently practiced, the risk is great even in domesticated animals. The virus is carried in saliva and is transmitted by bite or lick (if the skin is broken). It has been transmitted in aerosolized saliva from bats in caves. Raccoons, dogs, cats, foxes, coyotes, skunks, wolves, bats, woodchucks, and groundhogs are the most common carriers. Rabies has not been reported in bears. Although rabbits, mice, squirrels, chipmunks, rats, guinea pigs, and ferrets may be rabid, they are rarely involved in the transmission of rabies to humans. Domestic animals such as cattle, horses, and sheep become infected in regions where skunk or raccoon rabies is found.

Animals with rabies show abnormal behavior. In the "furious" phase, they are hyperactive, may have a fever, are overtly aggressive, and salivate excessively. With "dumb" rabies, they appear tired, lack coordination, and may become paralyzed.

Because of rabies risk, all wild animal bites or scratches, and bites or scratches of unregistered or strangely behaving cats and dogs, should be reported to the appropriate public health authority. If the animal is a pet with otherwise normal behavior, it should be observed for 10 days. If the animal is rabid, it will become very ill or die during that time, and its brain tissue can be analyzed for the presence of rabies. If the animal is a pet with unusual behavior, or a captured high-risk wild animal, it should be killed and examined. *If it is a high-risk animal and cannot be captured, it must be presumed to be rabid.*

Immediately scrub an animal bite wound or a wound that has been licked by a potentially rabid animal vigorously with soap and water. If benzalkonium chloride 1% (Zephiran); 10% povidone iodine (Betadine) solution (less effective); or, in a pinch, Bactine (benzalkonium 0.13%) antiseptic is available, one of these should be used to irrigate and deeply swab the wound, since they may kill rabies virus.

If rabies is a consideration, the victim should seek the assistance of a physician, who will determine the need for postexposure rabies vaccination (a series of five injections) and injections of antirabies serum (human rabies immune globulin; half is injected around the bite wound, and half intramuscularly). A person who has been previously immunized against rabies still needs two booster doses of rabies vaccine after high-risk contact with a rabid animal.

Preexposure vaccination against rabies should be administered to people at high risk of exposure (animal handlers, cavers, hunters, and trappers in rabies-endemic areas, along with travelers to certain foreign countries). This is given as a series of three injections over 30 days.

The incubation period of rabies ranges from 9 days to more than 1 year, but is usually between 2 and 16 weeks. The first symptoms are fatigue, weakness, anxiety, irritability, fever, headache, nausea and vomiting, sore throat, abdominal pain, and loss of appetite. Some victims complain of numbness and tingling where they were initially bitten. After a few days to 2 weeks, the virus shows its devastating effect upon the nervous system, with symptoms of increased agitation, hyperactivity, seizures, hallucinations, uncontrollable behavior, and inability to drink (hydrophobia) due to muscle spasms in the throat. This constellation is called "furious rabies." With "dumb" rabies, a person becomes progressively weak, uncoordinated, and paralyzed. Unfortunately, rabies is virtually always fatal, with the terminal events being one or more of coma, respiratory failure, seizures, abnormal heart rhythms, paralysis, and pneumonia.

Skunks

In addition to biting a person and inoculating him with rabies virus, a skunk can spray secretions from its anal sacs. The main component of skunk musk is butyl mercaptan, which carries a horrible odor and causes skin irritation, eye redness and temporary blindness, and occasional seizures or loss of consciousness. The odor can be neutralized by strong oxidizing agents, such as household bleach diluted 1:5 with water. This solution can then be washed away with tincture of green soap, followed by a more dilute bleach rinse. Tomato juice has been recommended to deodorize hair, which may need to be bleached or cut short.

Bubonic Plague

Cases of bubonic plague are still reported in the United States. The disease is transmitted by the bites of fleas that have acquired the plague bacillus, *Yersinia pestis,* from infected squirrels, rats, prairie dogs, chipmunks, marmots, rabbits, and mice. Rarely, the disease can be contracted from direct contact with infected pets, particularly cats. It can also be contracted from skinning an infected wild animal, such as a coyote or bobcat.

The incubation period for bubonic plague is 2 to 6 days after exposure. At first, the victim complains of high fever, chills, severe fatigue, abdominal pain, vomiting, diarrhea, muscle aches, and headache. At the same time, he develops extremely enlarged and tender lymph nodes associated with the entry point for the disease, such as in the groin if an insect bite has occurred on the leg. Thereafter, as the bacteria overwhelm the victim, he may collapse and develop a skin rash with large dark patches of hemorrhage ("Black Death"). If pneumonia develops, the victim coughs bloody sputum.

Treatment should be initiated promptly, and requires intramuscular or intravenous antibiotics. If you are isolated away from a hospital, start the victim on tetracycline 1 g for the first dose, then 50 mg per kg (2.2 lb) of body weight in six divided doses every 4 hours for the first day, then 30 mg per kg of body weight in four divided doses every 6 hours for 14 days. This is extremely suboptimal therapy; the victim needs to get to a hospital as soon as possible.

The disease is contagious. All adults in direct face-to-face contact with a victim suffering from plague pneumonia (cough productive of sputum) should take tetracycline 500 mg four times a day, or trimethoprim-sulfamethoxazole one double-strength tablet twice a day, for 8 days. Children should take a pediatric dose of trimethoprim-sulfamethoxazole for 8 days. All contact people should have their temperature measured twice a day. If anyone develops a fever greater than 100° F (37.7° C), he should begin taking an antibiotic and be taken immediately to a physician.

With regard to prevention, pay attention to local public health warnings and do not travel with pets in areas of plague infestation. Take care to spray or dust your canine and feline companions with flea repellent regularly (after each time they get wet) when traveling in wooded areas. Do not allow children to handle small dead animals.

Preexposure immunization against plague is available (see page 401). If you have not been immunized against plague and will be actively exposed to plague-infected animals, ingest tetracycline 500 mg four times a day during the period of exposure.

Hantavirus Pulmonary (Lung) Syndrome

Hantaviruses (such as the sin nombre virus) cause a syndrome characterized by a combination of fever, lung failure, kidney failure, shock, and bleeding. The viruses are spread in the excreta of rodents; in the United States, hantavirus pulmonary syndrome (HPS) has been linked to the deer mouse, *Peromyscus maniculatus*, as well as to the cotton mouse. The animals shed the virus in saliva, urine, and feces.

HPS has now been reported in most states west of the Mississippi River, as well as in a few eastern states. In Louisiana and Florida, two new hantavirus species, bayou virus and Black Creek virus, have been identified. A person infected by the virus first suffers from fever, muscle aches, headache, cough, dizziness, abdominal pain, nausea and vomiting, and diarrhea for a few days; this is followed by difficulty breathing, mottled skin on the limbs, shock, and, sometimes, bleeding. Up to 75% of victims may die.

Most victims have had an interaction with rodents, such as when cleaning a barn or capturing the animals. Unfortunately, there is not yet any specific therapy beyond supportive care, although the antiviral agent ribavirin may prove useful.

To avoid unnecessary exposure to hantavirus, it is recommended that wilderness enthusiasts observe the following precautions: Keep food and water covered and stored in rodent-proof containers; dispose of food clutter; spray dead rodents, nests, and droppings with disinfectant prior to handling (wear gloves); clean and disinfect cabins and other shelters thoroughly before using; don't make camp near rodent sites; don't sleep on bare ground; burn or bury garbage promptly; and use only bottled or disinfected water for campsite purposes.

Avoidance of Hazardous Animals

Most wild animal encounters can be avoided with caution and a little common sense. Follow these rules:

1. Do not provoke animals. Unless they are apex predators, starving, senile, or ill, most animals will not attack humans without provocation. Do not corner or provoke a carnivore, and do not tease an animal by handling it or approaching its young.
2. Do not disturb a feeding animal. Do not explore into its feeding territory or disrupt mating patterns.

3. Do not separate fighting animals using your bare hands. If possible, drive animals apart using a long stick or club.
4. In bear country, hang all food off the ground in trees away from the campsite. Never keep food or captured game inside a tent. Make noise when hiking, particularly on narrow paths or through tall grass. If attacked by a bear, do not try to outrun it; you can't. Cover your head and the back of your neck with your arms and curl into a fetal position.
5. Never leave a small child alone with an animal, regardless of the animal's demeanor.

WILD PLANT AND MUSHROOM POISONING

Toxic plants and mushrooms may be eaten by curious children, or by hikers and amateur herbalists who mistake their selections for edible species. *Never eat wild plants, mushrooms, roots, or berries unless you know what you're doing.*

Medical History

Although the narrative description of the ingestion will have little bearing on the immediate management of a toxic ingestion, it is important to gather as much information as possible for the benefit of the physician who will ultimately care for the victim:

1. When was the plant eaten?
2. What parts of the plant were eaten? How many different plants were eaten?
3. What symptoms does the victim have? What were the initial symptoms (sweating, hallucinations, vomiting, abdominal pain)? What was the time interval between the ingestion and the onset of symptoms? Did anyone who did not eat the plant(s) develop similar symptoms? Did everyone who ate the plant(s) become ill?
4. Was the plant eaten raw or was it cooked? How was it cooked? Was alcohol consumed within 72 hours of the plant ingestion?

It is also important to obtain as much of the original plant as possible for identification. If the patient vomits, save his vomitus, because it may contain part of the plant or spores that can be identified by an expert.

There are few specific antidotes for toxic plant ingestions, so most victims are managed according to their symptoms, which may include sweating, nausea, vomiting, diarrhea, shortness of breath, slow or rapid heartbeat, pinpoint or dilated pupils, salivation, increased frequency of urination, weakness, difficulty breathing, hallucinations, and many others.

Treatment for Poisonings

If it is known that someone has ingested a toxic plant or mushroom within the last 2 hours, he should immediately be forced to vomit (if he has not already done so). This may be done by administering syrup of ipecac (adult or child older than 6 years—dose 2 tbsp, or 30 ml; pediatric dose, age between 12 months and 6 years, 1 tbsp, or 15 ml) followed by at least a pint (473 ml) of warm water (½ pint, or 237 ml, for a small child). If ipecac is not available, have the victim ingest 2 tbsp (15 ml) of dishwashing soap, such as Ivory or Joy (not automatic dishwasher soap), followed by the water. If the victim is drowsy, do not induce vomiting. After vomiting is induced, immediately seek the attention of a physician.

Children will eat just about anything. Nontoxic ingestions include stones, dirt, sand, candles, sunscreen, shampoo, and single doses of birth control pills, antacids, laxatives, and vitamins (without iron). Keep all toxic substances, particularly camp-stove fuel, kerosene, iodine crystals (for water disinfection), and prescription drugs, out of the reach of small children.

Commonly Ingested Toxic Plants and Mushrooms

1. Oleander (see figure 200) is a shrub, up to 20' (6 m) tall, commonly found along highways and in gardens. It carries attractive clusters of red, pink, or white flowers. The entire plant is toxic, including smoke from burning cuttings and water in which the flowers are placed. There have been deaths from use of the branches as skewers for roasting hot dogs. Symptoms begin 1 to 2 hours after ingestion and include nausea, vomiting, abdominal cramps, diarrhea, confusion, and blurred vision. In serious ingestions, the heart's rhythm may be disturbed.

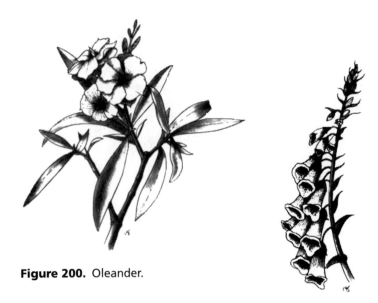

Figure 200. Oleander.

Figure 201. Foxglove.

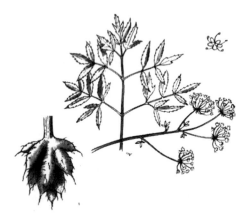

Figure 202. Water hemlock, with tuberous roots.

2. Foxglove (figure 201) is a European import that has toxic leaves and toxic tubular pink or purple flowers. Poisonings occur from ingestion of the plant parts or from foxglove tea. The symptoms are the same as those of oleander ingestion.

3. Water hemlock ("beaver poison") (figure 202) is found in salt- and freshwater marshes and along riverbanks. A member of the carrot family, the plant grows to 6' (1.8 m) and has clusters of whitish, heavily scented flowers, along with a bundle of tuberous roots. It is easily

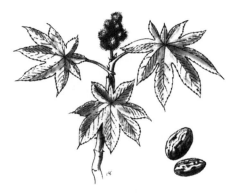

Figure 203. Castor bean.

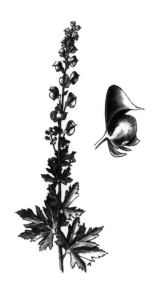

Figure 204. Monkshood.

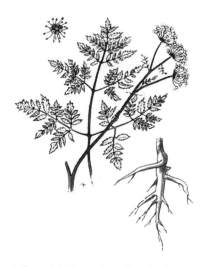

Figure 205. Poison hemlock.

confused with wild parsnip, celery, or sweet anise. When injured, the stem and trunk exude a yellow oil that smells like celery or raw parsnip. The entire plant is toxic. Symptoms begin 15 to 60 minutes after ingestion and include excessive salivation, abdominal pain, diarrhea, and vomiting. In a serious ingestion, the victim may suffer seizures and collapse, while having difficulty breathing. Death may occur.

4. Castor bean (figure 203) is a treelike shrub that may grow to 15' (4.6 m) with clusters of spiny seedpods, which contain seeds with coats that resemble pinto beans. The seeds contain a potent toxin (ricin) that

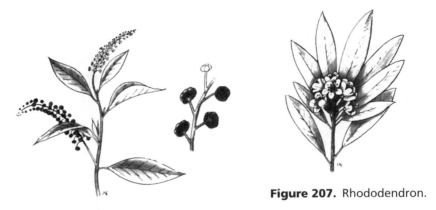

Figure 206. Pokeweed.

Figure 207. Rhododendron.

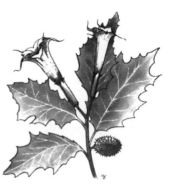

Figure 208. Jimsonweed.

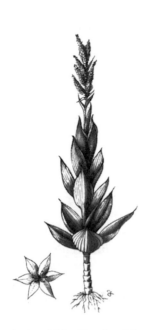

Figure 209. Skunk cabbage.

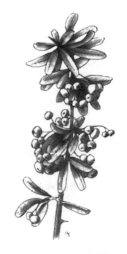

Figure 210. Pyracantha.

causes immediate mouth burning and abdominal pain, followed by vomiting, diarrhea, abnormal heart rhythms, and collapse.

5. Monkshood (figure 204) is a flowering plant with tuberous roots and blue helmet-shaped flowers. The leaves and roots are particularly toxic. Ingestion causes immediate mouth and throat burning, followed by vomiting, diarrhea, headache, muscle cramps, sweating, drooling, blurred vision, and confusion. In a serious ingestion, there may be abnormal heart rhythms and collapse.

6. Poison hemlock (figure 205) is a marsh plant that grows to 9' (2.7 m) with leaves that resemble a carrot top. The white flowers are clustered and smell like urine if they are crushed. The seeds and white unbranched tuberous roots are also toxic. The symptoms are similar to those of water hemlock ingestion, without significant abdominal pain or diarrhea. Death may follow seizures or paralysis with breathing failure.

7. Pokeweed (figure 206) is a widely distributed plant with clusters of white flowers and plentiful round purple berries. Ingestion of the root (commonly mistaken for horseradish) or the berries (a favorite of children) causes the intoxication. Symptoms include sore mouth, tongue, and throat (delayed by 2 to 3 hours); thirst; nausea; vomiting; abdominal cramps; and diarrhea, which may become bloody. The illness can be severe and last for up to 2 days, particularly if the roots were ingested.

8. Rhododendrons (figure 207) are common flowering plants that contain a number of toxins. Poisoning has occurred following ingestion of honey made from the flower nectar. Symptoms include mouth burning, followed by drooling, vomiting, diarrhea, headache, and numbness and tingling. Serious ingestions cause weakness, blurred vision, seizures, and collapse.

9. Jimsonweed (figure 208) has white or purple flowers, with prickly seedpods. Adults sometimes ingest a tea made from the leaves or flowers. The entire plant is toxic. Symptoms include dry mouth, rapid heartbeat, hot and dry skin, weakness, difficulty in walking, dilated pupils, and inability to urinate. Severe poisonings cause fever and collapse.

10. Skunk cabbage (figure 209) is a marsh and forest plant that grows to 6' (1.8 m) and has broad pleated leaves. The entire plant is toxic and causes symptoms similar to those that follow ingestion of monkshood, but generally much less severe.

11. Pyracantha (figure 210) is a thorned shrub with white flowers and clusters of small red berries. Ingestion of the berries in large quantities causes nausea and diarrhea. Birds sometimes eat fermented

pyracantha berries and become intoxicated. Scratches from the thorns may cause a burning skin irritation.

12. *Amanita phalloides* (death cap) is a gilled mushroom (figure 211) with a shiny yellow to greenish cap found in the western United States. The entire mushroom is toxic and cannot be detoxified by cooking. Symptoms occur 6 to 12 hours after ingestion and include abdominal pain; persistent nausea, vomiting, or diarrhea; low blood pressure; and rapid heartbeat. The victim may appear normal for the next few days, but then rapidly shows signs of massive liver inflammation and destruction, which include jaundice (yellow skin and eyeballs, darkened urine), easy bleeding, and altered mental status. Fatalities are frequent with this species, as well as with *Galerina autumnalis*.

Most nonfatal mushroom toxins act rapidly, producing symptoms of nausea, vomiting, diarrhea, and headache within 1 to 4 hours. Severe abdominal pain and headache approximately 6 hours after ingestion are likely due to *Gyrometra esculenta*. Typically, diarrhea and vomiting caused by ingestion of *Amanita phalloides* are delayed by 6 to 12 hours. However, because most unknowledgeable mushroom foragers eat a mixture of species, a rapid onset of symptoms does not rule out a potentially disastrous ingestion. Approximately 7 to 10 species of the several thousand varieties of wild mushrooms in the United States can cause death by ingestion.

13. *Amanita muscaria* (fly agaric) is a gilled mushroom (figure 212) with a variably colored (yellow, red, warty, and so on) cap. Most poisonings are intentional, because people brew and drink *Amanita* tea for its hallucinogenic effects. Symptoms occur 30 minutes to 2 hours after ingestion and include euphoria, difficulty walking, dizziness, hallucinations, and blurred vision. Severe ingestions can result in seizures and death.

14. *Coprinus atramentarius* (inky cap) is a gilled fungus (figure 213) with a conical cap that liquefies and turns black when picked. If alcohol is consumed within 24 to 72 hours after ingestion of the fungus, the victim suffers abdominal pain, vomiting, sweating, facial flushing, and headaches. *Cortinarius rainierensis* may cause the victim to have enormous thirst and increased urination 3 to 17 days after ingestion, due to a toxic effect on the kidneys.

Many other plants (wild and houseplants) can cause illnesses if consumed in sufficient quantities (one apple seed will not poison you). When in doubt as to the identity of a plant ingested, its quantity, or its potential toxicity, it is wisest to immediately consult a certified Poison (Control) Center or a physician.

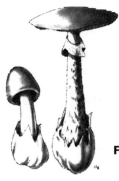

Figure 211. *Amanita phalloides* (death cap).

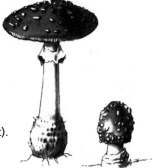

Figure 212. *Amanita muscaria* (fly agaric).

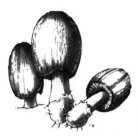

Figure 213. *Coprinus atramentarius* (inky cap).

Toxicity of Common Plants

The following list divides common plants into four groups:

T: TOXIC
O: TOXIC OXALATE (plant juices contain oxalates; ingestion may cause irritation of the mouth and throat, nausea, diarrhea, and difficulty breathing)
I: IRRITANT (ingestion may cause abdominal pain, nausea, vomiting, and diarrhea; contact with the skin may cause irritation)
N: NONTOXIC

Acorn (T)
Akee unripe fruit (T)
Algerian ivy (I)
Alocasia (O)
Aloe vera (I)
Amaryllis, common (I)
American ivy (O)
Amorphophallus (O)
Angel's-trumpet (T)
Anthurium (O)
Apple pits (T)
Apricot pits (T)
Aralia (N)
Arnica flowers and roots (T)
Arrowhead vine (O)
Asparagus fern (N)
Asparagus fern berries (I)
Autumn crocus bulbs (T)
Avocado leaves (T)
Azalea (T)
Baby's-breath (N)
Bamboo palm (N)
Baneberry berries, roots, stalk,
    and sap (T)
Barberry (I)
Beaver poison (T)
Beechnut seeds (I)
Begonia (N)
Belladonna (T)
Betel nut seeds (T)
Bird-of-paradise seeds and pods (I)
Bird's-nest fern (N)
Bittersweet (T)
Black alder berries (I)
Black cherry bark, leaves, and
    seeds (T)
Black locust (I)
Black nightshade leaves and green
    fruit (T)
Bleeding-heart (T)
Bloodroot (T)
Blue cohosh (T)

Boston ivy (O)
Boxwood leaves and twigs (I)
Buckeye flowers, seeds, and
    nuts (T)
Buckthorn (T)
Bull nettle green fruit (T)
Bunchberry (I)
Burning bush (T)
Buttercup (T)
Cactus thorn (I)
Calabar bean (T)
Caladium (O)
California poppy (N)
Calla lily (O)
Camellia (N)
Cardinal flower (T)
Carnation (I)
Cassava root (T)
Cast-iron plant (N)
Castor bean seeds (T)
Celandine (I)
Century plant (I)
Cherry pits (T)
Chinaberry (T)
Chinese evergreen (N)
Chokecherry (T)
Christmas rose (T)
Chrysanthemum (T)
Clematis (T)
Climbing lily (T)
Coffee senna (I)
Coffee tree (N)
Coleus (N)
Colocasia (O)
Coralberry (I)
Corn cockle seeds (T)
Cornstalk plant (N)
Cotoneaster (T)
Cowbane (T)
Crape myrtle (N)
Creeping Charlie (T)
Crocus: autumn, meadow (T)

Croton (N)
Croton seeds (T)
Crowfoot (T)
Crown-of-thorns (I)
Cyclamen (I)
Daffodil bulbs (I)
Dahlia (N)
Daisy (I)
Daphne (T)
Deadly nightshade (T)
Death camas bulbs and roots (T)
Delphinium (T)
Desert rose (T)
Devil's ivy (O)
Dieffenbachia (O)
Dogwood (N)
Donkey's-tail (N)
Dracunculus (O)
Dragon tree (N)
Dumb cane (O)
Dutchman's-breeches (T)
Easter cactus (N)
Easter lily (N)
Elderberry (T)
Elephant's-ear (O)
Emerald duke (O)
Emerald ripple (N)
English ivy (I)
European bittersweet (T)
European spindle tree (T)
False hellebore (T)
Fava beans and pollen (T)
Fetterbush (T)
Fiddle-leaf fig (N)
Fig tree (N)
Fishberry dried fruit (T)
Fishtail palm (O)
Fool's parsley (T)
Forget-me-not (N)
Forsythia (N)
Four-o'clock roots and seeds (I)
Foxglove (T)

Fuchsia (N)
Garden sorrel (O)
Gardenia (N)
Geranium, California (I)
Glacier ivy (I)
Gloriosa (T)
Glory lily (T)
Gloxinia (N)
Golden-chain tree (T)
Goldenseal (T)
Golden-shower (I)
Grape ivy (N)
Groundsel (T)
Hawaiian ti plant (N)
Hawthorn berries (N)
Heart ivy (I)
Heart leaf (O)
Hemlock tree (N)
Henbane, black (T)
Hibiscus (N)
Holly berries (I)
Honeysuckle berries (N)
Horse beans and pollen (T)
Horse chestnut (T)
Horse nettle green fruit (T)
Hyacinth bulb (I)
Hydrangea (T)
Ice plant (N)
Indian tobacco (T)
Inkberry (T)
Iris roots (I)
Jack-in-the-pulpit (O)
Jade plant (N)
Jasmine (N)
Jequirity bean (T)
Jerusalem cherry leaves and unripe
    fruit (T)
Jessamine (T)
Jimsonweed (T)
Jonquil bulbs (I)
Kentucky coffee tree (I)
Laburnum leaves and seeds (T)

Lady's-slipper (N)
Lantana (T)
Larkspur (T)
Laurel, American (T)
Laurel, black (T)
Laurel, English (T)
Laurel, mountain (T)
Laurel, sheep (T)
Lichen (T)
Lily-of-the-valley (T)
Lipstick plant (N)
Lupine (T)
Maidenhair fern (N)
Majesty (O)
Manchineel fruit (I)
Mandrake (I)
Mango skin and sap (I)
Marble queen (O)
Marigold, cowslip (I)
Marijuana (T)
Marsh marigold (T)
Mayapple (I)
Meadow saffron (T)
Mescal (T)
Mexican jumping bean (T)
Mexican prickle poppy seeds and
    oil (T)
Mimosa (T)
Mistletoe berries (T)
Monkeypod nuts (I)
Monkshood (T)
Moon cactus (N)
Moonseed roots and fruit (I)
Morning-glory seeds (T)
Mother-in-law's-tongue (N)
Mother-of-pearl (N)
Mountain ash berries (N)
Mountain laurel (T)
Mulberry, red (green berries and
    sap) (T)
Narcissus bulbs (I)
Nephthytis (O)

Nerve plant (N)
Nightshade (T)
Norfolk Island pine (N)
Nutmeg seeds (T)
Old-man cactus (N)
Oleander leaves (T)
Olive tree (N)
Orchid (N)
Oregon grape (N)
Pansy flowers (N)
Paradise palm (N)
Parlor ivy (O)
Parlor palm (N)
Passion vine (N)
Peach pits (T)
Peanut cactus (N)
Pear pits (T)
Pellionia (N)
Peony flower (N)
Peperomia (N)
Periwinkle (T)
Petunia (N)
Peyote (T)
Pheasant's-eye (T)
Philodendron (O)
Phlox (N)
Physic nut seeds (T)
Plum pits (T)
Poinsettia (I)
Poison hemlock (T)
Poison ivy (I)
Poison oak (I)
Poison sumac (I)
Pokeberry (T)
Pokeweed (T)
Potato (except tuber) (T)
Pothos (O)
Prayer bean (T)
Privet: common, California (T)
Pussy willow (N)
Pyracantha (I)
Rabbit's-foot fern (N)

Ragwort (T)
Rainbow plant (N)
Red sage (T)
Rhododendron (T)
Rhubarb leaves (O)
Ripple ivy (I)
Rosary bean/pea (T)
Rose (N)
Rubber plant (N)
Scotch broom seeds and leaves (T)
Sentry palm (N)
Shamrock plant (O)
Skunk cabbage (O)
Snakeberry berries, roots, stock, and sap (T)
Snakeroot, white (T)
Snapdragon (N)
Snowberry berries (I)
Snowdrop (I)
Soapberry (I)
Spanish broom seeds and leaves (T)
Spider plant (N)
Sprengeri fern (I)
Squill (T)
Staghorn fern (N)
Star anise, Japanese (T)
Star-of-Bethlehem (I)
Stinkweed (T)
Swedish ivy (N)
Sweet pea (T)
Swiss-cheese plant (O)
Sword fern (N)

Thorn apple (T)
Tobacco, green (T)
Tomato leaves (T)
Toyon leaves (T)
Tulip bulbs (O)
Tung nut seeds (T)
Umbrella plant (T)
Venus's-flytrap (N)
Vinca (T)
Virginia creeper (O)
Wahoo (T)
Walnut, green shells (T)
Wandering Jew (inch plant) (N)
Water arum (O)
Water hemlock (T)
Wild cherry (T)
Wild garlic (I)
Wild grape roots (T)
Wild onion (I)
Wild sage (T)
Wild tobacco (T)
Wild tomato green fruit (T)
Windsor beans and pollen (T)
Wintersweet (T)
Wisteria pods (I)
Witch hazel (T)
Wood rose (T)
Yellow jessamine (T)
Yellow nightshade fruit (T)
Yew (T)
Yucca (N)
Zinnia (N)

PART FIVE

Miscellaneous Information

OXYGEN ADMINISTRATION

It may be advisable or necessary under certain circumstances to administer supplemental oxygen gas (O_2) to a person who would benefit from such therapy. Examples include those stricken with severe high-altitude pulmonary edema, acute severe congestive heart failure, decompression sickness (the bends), and so forth. Anyone who may be called upon to use oxygen delivery equipment should be properly trained in its use ahead of time.

The equipment required to deliver oxygen includes a medical oxygen cylinder (tank), pressure gauge, pressure-reducing valve, flowmeter, tubing, and nasal cannula (tube) or face mask (with or without a reservoir bag).

Oxygen cylinders in the United States are usually painted green or have distinctive green markings. They come in two practical field sizes: D (20", or 50.8 cm, in length; carries 360 liters of oxygen) and E (30", or 76.2 cm, in length; carries 625 liters of oxygen). The length of time that oxygen can be delivered is calculated by dividing the tank capacity by the flow rate. For instance, a D cylinder can deliver 10 liters per minute for 36 minutes. To make the oxygen last longer, keep the flow rate to the lowest effective number.

The pressure gauge reading indicates how much oxygen remains in the cylinder. At full capacity, an oxygen tank is pressurized to 2,000 lb per square inch (psi). Thus, when the gauge indicates a pressure of 500 psi, one-quarter of the tank's capacity for oxygen remains. At a reading of 200 psi, a tank is near empty.

The pressure gauge, pressure-reducing valve, and flowmeter combine to create the regulator, which reduces the pressure of the oxygen from that inside the tank to approximately 50 psi. This allows delivery to the victim at flow rates between 1 and 15 liters per minute.

The delivery device attached to the victim is either a two-pronged (one for each nostril) nasal cannula, or a mask, the latter with or without a reservoir bag. A nonrebreather is a mask with a reservoir bag attached by a one-way valve such that the victim can breathe oxygen that is delivered into the bag, but cannot exhale carbon dioxide back into the bag (he cannot "rebreathe" from the bag). The nonrebreather is used to deliver high concentrations (as a percent of inspired air, 80 to 90% oxygen at flow rates of 10 to 15 liters per minute) of oxygen. The reservoir bag should be kept at least half full of oxygen. This can be accomplished with flow rates of 6 liters per minute or greater.

If lesser concentrations of oxygen are adequate or desired, as with a patient who has chronic obstructive pulmonary disease (see page 42), a nasal cannula can be used. The cannula will deliver 25 to 40% oxygen at flow rates of 2 to 6 liters per minute. The nasal cannula is less confining in that the victim can speak, drink, and eat without having to remove a mask.

Since O_2 is dry, it is often desirable to interpose a humidifying device when O_2 delivery will be prolonged.

To administer oxygen:

1. Place the cylinder upright. Open and close the tank valve slowly ("crack the tank") with a wrench to clean debris from the outlet.
2. Close the regulator flow valve and attach the regulator to the tank. Tighten securely by hand. Never use a regulator without the proper O-ring fitting. Never use tape to hold a loose regulator in place.
3. Open the tank valve slowly to half a turn beyond where the regulator becomes pressurized and there is a maximum reading on the pressure gauge.
4. Attach the plastic delivery tubing to the regulator outflow nipple. Attach the breathing mask or nasal cannula to the other end of the tubing, if it's not already attached.
5. Open the regulator flow valve to the desired flow rate in liters per minute (LPM). A regulator marking of "low" indicates 2 to 4 LPM, "medium" is 4 to 8 LPM, and "high" is 10 to 15 LPM. The flow rate for a nonrebreather mask should not be less than 6 LPM; the flow rate for a nasal cannula should not be more than 6 LPM.
6. Position the mask or cannula on the victim's face. Adjust for comfort. Observe the victim to be certain that the device is tolerated, and that the reservoir bag fills properly.

Precautions

1. Never allow an open flame near an oxygen-delivery system.
2. Do not expose an oxygen tank to excessive heat (125° F, or 52° C) or freezing cold.
3. Do not position any part of a person directly over a tank valve—a loose regulator can be blown off the top of the cylinder with tremendous force.
4. Do not drop a cylinder; do not roll a cylinder.
5. Close all valves when the cylinder is not in use.

WATER DISINFECTION

Water *purification* is the removal of chemical pollutants by filtration through activated charcoal or active resin compounds. This usually improves the taste, but does not decrease the incidence of infectious disease, because microorganisms are not removed. Water *disinfection* is the treatment of water with chemicals, boiling, or filtration to remove agents of infectious disease, such as bacteria and cysts. *Sterilization* is the removal of all life forms.

If at all possible, carry disinfected water with you. If you must drink water from a stream or lake that you cannot disinfect, try to use small tributaries that descend at right angles to the main direction of valley drainage. Clean melted snow is of less risk than ice taken from the surface of a lake or stream. Most bacteria that cause diarrhea can survive for months in ice.

The principal offending agents in contaminated water or on unwashed food that cause illness and diarrhea are the bacteria *Salmonella, Shigella, E. coli,* and *Campylobacter,* and the flagellate protozoan *Giardia lamblia* (see page 190). Drinking nondisinfected water in parts of Africa, India, and Pakistan can cause dracunculiasis (guinea worm disease). In countries where water is improperly disinfected, stick to bottled or canned carbonated beverages, beer, and wine. All containers should be wiped clean to remove external moisture and dirt. All ice should be considered contaminated.

Do not urinate or defecate (inadvertently) into or near your water supply. Build a latrine 8 to 10" (20 to 25 cm) deep into the ground at least 100' (31 m) and downhill from the water supply. Try to keep the latrine away from a gully or other formation that might become a runoff stream during a thaw or after heavy rainfall.

"Raw" drinking water should be allowed to rest for several hours in order for large particles to settle to the bottom. The top portion can be poured off. Coagulation and flocculation techniques remove smaller suspended particles. Add a pinch of alum (an aluminum salt) to a gallon (3.8 liters) of water and mix well, then stir occasionally for 60 minutes. Allow the water to rest while the aggregated particles settle, then pour off the upper (hopefully clearer) part through a paper filter (such as a laboratory-grade filter with a pore size of 20 to 30 microns).

Water may be disinfected by any of the following methods:

1. The usual advice—to boil water for 5 to 10 minutes plus 1 minute for each 1,000' (305 m) of altitude above sea level—is probably overkill.

Giardia cysts are instantly killed in water heated to 158° F (70° C). To play it safe, bacteria and most viruses require a few minutes at this temperature. Hepatitis A virus requires a full minute of boiling to assure inactivation.

Time and temperature have an inverse relationship with respect to water disinfection: The higher the temperature, the less time is required, and vice versa. For instance, pasteurization of food products can occur at a lower temperature (158° F, or 70° C) if 30 minutes at this temperature are allowed. Sterilization (killing of all microorganisms) occurs after 5 to 10 minutes of boiling at sea level.

The temperature at which water boils varies with altitude because of the surrounding barometric pressure. Barometric pressure is expressed in terms of the height (in inches or millimeters) of a column of mercury (Hg) that exerts a pressure equal to that of a column of air with the same size base. At sea level (barometric pressure 760 mm Hg), water boils at 212° F (100° C); at 5,000', or 1,525 m (632 mm Hg), 203° F (95° C); at 10,000', or 3,050 m (522 mm Hg), 194° F (90° C); at 14,000', or 4,270 m (446 mm Hg), 187° F (86° C).

Thus, boiling water is effective for disinfection at any altitude below 18,000' (5,490 m) likely to be attained by a wilderness enthusiast. The time required to heat the water to boiling contributes to the disinfection process. To provide a wide margin of safety, boil the water for 3 minutes.

Halogens, such as iodine and chlorine, are effective chemical disinfectants. The rate at which they kill microorganisms depends upon the concentration (measured in mg per liter, or parts per million [ppm], which are equivalent) of halogen and time allowed for disinfection. At a given water temperature and pH, contact time is inversely related to concentration. Thus, you double the contact time if half the concentration of halogen is present. Decreased (cold) water temperature or cloudy (more organic material) water requires a longer contact time or higher halogen concentration. Halogens can create an unpleasant taste if the concentration exceeds 4 mg/liter. They can lose effectiveness after prolonged exposure to moisture, heat, or air, and may be corrosive or stain clothing. In general, to improve taste, use a lower concentration of halogen for a longer contact time. Eight mg/liter (or ppm) is considered the concentration of iodine effective for water disinfection in room-temperature, clear water. A pregnant woman or a person with thyroid disease or iodine allergy should consult a physician before using any iodine compound for water disinfection.

2. Add one tablet of fresh tetraglycine hydroperiodide (Potable Aqua, Globaline, Coughlan's, EDWGT) to 1 quart (liter) of water and allow the water to stand for 15 minutes. If the water is cloudy, use two tablets. If the water is cold, allow 1 hour after adding the tablets before drinking. Each tablet releases approximately 8 mg/liter of iodine. Do not leave an open bottle exposed to high heat and/or humidity. Potable Aqua Plus includes oxidizing tablets to remove the iodine taste after disinfection.

ADD TO 1 QUART (LITER) OF WATER:

water	clear	cloudy
warm (>15° C, 59° F)	1 tab for 15 minutes	2 tabs for 30 minutes
cold	1 tab for 60 minutes	2 tabs for 60 minutes

After adequate time for disinfection has elapsed, add a few grains of sodium thiosulfate per quart (liter) of water; this kills the iodine taste. Ascorbic acid (vitamin C) is also effective. Any fruit flavorings that contain vitamin C should be mixed in after full time for disinfection has elapsed. Potable Aqua Plus treatment includes an oxidizing tablet to remove the iodine taste. Granular activated charcoal removes organic material, chemicals, and radioactive particles by adsorption, but does not remove all microorganisms, and thus cannot be relied upon to disinfect water. Rather, it should be used to improve taste and clarity. Use it after water has been properly disinfected.

Zinc metal reduces free chlorine or iodine in solution through a chemical reaction. A wand of zinc bristles stirred into a quart (liter) of water for 4 minutes will remove 10 mg/liter of residual chlorine.

Because a 50-tablet bottle of tetraglycine hydroperiodide contains only 0.4 g of iodine (⅟₅₀ the lethal dose), the tablet method is very safe. If you use military surplus iodine tablets, they should be steel gray in color and not crumble when pinched by two fingers; discard older, crumbled tablets. Also, no matter what chemical disinfection system you use, allow disinfected water to seep around the cap and threads of your canteen or water bottle, in order to disinfect them.

3. Add 8 to 10 drops (0.5 ml in each drop) of standard 2% iodine tincture per quart (liter) of water and allow it to stand for 15 minutes. Use a dropper for measurement. If the water is not at least 68° F (20° C), this technique may not eliminate *Giardia*. If the water is cold, allow it to stand for 1 hour before drinking. If you have extra time and do not like the iodine taste, use four to five drops of iodine and allow the water to stand for 8 hours or overnight. Five drops of tincture of iodine disperses to approximately 4 mg/liter.

ADD TO 1 QUART (LITER) OF WATER:

water	clear	cloudy
warm (>15° C, 59° F)	5 drops for 15 minutes	10 drops for 30 minutes
cold	5 drops for 60 minutes	10 drops for 60 minutes

Another iodine product that can be used to disinfect water, but has not definitively been proven effective for this purpose, is 10% povidone iodine (Betadine) solution (not "scrub"):

ADD TO 1 QUART (LITER) OF WATER:

water	clear	cloudy
warm (>15° C, 59° F)	8 drops for 15 minutes	16 drops for 30 minutes
cold	8 drops for 60 minutes	16 drops for 60 minutes

4. Fill a 1 oz (30 ml) glass bottle with iodine crystals (U.S. Pharmacopoeia [USP] grade, resublimed: 2 to 8 grams), then fill the bottle with water. The bottle should have a paper-lined Bakelite cap. Warm the water to 68 to 77° F (20 to 25° C). Shake vigorously, then allow the crystals to settle to the bottom for 1 hour. This will create a saturated solution of iodine. As a crude measure, pour at least half of this liquid (not the remaining crystals), or approximately 12.5 to 15 ml, through a fine filter (such as Teflon) into a quart (liter) of water and allow it to stand for 30 minutes. If the water temperature is not at least 68° F (20° C), this technique may not eliminate *Giardia*. The crystals may be reused up to 1,000 times. Remember that 2 g (0.07 oz) of iodine represents a potentially lethal dose if ingested, so it is absolutely essential to keep the iodine crystals out of the hands of children. A commercial iodine crystal system that can be reused to disinfect up to 2,000 quarts (liters) of drinking water is sold as Polar Pure Water Disinfectant (Saratoga, California).

If one capful from a 2 oz (59 ml) bottle equals approximately 2.5 ml, then using a saturated solution prepared from iodine crystals in water:

ADD TO 1 QUART (LITER) OF WATER:

water	clear	cloudy
warm (>15° C, 59° F)	5 capfuls for 15 minutes	10 capfuls for 30 minutes
cold	5 capfuls for 60 minutes	10 capfuls for 60 minutes

An alcohol-iodine solution can be prepared by adding 8 g of iodine crystals to 100 ml of 95% ethanol. The resulting supernatant yields 8 mg iodine per 0.1 ml. To add to water, measure with an eyedropper:

ADD TO 1 QUART (LITER) OF WATER:

water	clear	cloudy
warm (>15° C, 59° F)	0.1 ml for 15 minutes	0.2 ml for 30 minutes
cold	0.1 ml for 60 minutes	0.2 ml for 60 minutes

5. Filter the water through a category-three (as set for purification by the Environmental Protection Agency) water treatment device. Representative devices are the Mountain Safety Research 0.1 micron filter, Recovery Engineering (PUR) 0.1 micron filter (with tri-iodine resin matrix), General Ecology 0.4 micron filter, Katadyn 0.2 micron filter (silver impregnated), and Timberline 0.2 micron filter. These have pores small enough to filter out *Giardia* cysts and some bacteria, but not viruses (which are 0.03 micron in diameter). If the filter doesn't come with a "prefilter" (nylon mesh or screen) to remove large particles, pour the water through filter paper (see below) or fine cheesecloth. This helps keep your expensive water filter from clogging up, allows it to work more efficiently, and will improve the appearance and taste of the water.

   Filter pore sizes (in microns) for removing microorganisms are: parasitic eggs and larvae—20; *Giardia lamblia, Entamoeba histolytica*—1 to 5; enteric bacteria (such as *E. coli*)—0.1 to 0.2; and viruses—0.004 to 0.01.

6. Halazone (a mixture of monochloraminobenzoic and dichloraminobenzoic acids) or other chlorine (bleach) products have been considered less effective for field water disinfection. Halazone has been characterized as losing 75% of activity after 2 days' continuous exposure to air with high heat and humidity; having a shelf life of 6 months; and decreasing potency by 50% after storage above 104° F (40° C). Therefore, you should obtain a new bottle every 3 to 6 months.

   Each Halazone tablet releases 2.3 to 2.5 mg/liter of chlorine. To disinfect water:

ADD TO 1 QUART (LITER) OF WATER:

water	clear	cloudy
warm (>15° C, 59° F)	5 tablets for 15 minutes	7 tablets for 15 minutes
	2.5 tablets for 30 minutes	5 tablets for 30 minutes
cold	5 tablets for 60 minutes	7 tablets for 60 minutes

Liquid bleach (hypochlorite solution; household bleach, usually 5.25%) can be used to disinfect water via chlorination.

FOR 5.25% BLEACH, ADD TO 1 QUART (LITER) OF WATER:

water	clear	cloudy
warm (>15° C, 59° F)	2 drops (0.1 ml) for 30 minutes	4 drops (0.2 ml) for 30 minutes
cold	2 drops (0.1 ml) for 60 minutes	4 drops (0.2 ml) for 60 minutes

FOR 1% BLEACH, ADD TO 1 QUART (LITER) OF WATER:

water	clear	cloudy
warm (>15° C, 59° F)	10 drops (0.5 ml) for 30 minutes	20 drops (1 ml) for 30 minutes
cold	10 drops (0.5 ml) for 60 minutes	20 drops (1 ml) for 60 minutes

7. Superchlorination followed by dechlorination (available as The Sanitizer) is an effective technique. This is a more complicated method that requires understanding and experience. Add 27 g or more of calcium hypochlorite crystals to a gallon (3.8 liters) of water to attain a chlorine concentration of 27 to 30 parts per million. After the requisite disinfection time (10 to 30 minutes), add six drops of concentrated (30%, caustic) hydrogen peroxide to dechlorinate the water. The chemical reaction produces calcium chloride (which remains in solution), water, and oxygen.

8. Chlorination can be combined with flocculation. AquaCure tablets contain alum and sodium dichloro-s-triazinetrione. Dropped into a liter of cloudy water, a tablet releases 8 mg/liter of free chlorine. If a tablet is dropped into clear water where the flocculation capability isn't exhausted, the alum causes a bit of cloudiness, and there is a stronger chlorine taste.

MOTION SICKNESS

Motion sickness (seasickness) can be a disabling problem for sailors, fishermen, divers, and air travelers. It is caused by fluid movement in the labyrinth of the inner ear, which plays a major part in the control of equilibrium. It is made worse by alcohol ingestion, emotional upset, noxious odors (such as diesel exhaust fumes), and inner-ear injury or infection. Most people adapt to motion after a few days, but may require medication until they are adjusted to the environment.

Signs and symptoms of motion sickness include pale skin color, sweating, nausea, weakness, yawning, and increased salivation. Vomiting may provide temporary relief, but prolonged salvation does not occur until the inner-ear labyrinth acclimatizes to motion or someone intervenes with medication.

To manage motion sickness:

1. Keep your eyes fixed on a steady point in the distance. If on board a ship, stay on deck. Splash your face with cold water.

2. Take meclizine (Antivert, Bonine) or cyclizine (Marezine) 25 mg orally, or dimenhydrinate (Dramamine) 50 mg orally, every 6 to 12 hours as necessary to control motion sickness. To be most effective, the first dose of medication should precede the environmental change by 1 hour. Astemizole (Hismanal) is a nonsedating antihistamine that appears to suppress motion sickness as a side effect in some individuals. The dose is 10 mg by mouth every 24 hours. Those with impaired liver function or who are taking ketoconazole, itraconazole, erythromycin, clarithromycin, or troleandomycin should not take this drug.

3. Place a transdermal scopolamine patch (Transderm Scōp) on the skin behind the ear. This patch releases the drug slowly through the skin and is effective against motion sickness for up to 3 days. Side effects include drowsiness, blurred vision (sometimes with a dilated pupil in the eye on the side of the patch), decreased sweating, dry mouth, and a propensity to be susceptible to heat illness during times of heat exposure. The patch should be positioned at least 3 hours before rough seas are encountered.

4. Some persons report that wearing a "sea band" is helpful. This is a knitted, elastic stretch band with a button(s) that applies pressure to an acupuncture point(s).

FIRST-AID KITS

First-aid kits should be designed according to the environment to be encountered, number of travelers, medical training of the party leaders, and distance from sophisticated medical care. The following lists include items that should be included to deal effectively with the most common problems. They are not camping lists (shelter, food, toiletries, and the like). Basic survival supplies must be adequate. The more multipurpose your selections, the less the weight of your pack.

In all cases, what you should carry depends upon your predetermined needs. For instance, a day hiker need not carry a portable traction splint, but a rock climber on a lengthy expedition should consider bringing one along. A scuba diver should carry a bottle of vinegar to pour on a jellyfish sting. Select the items that make sense for your group or expedition. Carry a realistic quantity of supplies; you should be prepared to treat more than one person at a time. Specific medications to choose from are described in Appendix 1 and throughout the book. Remember to bring along pediatric doses (in liquid form, if necessary) when traveling with children.

First-aid supplies should be packed to be readily accessible, and marked clearly to allow rapid identification. On boating, rafting, or diving adventures, carry medical supplies in a plastic (a Pelican case, for example) or metal container equipped with a rubber O-ring gasket for a tight, waterproof seal, or store the supplies in a "dry bag." Use Ziploc-type bags within the kit for extra material and to sort your supplies. For instance, it is helpful to partition supplies into modules "for wound care," "for an allergic reaction," and so forth.

A preprinted first-aid report form, designed for use on mountain or backcountry expeditions, is a convenient way to record a victim's medical condition and treatment, while serving as a good checklist for proper evaluation. Space is usually provided for a written rescue request to be carried by a messenger in an emergency.

Before the trip, show all members of the expedition where the medical supplies are stored and explain how they are to be used.

An excellent selection of first-aid kits is available in stores and by mail order from Adventure Medical Kits (P.O. Box 2586, Berkeley, CA 94702; telephone 1-800-324-3517) or Atwater Carey, Ltd. (339 East Rainbow Blvd., Salida, CO 81201; telephone 1-800-359-1646). Chinook Medical Gear, Inc. (P.O. Box 1736, Edwards, CO 81632; telephone 1-800-766-1365; www.chinookmed.com) is a mail-order company that specializes in first-aid kits and a complete line of medical and survival equipment and supplies.

Basic Supplies

Brand names are shown to indicate representative products, not to indicate that these are the only products that may be used. Quality, availability, cost, and preference will influence which specific products you choose. Before you embark on an outdoor expedition, go through this list carefully, and make a decision to include or exclude these items from your medical kit.

General Supplies
> medical guidebook
> first-aid report form
> pencil or pen with small notepad
> steel sewing needle
> paper clip
> safety pins
> needle-nose pliers with wire cutter
> sharp folding knife
> disposable scalpels (#11 and/or #12 blades)
> paramedic or EMT shears (scissors)
> sharp-pointed surgical scissors
> bandage scissors
> splinter forceps (tweezers)
> standard oral thermometer: digital, mercury, or alcohol
> low-reading hypothermia thermometer
> wooden tongue depressors ("tongue blades")
> rolled duct tape (3" x 1 yd, or 91 cm)
> ⅛- to ¼-inch diameter braided nylon cord (minimum 10', or 3 m)
> water bottle (such as Nalgene ½ to 1 liter)
> blue "baby bulb" or "turkey baster" suction device
> waterproof flashlight (such as Pelican MityLite) or headlamp (and spare batteries)
> CYALUME fluorescent light sticks
> CPR mouth barrier or pocket mask (such as a Microshield X-L Mouth Barrier)
> sterile (hypoallergenic or latex) surgical gloves; if you are allergic to latex, bring other (such as nonlatex synthetic) nonpermeable gloves
> signal mirror
> waterproof matches
> fine-mesh head net or travel tent to repel insects
> Oral Rehydration Salts or Cera Lyte 70 oral rehydration salts

Wound Care—Preparations and Dressings
> elastic bandages (Band-Aid or Coverlet), assorted sizes (strip, knuckle, and broad); cloth with adhesive is preferable
> butterfly bandages

adhesive strips for wound closure (Steri-Strip or Cover-Strip II), assorted sizes (such as ¼" x 4", ⅛" x 3", ½" x 4"), reinforced [plain or impregnated with an antimicrobial] or elastic

3" x 3" or 4" x 4" sterile gauze pads (packets of 2 to 5) (such as Nu-Gauze highly absorbent)

5" x 9" or 8" x 10" sterile gauze ("trauma") pads (packets of 2 to 5)

nonstick sterile bandages (Telfa or Metalline), assorted sizes

1", 2", 3", and 4" rolled conforming gauze (C-wrap or Elastomull)

1" x 10 yds (9.1 m) rolled cloth adhesive tape

1" x 10 yds (9.1 m) rolled paper or silk (hypoallergenic) adhesive tape

1" x 10 yds (9.1 m) rolled waterproof adhesive tape

½" x 10 yds (9.1 m) rolled waterproof adhesive tape

Molefoam (4 ⅛" x 3 ⅜")

Moleskin Plus (4 ⅛" x 3 ⅜")

Spenco 2nd Skin (1.5" x 2", 3" x 4", 3" x 6.5") and Spenco Adhesive Knit Bandage (3" x 5")

Aquaphor moist nonadherent (petrolatum-impregnated) dressing (3" x 3")

Hydrogel occlusive absorbent dressing (4" x 4" x ¼")

Tegaderm transparent wound dressing (also comes in combination with a Steri-Strip in a Wound Closure System)

liquid soap

sterile disposable surgical scrub brush

cotton-tipped swabs or applicators, sterile, 2 per package

safety razor

syringe (10 ml or 12 ml) and 18-gauge intravenous catheter (plastic portion), for wound irrigation

Zerowet Splashield (2)

tincture of benzoin, bottle or swabsticks

benzalkonium chloride 1:750 solution (Zephiran)

povidone iodine 10% solution (Betadine), 1 oz bottle or swabsticks

suture material (nonabsorbable monfilament nylon on curved needle, suture sizes 3–0 and 4–0; consider sizes 2–0 (thicker) and 5–0 (finer)

stainless-steel needle driver

disposable skin stapler (15 staples)

disposable staple remover

tissue glue

Splinting and Sling Material

cravat cloth (triangular bandage)

2", 3", and 4" elastic wrap (Ace)

4 ¼" x 36" SAM Splints (2)
aluminum finger splints
Kendrick femur traction device

Eye Medications and Dressings
prepackaged individual sterile oval eye pads
prepackaged eye bandages (Coverlet Eye Occlusor)
metal or plastic eye shield
sterile eyewash, 1 oz (30 ml)
contact lens remover
sodium sulamyd, tobramycin, or gentamicin eye drops
oxymetazoline hydrochloride 0.025% eye drops

Dental Supplies
oil of cloves (eugenol), 3.5 ml
Cavit, 7 g tube
IRM (Intermediate Restorative Material)
Express Putty
zinc oxide powder
dental floss
mouth mirror
paraffin (dental wax) stick
wooden spatulas
cotton (rolls and pellets)

Topical Skin Preparations
hydrocortisone cream, ointment, or lotion (0.5 to 1%)
potent corticosteroid ointment
bacitracin ointment
mupirocin ointment
mupirocin calcium 2% cream
bacitracin-neomycin polymyxin B sulphate ointment
miconazole nitrate 2% antifungal cream
silver sulfadiazine 1% (Silvadene) cream
insect repellent
sunscreen lotion or cream
lip balm or sunscreen
sunblock
Adolph's meat tenderizer (unseasoned)
Kenalog in Orabase (oral adhesive steroid for canker [mouth] sores),
    5 g container

aloe vera gel
hemorrhoidal ointment with pramoxine 1%

Nonprescription Medications
buffered aspirin, 325 mg tablets
ibuprofen, 200 mg tablets
acetaminophen, 325 mg tablets
antacid
decongestant (such as pseudoephedrine) tablets
decongestant (such as oxymetazoline) nasal spray
loperamide (Imodium AD), 2 mg caplets
Glutose (liquid glucose) paste tube
stool softener (such as docusate calcium, 240 mg gel caps)

Prescription Medications
codeine, 30 mg tablets (with or without acetaminophen)
metered-dose bronchodilator (albuterol)
prednisone, 10 mg tablets
penicillin Vee K, 250 mg tablets
dicloxacillin, 250 mg tablets
ampicillin, 250 mg tablets
amoxicillin-clavulanate, 500 mg tablets
erythromycin, 250 mg tablets
cephalexin, 250 mg tablets
ciprofloxacin, 500 mg tablets
tetracycline, 500 mg tablets; or doxycycline, 100 mg tablets
trimethoprim-sulfamethoxazole, double-strength tablets
prochlorperazine (Compazine) suppositories, 25 mg
promethazine (Phenergan) suppositories, 25 mg

Allergy Kit
allergy kit with injectable epinephrine (EpiPen
[0.3 mg] and EpiPen Jr. [0.15 mg])
diphenhydramine, 25 mg capsules

Forest and Mountain Environments

water disinfection equipment or chemicals (such as Potable Aqua
tablets or Polar Pure iodine crystals)
Sawyer Extractor suction device

calamine lotion
Space Emergency Blanket (2 oz, 56" x 84")
hypothermia thermometer
hyperthermia thermometer
whistle
acetazolamide (Diamox), 250 mg tablets
dexamethasone (Decadron), 4 mg tablets
nifedipine (Adalat CC), extended-release 30 preparation
powdered electrolyte beverage mix (Oral Rehydration Salts)
instant chemical cold pack(s)
hand warmer (mechanical or chemical)
Kendrick Traction Device (leg splint)

Aquatic Environments

waterproof dry bag or hard case (such as Pelican), to carry first-aid
    supplies
motion sickness medicine
acetic acid (vinegar) 5%
isopropyl alcohol 40%
hydrogen peroxide
VōSoL otic solution

IMMUNIZATIONS

Because the spectrum of infectious diseases changes with time and location, travelers to or between foreign countries should be aware of the
necessity for immunizations. A detailed, updated list of required immunizations by country can be obtained in the annual publication *Health
Information for International Travel* (Centers for Disease Control, 1600
Clifton Road NE, Atlanta, GA 30333; or U.S. Government Printing Office,
Washington, D.C. 20402—HHS Pub. No. [CDC] 85–8280). In this mono-
graph, specific vaccinations (cholera, yellow fever) are listed as "required
by country" in three categories: I) vaccination certificate required of travelers arriving from countries; II) vaccination certificate required of travelers arriving from infected areas; and III) vaccination certificate required
of travelers arriving from a country any part of which is infected. Also

noted by country is malaria risk. General rules and standards for vaccination are discussed, including special topics such as vaccination during pregnancy, vaccination of people with altered immunocompetence (ability to fight infections), and vaccination of those with severe febrile (fever) illnesses.

Vaccinations may be given under the supervision of any licensed physician. All travelers should carry a completed International Certificate of Vaccination with proper signature and validation for all vaccinations administered. Yellow fever and cholera vaccinations must be officially recorded and stamped. Failure to secure validation at an authorized city, county, or state health department renders the certificate invalid, and may force you to be revaccinated or quarantined. The form (stock number 017-001-004405) is available from the Superintendent of Documents, U.S. Government Printing Office, Washington, D.C. 20402.

It is extremely important to plan immunizations as far in advance of an expedition as possible, since some vaccines interact in ways that diminish effectiveness. For instance, yellow fever and cholera vaccines need to be given either on the same day or at least 3 weeks apart.

Tetanus

Any traveler who will be away from medical care for more than 48 hours should have adequate tetanus immunization. The recommendations are as follows:

1. A person previously immunized should receive a booster dose of tetanus toxoid if his last dose was not administered within the past 10 years. If there is a good chance that the traveler will suffer an injury during the trip, he should take a booster if the last dose was not administered within the past 5 years.

2. Nonimmunized individuals should become immunized with a series of three injections (this requires 3 to 6 months).

3. Low-risk (for tetanus infection) wounds are those that are recent (less than 6 hours old), simple (linear), superficial (less than ½", or 1.3 cm, deep), cut with a sharp edge (knife or glass), without signs of infection, and free of contamination with dirt, soil, or body secretions. High-risk wounds are those that are old (greater than 6 hours), crushed or gouged, deep (greater than ½" deep), burns, frostbite, with signs of infection, and contaminated. If someone suffers a wound, here are standard recommendations:

Victim	Low-Risk Wound (not heavily contaminated)	Contaminated Wound (tetanus-prone)
NEVER IMMUNIZED	*Tetanus toxoid* *Tetanus immune globulin*	*Tetanus toxoid* *Tetanus immune globulin*
IMMUNIZED Last booster within 5 yr	*No shot*	*No shot*
Last booster within 10 yr	*No shot*	*Tetanus toxoid* *Tetanus immune globulin*
Last booster over 10 yr	*Tetanus toxoid*	*Tetanus toxoid* *Tetanus immune globulin*

Poliovirus, Diphtheria, Pertussis (Whooping Cough), Measles, Mumps, Rubella (German Measles), Chicken Pox, Haemophilus b

Immunization against poliomyelitis, diphtheria, pertussis, measles, mumps, and rubella should be obtained prior to travel. These are routinely administered during childhood in the United States. Because of the incidence of these infectious diseases in developing countries, such immunizations are mandatory prior to travel. Immunizations against Haemophilus type b (which causes middle ear infections and meningitis) and the virus that causes chicken pox are available, and should be considered under recommendation from your physician.

Polio is still common in developing nations. Unimmunized adults (age greater than 18 years) should receive a series of three injections of the inactivated (virus) Salk vaccine, not the oral (Sabin) vaccine, which is recommended for children. Those under 18 who have never been immunized should receive three doses of oral polio vaccine 1 month apart. People who travel to high-risk areas who were immunized as children should receive one booster dose of oral polio vaccine.

Smallpox

The last reported case of smallpox (caused by the *Variola* virus) was in 1977. Therefore, smallpox immunization is no longer required for international travel, and the vaccine is not commercially available. However, there is a chance that isolated cases still occur (without reporting) in India, the Himalayas, and equatorial Africa. Travelers to these areas should inquire about the latest recommendations from the Centers for Disease Control in Atlanta.

Monkeypox is endemic to forested areas of western and central Africa, but *does not* as yet pose a significant public health risk; there is no vaccine against the causative agent.

Cholera

Cholera is an intestinal infection caused by the microorganism *Vibrio cholerae*, which induces painful diarrhea and extreme fluid losses through the gastrointestinal tract; it can reach epidemic proportions. A person whose stomach contains normal gastric acid is not at much risk for acquiring cholera. Most countries do not require immunization. However, some countries require cholera immunization for travelers entering from a territory that still reports the disease. Two injections are administered 1 week apart, and partial (the vaccine is not extremely efficient) immunity is acquired after a 6-day waiting period. In special, high-risk cases—by virtue of living in unsanitary conditions, or for people with insufficient gastric acid—an additional booster injection may be required a month after the primary series. The vaccine is good for 6 months, so frequent booster shots are necessary. Infants should not be immunized. The vaccine appears to provide 50% effectiveness in reduction of the disease. To be maximally effective, cholera and yellow fever vaccines should be administered either at the same time or at least 3 weeks apart.

Yellow Fever

Yellow fever is acquired in tropical Africa and South America, where victims may suffer the bite of the *Aedes aegypti* mosquito (urban environment) or other mosquitoes (jungle environment). Immunization is effective in preventing the disease; a single injection is administered and immunity is acquired after a 10-day waiting period. The vaccine is good for 10 years, after which time a booster is required to maintain immunity. Infants younger than 9 months and pregnant women should not be routinely immunized, unless they are at high risk for contracting the disease. It is also contraindicated in people with immunosuppression (such as HIV infection) or with an allergy to eggs. Yellow fever vaccinations must be given at an officially designated Yellow Fever Vaccination Center, and the certificate validated at the same center. The vaccine is not required for travel from the United States into Canada, Mexico, Europe, or Caribbean countries. To be maximally effective, cholera and yellow fever vaccines should be administered either at the same time or at least 3 weeks apart.

Meningococcus

The meningococcus is a bacterium (*Neisseria meningitidis*) that can cause meningitis, particularly in children and young adults. It is a wise idea for travelers to Nepal—particularly hikers and backpackers—to be immunized. The vaccine is given in one injection; protection for 3 years is achieved 1 to 2 weeks after administration.

Hepatitis

A recombinant DNA vaccine (Recombivax, *not* derived from human plasma) for immunization against viral hepatitis Type B is recommended for travelers to underdeveloped countries. A series of three injections requires 6 months to complete. Another recombinant vaccine is Engerix-B, which can be given on an accelerated schedule over 2 months.

Hepatitis A virus is spread through contamination of water and food, and is often encountered in developing nations and areas of poor hygiene. A new hepatitis A vaccine (Vaqta), inactivated, is available. It is administered intramuscularly to those age 2 years or older at least 2 weeks prior to exposure to hepatitis A virus. The dose is 0.5 ml (25 units) up to the age of 17 years, and 1 ml (50 units) in people older than 17 years. It is given in a series of two injections.

Pooled immune serum globulin (ISG, or gamma globulin) can be administered to prevent or diminish the effects of viral hepatitis Type A in unimmunized people. The administration of ISG interferes with the antibody response stimulated by other live-virus vaccines, so it should be administered 2 to 4 weeks after any other vaccines. Because the effects of ISG disappear after 6 months, it should be administered just prior to the trip, and at appropriate booster intervals during prolonged travel in endemic areas.

Bubonic Plague

A preexposure vaccine is available for immunization against bubonic plague caused by *Yersinia pestis*. This is administered only to people whose travels or occupations place them at high risk. In most countries where plague is reported, the risk is greatest in rural mountain or upland regions. Vaccination is generally considered for those who will reside in regions where plague is endemic, and where avoidance of rodents and fleas is impossible. The vaccine is injected in two doses 1 month apart, followed by a booster dose after 6 months.

Rabies

Pre- and postexposure rabies vaccinations are discussed on page 364.

Malaria

Malaria is discussed on page 131.

Typhoid Fever

A vaccine is available for immunization against typhoid fever caused by *Salmonella typhi*. Immunization is recommended only for travelers who visit tropical regions known to harbor the disease. A two-injection series given 4 or more weeks apart is required, followed by booster injections at 1- to 3-year intervals, depending on the local disease risk. An oral vaccine is given as one capsule every other day for four doses in those people age 6 years or older. A booster series is necessary every 5 years. Side effects, which include fever, headache, and flulike symptoms, are more commonly associated with the injections.

Typhus Fever

Typhus vaccine is no longer available in the United States and is not recommended for the foreign traveler.

Influenza

Influenza vaccine is administered in one or two injections to children (particularly those receiving long-term aspirin therapy) and adults in October and November (in the Northern Hemisphere) prior to the flu season

(December through March), with a maximum duration of effect of 6 months.

Vaccination of high-risk people (older than 65 years or with chronic illness) prior to flu season is essential. Each year, the vaccine contains the influenza virus strains that are felt to be most prevalent in the United States. Inactivated (killed-virus) influenza vaccine should not be given to those who are sensitive to egg products. "Whole" vaccines should not be given to children under the age of 13 years. Children should be given "split" vaccines, which have been chemically treated to reduce adverse reactions.

A new nasal spray vaccine is currently being tested. It appears to be as effective as injected vaccine.

Amantadine hydrochloride (Symmetrel) is a prescription oral drug that is moderately effective in preventing influenza A. However, because it confers no protection against influenza B, it is not considered a substitute for appropriate immunization.

Pneumococcal Pneumonia

A polyvalent pneumococcal polysaccharide vaccine is available against pneumonia caused by *Streptococcus pneumoniae* (pneumococcus). In general, this vaccine is recommended for elderly (over 65 years) or infirm (those with cancer or with chronic heart, kidney, liver, or lung disease; people without a spleen; alcoholics; diabetics; those with sickle cell anemia) travelers who would be debilitated by a bout of pneumonia. The vaccine is not routinely recommended for children.

Japanese B Encephalitis

Japanese B encephalitis is a viral disease transmitted by *Culex* mosquitoes in Asia and Southeast Asia. The victim first suffers a mild, nonspecific viral illness accompanied by fever and headache. Most infections remain mild. However, in an extremely small number of cases, the victim goes on to develop severe headache, weakness, fatigue, fever, confusion, seizures, and altered mental status ("encephalitis"). There is no specific therapy beyond supportive care.

Travelers for more than 1 month to tropical Asia, particularly into rural rice-growing settings, are candidates for Japanese B encephalitis vaccine, which is given in a series of three injections over 2 weeks to 1 month. A booster dose may be given after 2 to 3 years. The vaccine is obtained from the Vector-Borne Viral Disease Branch of the Centers for Disease Control in Atlanta.

Lyme Disease

See page 139.

Physicians Abroad

A traveler to a foreign country may become ill enough to require the services of a physician. The International Association for Medical Assistance to Travelers (IAMAT) is a nonprofit organization that provides a list of approved doctors who adhere to international standards, which include standard fees. IAMAT also distributes, free of charge, updated material on immunization requirements, malaria and other tropical diseases, and sanitary (food and water) and climatic conditions around the world. The directory of affiliated institutions can be obtained by calling or writing to IAMAT in Ontario, Canada. Other international medical assistance programs include the following (since specific street addresses and phone numbers are constantly changing, check with directory assistance):

Air Ambulance Network, Inc.
Miami, Florida

Divers Alert Network
Duke University Medical Center
Durham, North Carolina

Global Emergency Medical Service
Alpharetta, Georgia

International SOS Assistance
Philadelphia, Pennsylvania

Medex Assistance Corporation
Tinimiun, Maryland

Nationwide/Worldwide Emergency Ambulance Return (NEAR)
Oklahoma City, Oklahoma

Physicians Air Transport International
Northampton, Massachusetts

World Care Travel Assistance Association, Inc.
Washington, D.C.

TRANSPORT OF THE INJURED VICTIM

1. Never move a victim unless you know where you are going. If you are lost and caring for an injured victim (or yourself), prepare a shelter. Try to position yourself so that visual distress signals can be fashioned in an open field, in the snow, or near a visible riverbank. Keep the victim covered and warm. Remember that the victim is frightened and needs frequent reassurance. If he cannot walk, you must attend to his bodily functions. A urinal can be constructed from a widemouthed water bottle. Defecation is more complicated, but may be assisted by cutting a hole in a blanket or sleeping pad placed over a small pit dug in the ground.

2. Unless you are in danger, never leave a victim who is unconscious or confused.

3. If possible, send someone for help and wait with the victim, rather than perform an exhausting and time-consuming solo or duo extrication. If someone is to be sent for help, choose a strong traveler and provide him with a written request that details your situation (number of victims, injuries, need for supplies, specific evacuation method required). While you certainly don't want to underestimate the seriousness of the situation, don't request a helicopter evacuation for someone with a sprained ankle who can easily be carried out in a litter. Anyone sent to obtain assistance should contact the closest law enforcement agency, which will seek the appropriate rescue agency.

4. Conserve your strength. Don't create additional victims with heroic attempts at communication or feats of strength and exertion.

5. Attempt to transport a victim only if waiting for a rescue party will be of greater risk than immediate movement, if there are sufficient helpers to carry the victim (as a general rule, it takes six to eight adults to carry one injured victim), and if the distance is reasonable (under 5 miles, or 8 km). A victim who is carried on an improvised stretcher over difficult terrain usually gets a rough ride. Always test your carrying system on a noninjured person before you use it on the victim.

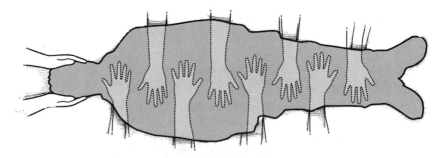

Figure 214. Proper hand positioning for straight lift.

Lifting and Moving Techniques

Straight Lift

If a person is seriously injured, profoundly weak, or unconscious, he should be lifted so that he remains motionless and with his spine in as straight an alignment as possible. This can be accomplished by five rescuers. The first kneels at the head, controls the victim's head and neck, and calls out commands. The other four rescuers kneel at the victim's sides, one at chest level and one at hip level on one side, and the others at lower back level and leg level on the opposite side (figure 214). In this way, they can slide their hands under the victim in a staggered fashion to provide a continuous chain of support. If necessary, the rescuer closest to the legs can free a hand to position a pad, backboard, or litter underneath the victim. The rescuers should lift the victim straight up into the air, taking care not to injure *their* backs.

Logrolling the Victim (See figure 19)

The best way to carry and immobilize a person who may have an injured spine is to use a scoop stretcher, or to slide a backboard underneath the victim. However, when these are not available and a spine-injured person must be turned, logrolling is the best alternative. It is also the preferred method to turn a victim on his side in order to slide a pad, board, or litter underneath him.

1. The first rescuer approaches the victim from the head, and keeps the head and shoulders in a fixed position (no neck movement).

2. The second rescuer extends the victim's arm (on the side over which the victim is to be rolled) above the victim's head. The first rescuer takes this arm and uses it to help support the head in proper position. If the arm is injured, it is maintained at the victim's side.

3. All rescuers work together to roll the victim, without moving his neck.

Carries and Litters

The method of evacuation used to transport a victim will depend upon the degree of disablement and what is available to the rescuer(s). To conserve the energy of all party members, victims of minor injuries should travel under their own power as much as possible, but should never travel unattended. One healthy and strong person should accompany anyone who must leave the group for medical reasons.

Carries

If the victim has suffered an injury that does not allow him to walk out, then mechanical transport must be improvised. A single person who cannot walk but who does not need to be on a litter (one with, for example, a broken ankle, mild exhaustion, or acute mountain sickness) may be carried on the back of a strong rescuer using a rope seat. This is fashioned by passing a long 1" (2.5 cm) rope or strap across the victim's back and under his arms, then crossing the rope in front of his chest. The victim is loaded piggyback onto the rescuer's back, and the rope ends are passed forward over the shoulders of the rescuer, under his arms, and around to the rescuer's back, then between and through the victim's legs from the front, and around the outside of the victim's legs just under the buttocks, to be tied snugly in front of the rescuer's waist (see figure 215). Such a rope seat is far preferable to a standard fireman's carry, which is very fatiguing (see figure 216). A blanket drag (see figure 217) is only good for very short distances, such as to pull a person quickly away from an immediate hazard.

Other simple ways to carry a victim include the four-hand seat, backpack carry, ski pole or tree limb backpack carry, and coiled rope seat. In the first method, two rescuers interlock hands. Each rescuer first grasps his right wrist with his left hand. Holding the palms down, each rescuer then firmly grasps the left wrist or forearm of the other rescuer with his right hand, interlocking all four hands (see figure 218). The victim sits on the four-hand seat. In the second method, leg holes can be cut into a

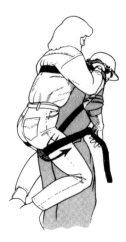

Figure 215. Fashioning a rope (webbing) seat.

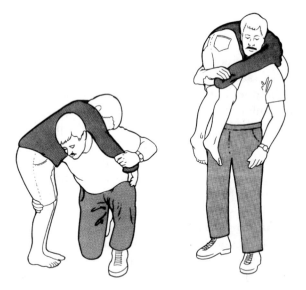

Figure 216. Fireman's carry.

large backpack, so that a victim can sit in it like a small child would in a baby carrier. In the third method, two rescuers with sturdy backpacks stand side by side. Pack straps are looped down from each pack, and ski poles or tree limbs are slung across through the loops, or the poles are placed to rest on the padded hip belts. The poles should be padded so that the victim can sit on the rigid seat, steadying himself by draping his

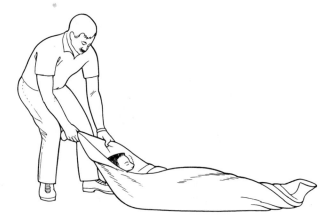

Figure 217. Blanket drag.

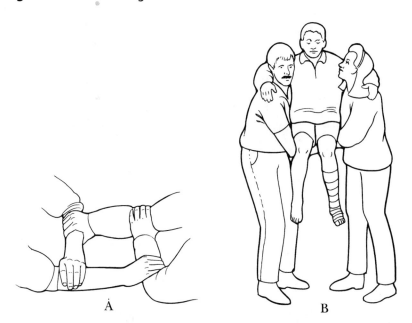

A   B

Figure 218. (A) Overlapping hands to create a four-hand seat. (B) Carrying the victim.

arms around the shoulders of his rescuers (see figure 219). The split-coil rope seat is created by coiling a rope, then fixing the coil at one segment. The coil's loops are split and used to position the victim upon the rescuer's back (see figure 220). A two-rescuer split-coil technique is also useful (see figure 221).

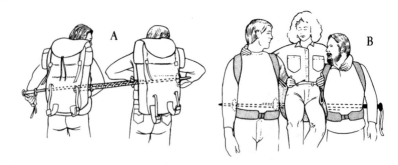

Figure 219. Fashioning a ski pole seat. (A) The poles are slung between rescuers wearing backpacks. (B) A victim can sit comfortably on the padded ski poles.

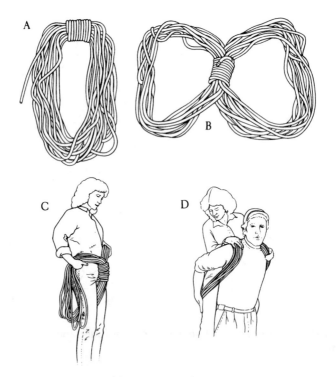

Figure 220. Creating a coiled rope seat. (A) The rope is coiled and the loops secured. (B) The loops of the coil are divided into equal sections at the point of fixation. (C) The victim can step through the split loops, so that (D) a single rescuer can carry the victim.

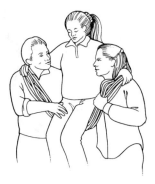

Figure 221. Two-rescuer split-coil rope seat.

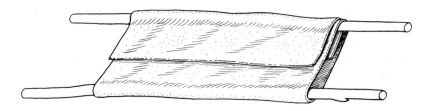

Figure 222. Blanket-pole litter.

Litters

The safest anatomical position for an injured victim (from a transport perspective) is supine with his back straight, eyes forward, and arms and legs straight with his hands at his sides. If the victim might vomit or is unconscious, he should be on his side, cushioned to protect against undue motion and to assure an open airway.

If a specialized litter or stretcher (such as a Stokes basket or split scoop frame) is not available, an improvised litter can be constructed from a blanket or sturdy drop cloth and two 6 to 7' (1.8 to 2.1 m) poles or sturdy tree limbs (saplings). Separate the poles by slightly more than the width necessary to carry the victim. Fold the blanket over one pole, then fold the edges over the other pole sequentially and back again over the first pole (figure 222). Secure the outside blanket flap with safety pins or stitches of cord. Test it to be sure that it can support the victim. Carry the victim so that his body secures the outside (free) blanket flap. Be sure to immobilize the victim on the litter, and cushion his head and neck.

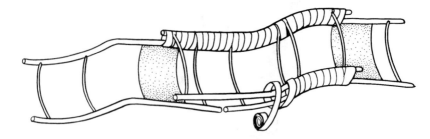

Figure 223. Construction of a backpack frame litter. Pads or a sleeping bag are placed on the litter.

Litters resembling ladders can be fashioned from tree limbs or ski poles fastened with twine, rope, clothing, or pack straps. Two backpack frames can be fastened together with tape or rope (figure 223) to form a ladderlike platform for a sleeping bag or pads and blankets.

A rope stretcher is constructed by stretching a 150 to 200' (46 to 61 m) rope on the ground and determining its midpoint. At the midpoint, fold the rope back upon itself. Measure 3' (91 cm) from the bend, and fold each half of the rope back again to the outside. This creates the central "rungs" of a "ladder" that will be 3' wide. Repeat the process of folding the rope back upon itself in 3' segments, moving away from the central rungs in each direction and laying out a series of evenly spaced parallel loops. About 16 or 18 loops (rungs) should create a ladder approximately the same length as the victim. Take the two remaining long ends of the rope and lay them perpendicular to the rungs, alongside the bends in the rope (figure 224). Use the long ends to secure the loops together (completing the long sides of the ladder) by tying a clove hitch (see figure 236) or other secure knot onto each consecutive bend in the rope 2 to 3" (5 to 7.5 cm) inside the bend, so that a small loop remains to the outside of the knot. Each pair of knots should be separated by 3 to 4" (7.5 to 10 cm). After all the knots are tied, the rope ends are threaded through the small outside loops as the remaining lengths are circled around the outside of the stretcher and finally tied off.

A mummy litter (also called a daisy chain or cocoon wrap) can be constructed of a long climbing rope, large tarp, sleeping pads, blankets or a sleeping bag, and stiffeners (skis, poles, tree limbs, or the like). The rope is laid out with even U-shaped loops (see figure 225) that are roughly twice the victim's width. Tie a small loop at the foot end of the rope. Lay a tarp on the rope. Upon the tarp, lay down foam pads, then lengthwise stiffening rods, then another layer of pads. Lay the victim on the pads, and cover with the sleeping bag or blankets. Pull the sides of the tarp up to wrap the

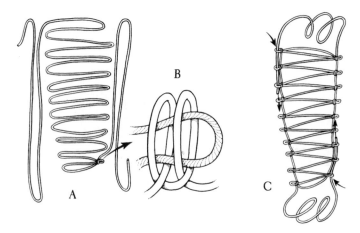

Figure 224. Making a rope stretcher. (A) Having laid a series of parallel loops, lay the lengthwise segments perpendicularly alongside. (B) Use a clove hitch to secure the loop ends. (C) The remaining long ends of the rope are passed through the outside loops to form the perimeter of the stretcher, and are tied off to complete the process.

victim. To secure him, bring the first untied loop above the tied end (foot) loop through the tied loop, and pull it toward the center. Moving toward the head, feed the next loop through the preceding loop, and so on until the armpits are reached. At this point, bring a loop up over each shoulder and tie the rope off in front of the victim.

Test any litter on an uninjured person before trusting it to bear the weight of the victim. Be certain to fasten the victim securely into the stretcher or litter, so that he doesn't fall out. Pad all injuries, and the head and neck in particular, to make the victim as comfortable as possible. Positioning on a litter is very important. In general, keep the injury uphill, to keep extra weight (pressure) and jostling from causing pain. If the chest is injured, keep the victim lying on his side with the wounded side (lung) down, to allow the good lung to expand more fully. If the victim has altered consciousness, is nauseated, or is vomiting, he should be kept on his side, to protect the airway (see page 17). If the victim has suffered a face, head, or neck injury, he should be transported with his head slightly elevated (see page 55). Victims with shock (see page 54), bleeding, or hypothermia (see page 269) should be carried with the head down and feet elevated. Victims with chest pain and/or difficulty breathing, which might indicate a heart attack or heart failure (see page 41), should be carried with the upper body elevated.

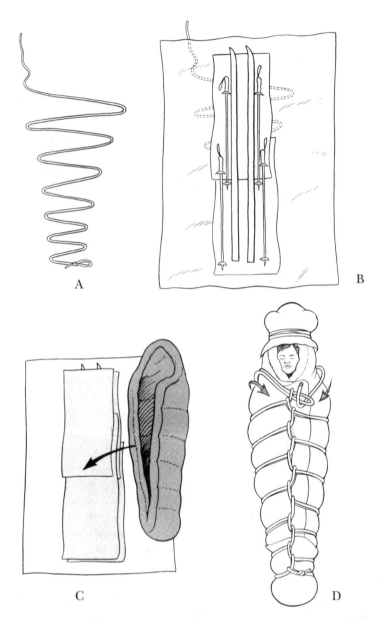

Figure 225. Mummy litter. (A) Lay out the rope in even loops. (B) Lay blankets or tarps over the loops, then long, rigid objects for stability. (C) Place a sleeping bag or blanket in the center to hold the victim. (D) Pass the first nontied loop through the tied loop and work your way to the top. Bring the finishing loops over the shoulders, and tie off.

All victims should be covered above and below with blankets, clothing, sleeping bags, or whatever else is available for warmth. Handle all suspected hypothermics gently. A victim secured to a stretcher should never be left unattended. Constantly reassure the victim. If the terrain is steep, keep his feet pointed downhill. Remember that litter transport is exhausting for the rescuers and should not be entertained if the distance to be covered is more than a few miles.

If possible, position at least one rescuer at the head of the victim, one at each shoulder, one at each hip, and one at the legs. This allows a litter to be carried and facilitates a quick action to turn the victim, should that be necessary. A leader should call out all activities of the team.

Helicopters

Most helicopters used for medical evacuation can land at altitudes of up to 10,000' (3,050 m) and are limited by visibility, landing space, and weather conditions. People on the ground should be aware of the limitations of maneuverability, and should obey certain rules when involved with a helicopter rescue:

1. Prepare and brightly mark a proper landing site. The ideal location is on level ground (bare rock is best; snow is worst) with no more than 10 degrees of incline and access from all sides. If possible, choose a site where the helicopter will be able to drop off during takeoff, rather than having to climb up. Ideally, there will be 360-degree access so that the helicopter can take off in any direction, depending upon wind conditions. Clear an area 100' (31 m) long by 100' wide of all debris that could interfere with landing or be scattered by gusts from the propellers. Although the absolute minimum ground dimensions for a "safety square" can, under ideal conditions, be somewhat less than this, you should clear the full area. A smoky fire or smoke signal should be placed near the landing site so that the pilot can judge the wind (pilots prefer takeoffs and landings to be directed into the wind). If this is not possible, stand away from the landing site where the pilot can see you, and hold up an improvised wind flag (such as streamers), or position yourself with the wind behind your back, and point with both arms at the landing site. At night, if you have lights, shine them on objects that will alert the pilot to unseen danger (such as the poles of power lines). If there is a danger at the last minute prior to landing, signal "do not land" to the helicopter pilot by lifting your arms from a horizontal (to-the-side) outstretch to straight overhead several times.

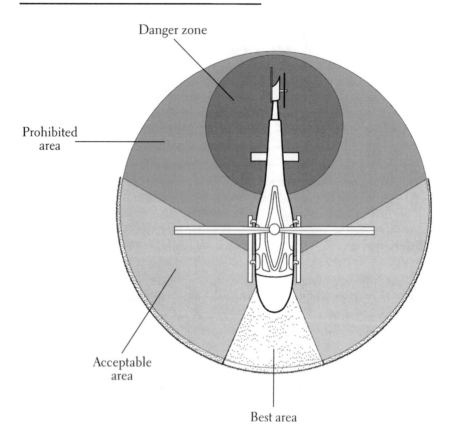

Danger zone

Prohibited area

Acceptable area

Best area

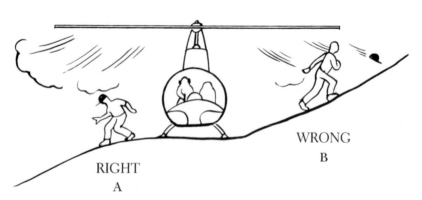

WRONG
B

RIGHT
A

Figure 226. Approach zones around a helicopter. (A) It is best to approach from the front. (B) Don't walk uphill into the helicopter rotor blades.

2. Unless otherwise instructed, stay at least 150' (46 m) from a helicopter with rotors spinning. Look away as the ship lands, so as not to be struck in the face or eyes by flying debris. Protect the victim. Secure all loose objects or clear them from the landing area. Coil and secure all ropes. Because of the strong gusts from the approaching helicopter (up to 100 mph, or 161 km per hour), do not stand near the edge of a cliff!

3. Always approach or leave a helicopter at a 30- to 45-degree angle from the front, in sight of the pilot and crew (figure 226). Never approach the helicopter from ground higher than the landing spot, to avoid walking into a rotor. Stay away from the tail rotor, because it is nearly invisible when rotating.

4. Keep your head down! You may not perceive that the rotor blade is dipping (up to 4', or 1.2 m, from the center attachment) until it chops your head off. Don't hold any objects (particularly not your arms) above your head. Protect your eyes from dust kicked up by the rotor wash.

5. Do not smoke a cigarette near a helicopter.

6. Follow the pilot's instructions. Do not enter, leave, or load a helicopter until he gives the command.

7. Do not stand under or anywhere near a helicopter during takeoff or landing. Everyone near the landing site should stay at a safe distance in a single group, clearly visible to the pilot.

8. If a cable or rope is lowered, allow it to touch the ground before you handle it, to avoid a shock from static electricity. Never tie the rope or cable to an immovable object on the ground; this could cause a crash.

9. All people should wear hard hats and eye protection, if available.

GROUND-TO-AIR DISTRESS SIGNALS

If a party is trapped or lost, and helicopter or airplane search parties are likely to be in the region, it may help to attempt to signal the aircraft. One way that this can be done is by creating ground-to-air distress signals, either by marking an open field or a riverbank that is visible from the air by stamping out large (8 to 10', or 2.4 to 3 m) designs in the snow (in an open area), or by attracting attention with display patterns of clothing, rocks, fire rings, or the like. Figure 227 illustrates some standard ground markings for communication.

The three signals that are recognized (and remembered) by most

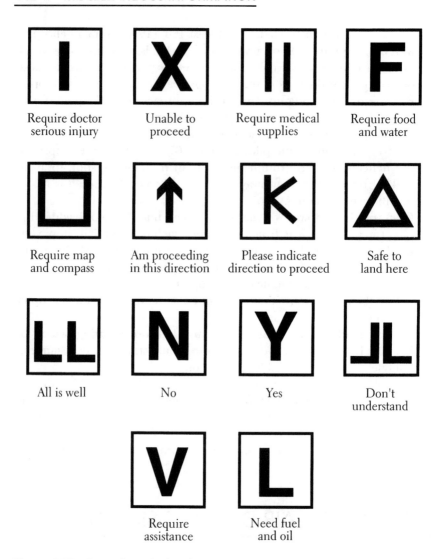

Figure 227. Ground-to-air signals.

pilots are: three of anything—"distress"; large X—"unable to proceed" or "need medical assistance"; and an arrow—"proceeding in this direction." Three fires (set 100', or 31 m, apart) placed in a triangular configuration is a sign of distress to a passing pilot. Ground-to-air patterns should be large, composed of straight lines, and made up of colors that contrast sharply with the natural colors of the environment (royal blue is best). Small battery-powered emergency strobes are also useful. A heliograph mirror is a small signal reflector that can be accurately aimed to reflect sunlight at a distant object (such as an aircraft).

LOST PEOPLE

People lost in the wilderness often act in a predictable manner. Rapid location of a lost person can make the difference between life and death. These general guidelines may assist you in a search. Remember:

1. Lost people tend to follow the path of least resistance (open fields, trails, roads, dry streambeds).
2. A person who is lost tends to travel downhill and to seek apparent shortcuts toward civilization or a familiar location.
3. People tend to avoid barriers and obstacles (lakes, large rivers, boulder fields, dense brush).
4. At night, a lost person tends to travel toward lights.
5. In bad weather, people tend to seek shelter with overhead protection.
6. Small children tend to seek shelter when tired.

PROCEDURES

Subcutaneous Injection

Subcutaneous (just below the skin) injection of epinephrine is used to manage a severe allergic reaction. The injection may be performed with a preloaded syringe (already containing the medicine in the barrel—see page 58) or may require that the medicine be drawn up for administration. After you wash your hands, follow these instructions:

1. Select the proper syringe and needle. For the treatment of an allergic reaction, a syringe that holds 1 milliliter (ml) is necessary, commonly equipped with a 25- or 27-gauge needle (the larger the gauge number, the smaller the diameter of the needle). Using a syringe (such as the NMT Safety Syringe, New Medical Technology, Inc., Zionsville, IN) in which the needle automatically retracts into the barrel of the syringe after its contents have been delivered may decrease accidental needle

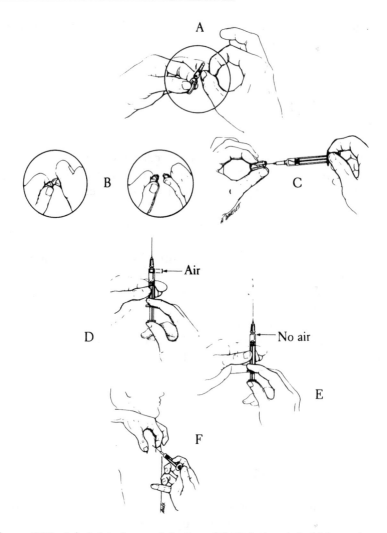

Figure 228. Administering an injection. (A) Flick the air bubble to the top of the vial. (B) Break off the top of the vial at the narrowing or line. (C) Draw the medicine into the syringe. (D) Holding the needle straight up, gently push the plunger until (E) no air is left. (F) Pinch up a fold of skin and briskly stick the needle through the skin.

stick injuries and make it easier to carry and dispose of used syringes and needles.

2. Never touch the metal of the needle with your hands.

3. Never share needles (use the same needle to inject multiple people).

4. If the medication is in a preloaded syringe, be sure to see that the amount of medicine does not exceed the dose you want to administer. Be certain not to inject too much medicine.

5. If the medicine is in a glass vial, flick the vial a few times with your finger to drive the air bubble to the top, and then snap the vial open at the line marked on the glass at the neck (figures 228A and B). Draw the proper amount of medicine to be administered up into the syringe (figure 228C). In the case of epinephrine, this will be 0.3 to 0.5 ml for an adult, and 0.01 ml per kg (2.2 lb) of body weight for a child, not to exceed 0.3 ml.

6. If the medication is in a glass bottle with a rubber top, wipe the top of the bottle with alcohol, stick the needle through the rubber, and draw up the desired amount of medication. If you cannot draw the medicine out of the bottle, you may need to inject some air into the bottle first (use the same entry into the bottle to inject air in and to draw medicine out).

7. Before injection, point the needle upward, tap the syringe a few times to float the air bubbles to the top, and squirt out any air that is in the syringe (figures 228D and E). You should be left with only medicine. Try not to inject any air.

8. Wipe off the skin with alcohol or with soap and water (if no alcohol is available) where you intend to administer the medicine. The easiest place to inject epinephrine is on the lateral arm at the shoulder.

9. Pinch the skin up between your fingers, and quickly plunge the needle in just under the skin at a 15- to 30-degree angle to the skin (figure 228F). With the needle in the skin, gently pull back on the plunger, to see if blood enters the syringe. If it does, you have inadvertently entered a blood vessel, and you should draw back the needle until no blood is returned. If no blood is returned, then firmly plush the plunger and inject the medicine. Quickly remove the needle from the skin, and gently massage the injection site.

Again, when administering an injection, *never* share needles between people.

Fishhook Removal

If a fishhook enters the skin, gently scrub the skin surrounding the entry point with soap and water. After the skin is clean, apply gentle pressure along the curve toward the point while pulling on the hook. If the hook is not easily removed, this means that the barb is caught in the tissue (see figure 229A).

If the hook has a barbed shank, the hook must usually be removed by pushing it through the skin. This should be done (because of the

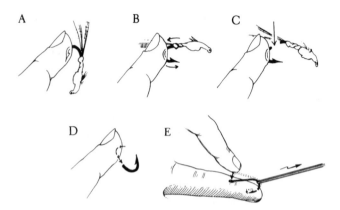

Figure 229. Fishhook removal. (A) The barb is embedded in the finger. (B) The hook and barb are pushed through the skin. (C) The shaft of the hook is cut. (D) Both pieces are easily extracted. (E) "Press-and-yank" method of fishhook removal.

increased risk of infection) if it will take more than 8 hours to get to a doctor. Grasp the shank of the hook with a pliers. With a steady, firm motion, push the hook through the skin so that the barb appears (see figure 229B). Cut off the shaft or the barb (take care to cover the area with a free hand to prevent the detached barb from flying into someone's eye) and then pull the remainder of the hook back out of the skin (see figures 229C and D).

A method of fishhook removal that has become extremely popular is the "string-pull" or "press-and-yank" technique (see figure 229E). Attach (tie) a shoelace or 2' (60 cm) length of string, fishing line, or rolled gauze around the bend of the hook. Push the shank of the hook down (toward the barb), parallel to the skin. This (hopefully) will disengage the barb from the tissue. Then use the string (at a 30-degree angle) to yank the hook from the skin in a snapping motion. Take care that the flying hook released from the skin does not impale anyone nearby.

Vigorously wash the wound and leave it open with a simple dry dressing. Do not seal in the dirt and bacteria with any grease or home remedies (see page 225). If the hook was dirty (or was holding a dirty worm), begin the victim on dicloxacillin, penicillin, erythromycin, or cephalexin. If the victim suffers from a depressed immune system, use an antibiotic that is effective against germs acquired in an aquatic environment (see page 308). If a hook enters the skin anywhere near the eye, do not attempt removal. Tape the hook in place so that it cannot be snagged and take the victim immediately to see a doctor.

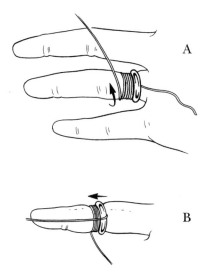

Figure 230. Ring removal. (A) Thread a string under the ring. Wrap the long portion to compress the finger next to the ring. (B) Unwrap the string to push the ring toward the end of the finger. The process is repeated until the ring is moved over the knuckle or swollen part of the finger.

Splinter Removal

A splinter can be removed by gently cutting away the skin near the entrance, until a firm grasp can be made with a small tweezers or with the fingers. If a splinter enters the finger under the fingernail, cut a small V-shaped wedge out of the nail, so that the splinter can be grasped. If a splinter cannot be removed for more than 24 hours, begin the victim on penicillin, erythromycin, or cephalexin.

If a splinter lies in full view longitudinally under the skin, it may be easier to take a sharp blade and carefully cut down through the skin directly over the splinter along its entire length, in order to avoid fragmenting it by dragging the (usually) wood out of a small opening.

Ring Removal

A ring should be removed if swelling of a finger underneath will cause the ring to become an inadvertent tourniquet. This is particularly true with broken fingers, burns, crush injuries, stings, and bites. The easiest method is to lubricate the skin with soap, ointment, or something greasy, and then apply a circular motion with traction on the ring. Keep the hand or foot (for a toe ring) elevated and cool (cold water or ice pack for 10 minutes) to minimize the swelling.

If swelling prevents easy removal, use the "string-wrap" technique (see figure 230). Take a 20"(50 cm) string and pass it under the ring so that the long portion is left on the fingernail side of the ring. Wrap the long portion around the finger in a spiral fashion, starting next to the ring and working out toward the fingernail, keeping the loops close together. (No tissue should bulge through between the loops.) The string is then unwrapped by unwinding on the side closer to the hand, which pushes the ring little by little off the finger. The process is repeated over and over until the ring can be forced over the swollen finger joint(s), which may be a bit painful. Take care between wraps not to lose ground by inadvertently pushing the ring back toward the hand.

Zipper Removal

If skin gets caught in a zipper (ouch!), the best way to solve the problem is to cut the diamond-shaped slider with a wire cutter so that the zipper falls apart. If you keep trying to slide the zipper, you may entrap more skin.

Knots and Hitches

One of the most useful wilderness skills is the ability to quickly tie a secure knot or hitch. This is particularly important when fashioning a litter or traction device. The following diagrams illustrate a selection of common useful knots and hitches: slip knot (figure 231), half hitch and double half hitch (figure 232), bowline (figure 233), loop knot and draw loop (figure 234), round turn with double half hitch (figure 235), clove hitch (figure 236), and double carrick bend (figure 237).

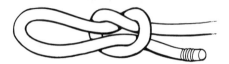

Figure 231. Slip knot.

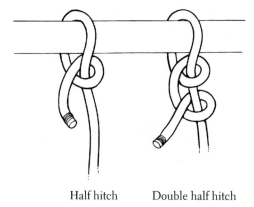

Half hitch   Double half hitch

Figure 232. Half hitch and double half hitch.

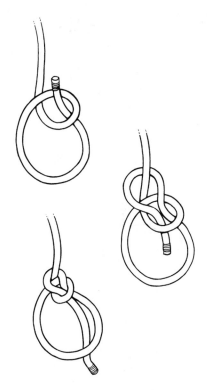

Figure 233. Bowline.

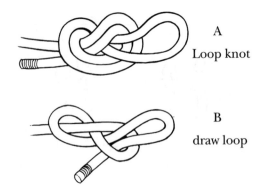

A
Loop knot

B
draw loop

Figure 234. (A) Loop knot. (B) Draw loop.

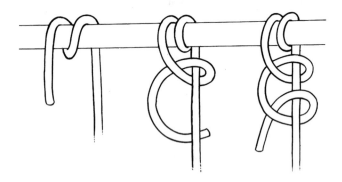

Figure 235. Round turn with double half hitch.

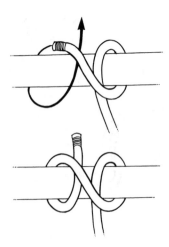

Figure 236. Clove hitch.

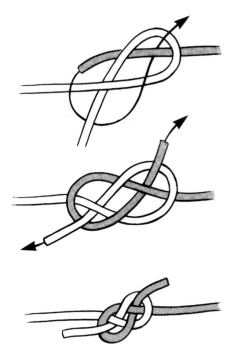

Figure 237. Double carrick bend.

APPENDIXES

Appendix One

COMMONLY USED DRUGS (MEDICATIONS) AND DOSES

Before administering a medication, always ask the recipient if he suffers from allergy to it. If so, do not administer the drug or anything that you feel is similar to it. Use medications only if you have a reasonable understanding of what you are treating.

Many drugs are used to suppress symptoms (such as abdominal pain, nausea and vomiting, and headache) of potentially serious disorders. In these cases, do not overmedicate the victim if you need to watch for a worsening condition.

Drugs are listed here by purpose. I have listed a number of products that are available over the counter; however, many of the drugs require a prescription.

Always have a doctor or pharmacist explain the actions and side effects of any drug you obtain. I have listed some drugs that people may carry for preexisting conditions, so that the rescuer may have a better understanding of his patient's medical history.

Doses are listed in absolute amount (generally, for adults) or in amount to be given per body weight or per age (generally, for children). For determination of weight, 1 kilogram (kg) equals 2.2 pounds (lb). The drug should be administered orally unless otherwise specified.

Because children generally require a fraction of the dose used for adults, they may need to have the drug in special tablet or liquid form. The average weights for children, according to age, are:

1 year—10 kg (22 lb)
3 years—15 kg (33 lb)
6 years—20 kg (44 lb)
8 years—25 kg (55 lb)
9½ years—30 kg (66 lb)
11 years—35 kg (77 lb)

Exercise extreme caution and do not administer drugs to pregnant women, infants, or small children unless absolutely necessary.

Drugs have many side effects. Some of the common ones are noted. Be familiar with the drugs you carry.

Corticosteroids ("steroids") are interchangeable to a certain degree. If you must substitute, here is a rough measure of equivalence: 20 mg prednisone equals 16 mg methylprednisolone equals 3 mg dexamethasone.

Drugs are listed in the following order:

Drugs and Pregnancy

In general, it is best to avoid taking any medication when pregnant in order to avoid the risk of fetal malformation, or illness or injury in the newly born child. A pregnant woman should be discouraged from taking over-the-counter drugs. However, women can certainly become ill during pregnancy, so it is important to know what can be administered safely and what should be absolutely avoided. Fortunately, many of the drugs that are labeled "potentially hazardous" have only been proven hazardous in laboratory animals, frequently in relative doses that far exceed their common usage in humans. Furthermore, some drugs formerly thought to cause malformation of the developing fetus have since been proven safe when administered in normal therapeutic doses.

The following list reflects recommendations compiled from the current medical literature. Whenever possible, a pregnant woman contemplating use of a medication should seek advice *in advance* from her physician.

Antibiotic, Antifungal, Antiviral, Antimalarial

NO RECOGNIZED HAZARD

amoxicillin-clavulanate
penicillin
cephalosporins
erythromycin
clotrimazole
miconazole
nystatin
proguanil
ampicillin/amoxicillin
paromomycin
mefloquine (apparently safe)
terconazole
gentamicin topical eye medication

AVOID IF POSSIBLE

chloramphenicol
chloroquine (apparently safe)
ciprofloxacin
gentamicin injection
trimethoprim-sulfamethoxazole
metronidazole
nitrofurantoin
quinine
primaquine
quinacrine
acyclovir

HAZARDOUS

tetracycline/doxycycline (causes staining of teeth and altered bone
    development in fetus)
norfloxacin
ofloxacin
fleroxacin

Pain Medication

NO RECOGNIZED HAZARD

acetaminophen
hydrocodone
meperidine
naproxen (use with caution in later pregnancy)
oxycodone

AVOID IF POSSIBLE

codeine
aspirin (but probably safe)
ibuprofen and most other nonsteroidal anti-inflammatory drugs
("NSAIDs") during later pregnancy

HAZARDOUS

indomethacin

Vaccine

NO RECOGNIZED HAZARD

hepatitis A
hepatitis B (killed)
tetanus toxoid
diphtheria toxoid
tetanus immunoglobulin
pooled serum immunoglobulin

AVOID IF POSSIBLE

influenza (inactivated virus)
polio (oral and injection)
typhus
tuberculosis (BCG)
typhoid
cholera
yellow fever
meningococcal vaccine
pneumococcal vaccine
rabies vaccine (preexposure; must be used for postexposure)

HAZARDOUS

smallpox

measles
mumps
varicella
rubella

Antiallergy
NO RECOGNIZED HAZARD

epinephrine (use only in a critical situation)
cimetidine
dimenhydrinate
famotidine
topical corticosteroids, decongestants (e.g., oxymetazoline)

AVOID IF POSSIBLE

chlorpheniramine
epinephrine (avoid in a noncritical situation)
hydroxyzine
prednisone

HAZARDOUS

diphenhydramine (during first trimester)
brompheniramine
dimenhydrinate
cyclizine

Antinausea, Anti-Motion-Sickness, Antidiarrheal, Anticonstipation
NO RECOGNIZED HAZARD

trimethobenzamide
prochlorperazine
promethazine
dimenhydrinate
docusate
bisacodyl
mineral oil
meclizine
metoclopramide (apparently safe)

AVOID IF POSSIBLE

scopolamine
anticholinergic drugs

Other

NO RECOGNIZED HAZARD

antacids

caffeine

cyproheptadine

prednisone

betamethasone

dextromethorphan

casanthranol

prednisolone

kaolin-pectin

loperamide

lindane (use with caution)

omeprazole

oxymetazoline

pyrethrins with piperonyl butoxide

ranitidine

simethicone

sucralfate

AVOID IF POSSIBLE

albuterol

amantadine

beclomethasone

bismuth subsalicylate

dexamethasone

furosemide

isoproterenol

acetazolamide

triazolam

loperamide

diphenoxylate

theophylline

metaproterenol

nifedipine

HAZARDOUS

Antithyroid

captopril (and all other angiotensin-converting
    enzyme ["ACE"] inhibitors

chlordiazepoxide

chlorothiazide
isotretinoin
phenacetin
phenytoin
dapsone
diazepam
hydrochlorothiazide
tolbutamide
midazolam

Allergic Reaction to a Drug

If a person develops an allergic reaction to a drug (itching, shortness of breath, swollen tongue, difficulty talking, skin rash, hives, and so on), immediately discontinue the drug and follow the instructions on page 58.

For Relief from a Severe Allergic Reaction

Epinephrine (adrenaline) 1:1,000 aqueous solution. Adult dose 0.3 to 0.5 ml injected subcutaneously (see page 419). This may be repeated two times at 20-minute intervals. The pediatric dose is 0.01 ml per kg (2.2 lb) of body weight, not to exceed 0.3 ml, injected subcutaneously. *Unless the situation is absolutely life threatening, do not use epinephrine if the victim is older than 45 years, has a known history of heart disease, or is a pregnant female.*

Side effects: rapid heartbeat, nervousness.

Epinephrine is available in preloaded syringes in certain allergy kits, which include the Ana-Kit (Hollister-Stier) and the EpiPen and EpiPen Jr. (Dey). Instructions for use accompany the kits. The EpiPen products are generally easier for laypeople to use, because they require less manual dexterity to accomplish the injection. The Ana-Kit preloaded syringe carries enough epinephrine for a second (repeat) adult dose.

For dosing purposes, the EpiPen should be used for adults and children over 66 lb (30 kg) in weight. Children 66 lb and under should be injected with the EpiPen Jr.

Take particular care to handle preloaded syringes properly, to avoid inadvertent injection into a finger or toe. Do not intentionally inject epinephrine into the buttocks or a vein. Epinephrine should not be exposed to heat or sun, but does not need to be kept refrigerated. If clear (liquid) epinephrine turns brown, it should be discarded.

When administering an injection, *never* share needles between people.

Diphenhydramine (Benadryl). Adult dose 25 to 50 mg every 4 to 6 hours; pediatric dose 1 mg per kg (2.2 lb) of body weight.

Side effects: drowsiness, paradoxical hyperactivity (children).

Albuterol (Ventolin) or metaproterenol (Alupent) metered-dose inhaler. Adult dose two puffs every 3 to 6 hours as needed.

Side effects: rapid heartbeat, nervousness ("jitters").

The proper technique for using a metered-dose inhaler device is:

1. Shake the inhaler vigorously.
2. Invert the inhaler so that the opening is downward. Hold the inhaler four finger widths in front of an open mouth, or place a spacer on the opening, around which the lips will be sealed.
3. Exhale fully.
4. Activate the inhaler at the beginning of inspiration.
5. Inhale slowly and deeply to full lung capacity.
6. Hold your breath for 10 seconds, then exhale slowly.

Prednisone. Adult dose 50 to 80 mg the first day. Each day, the dose is decreased by 10 mg. The pediatric dose is 1 mg per kg (2.2 lb) of body weight the first day, tapered every 4 days by halving the dose. Administer with food or with an antacid if possible.

For a severe skin reaction to poison ivy, oak, or sumac, see the instructions on page 205. For a severe sunburn, see the instructions on page 199.

Corticosteroids should always be taken with the understanding that a rare side effect is serious deterioration of the head ("ball" of the ball-and-socket joint) of the femur, the long bone of the thigh.

For Relief from a Mild Allergic Reaction or Hay Fever

Diphenhydramine (Benadryl). Same as "For Relief from a Severe Allergic Reaction."

Diphenhydramine (25 mg) with pseudoephedrine (60 mg) (Benadryl Decongestant). Adult dose one tablet every 8 hours.

Cetirizine hydrochloride (Zyrtec). Dose 5 to 10 mg a day; do not use in children under 6 years of age.

Fexofenadine (Allegra). Adult dose 60 mg every 12 hours. Rarely causes drowsiness. Do not use in children less than 12 years of age. This drug replaces terfenadine (Seldane), and should be used in preference to that medication. If for some reason terfenadine is used, observe the following precautions: a person with impaired liver function or who is taking ketoconazole, itraconazole, erythromycin, clarithromycin, or troleandomycin should not take terfenadine at the same time. Allegra-D: fexofenadine 60 mg with pseudoephedrine 120 mg extended-release tablet.

Loratadine (Claritin). Adult dose 10 mg every 24 hours. Rarely causes drowsiness. Do not use in children less than 12 years of age. Claritin-D: loratadine 5 mg with pseudoephedrine 120 mg. Claritin-D 24 Hour: loratidine 10 mg with pseudoephedrine 240 mg.

Astemizole (Hismanal). Adult dose 10 mg every 24 hours. Rarely causes drowsiness. Do not use in children less than 12 years of age. Those with impaired liver function or who are taking ketoconazole, itraconazole, erythromycin, clarithromycin, or troleandomycin should not take this drug. Do not administer with quinine (doses of 430 mg or higher). Up to 32 oz (1 liter) of tonic water, which contains 80 mg of quinine, may be consumed safely with this drug.

Prednisone. Adult dose 50 to 80 mg the first day for severe seasonal allergies that do not respond to other medications. Each day, the dose is decreased by 10 mg. The pediatric dose is 1 mg per kg (2.2 lb) of body weight the first day, tapered every 4 days by halving the dose. Administer with food or with an antacid, if possible. Corticosteroids should always be taken with the understanding that a rare side effect is serious deterioration of the head ("ball" of the ball-and-socket joint) of the femur, the long bone of the thigh.

Triprolidine with pseudoephedrine (Actifed). Adult dose 1 tablet every 8 hours; pediatric dose (6 to 12 years of age) half tablet every 8 hours.

Side effect: drowsiness.

For Relief from Severe Asthma/Chronic Obstructive Pulmonary Disease (COPD)

Many asthma/COPD medications are administered by metered-dose inhaler. The proper technique for using this device is:

1. Shake the inhaler vigorously.

2. Invert the inhaler so that the opening is downward. Hold the inhaler four finger widths in front of an open mouth, or place a spacer on the opening, around which the lips will be sealed.
3. Exhale fully.
4. Activate the inhaler at the beginning of inspiration.
5. Inhale slowly and deeply to full lung capacity.
6. Hold your breath for 10 seconds, then exhale slowly.

Epinephrine (adrenaline) 1:1,000 aqueous solution. Adult dose 0.3 to 0.5 ml injected subcutaneously (see page 419). This may be repeated two times at 20-minute intervals. The pediatric dose is 0.01 ml per kg (2.2 lb) of body weight, not to exceed 0.3 ml, injected subcutaneously. *Do not use epinephrine for treatment of COPD.*

The drug is available in preloaded syringes in certain allergy kits, which include the Ana-Kit (Hollister-Stier) and the EpiPen and EpiPen Jr. (Dey). Instructions for use accompany the kits. The EpiPen products are generally easier for laypeople to use, because they require less manual dexterity for injection.

For dosing purposes, the EpiPen should be used for adults and children over 66 lb (30 kg) in weight. Children 66 lb and under should be injected with the EpiPen Jr.

Take particular care to handle preloaded syringes properly, to avoid inadvertent injection into a finger or toe. Do not intentionally inject epinephrine into the buttocks or a vein. Epinephrine should not be exposed to heat or sun, but does not need to be kept refrigerated. If clear (liquid) epinephrine turns brown, it should be discarded.

Do not use epinephrine if the victim is older than 45 years, has a known history of heart disease, or is a pregnant female unless the situation is absolutely life threatening. Do not use epinephrine for treatment of COPD. When administering an injection, *never* share needles between people.

Primatene Mist (inhaler) is a mixture of epinephrine and alcohol available over the counter. This preparation should not be used in substitution for injected epinephrine in cases of severe asthma.

Side effects: rapid heartbeat, nervousness.

Terbutaline (Brethine) tablets. Adult dose 2.5 to 5 mg every 6 to 8 hours.

Terbutaline (Brethaire) metered-dose inhaler. Adult dose 2 puffs every 4 to 6 hours.

Flunisolide (Aerobid) metered-dose inhaler. Adult dose as directed.

Triamcinolone acetonide (Azmacort) metered-dose inhaler. Adult dose one puff twice a day for treatment of chronic asthma, equivalent to 10 mg per day of oral prednisone.

Albuterol (Ventolin) or metaproterenol (Alupent) metered-dose inhaler. Adult dose 2 puffs every 3 to 6 hours as needed.

Side effects: rapid heartbeat, nervousness ("jitters").

Combivent (ipratropium bromide and albuterol sulfate) metered-dose inhaler. Adult dose 2 puffs four to six times a day, not to exceed 12 puffs in 24 hours.

Bitolterol (Tornalate) metered-dose inhaler. Adult dose two puffs every 8 hours.

Pirbuterol (Maxair) metered-dose inhaler. Adult dose two puffs every 4 to 6 hours.

Salmeterol (Serevent). Adult dose two puffs every 12 hours.

Metaproterenol (Alupent) tablets. Adult dose 20 mg every 4 to 6 hours; pediatric dose (6 to 9 years of age or less than 60 lb, or 27.2 kg, of body weight) 10 mg.

Albuterol (Ventolin) tablets. Adult dose 2 to 4 mg three to four times a day.

Cromolyn sodium (Intal) metered-dose inhaler. Adult and pediatric dose two puffs every 4 to 6 hours; not for use in children less than 5 years of age.

Theophylline. Adult dose 100 to 200 mg every 6 to 8 hours; pediatric dose 4 mg per kg (2.2 lb) of body weight every 6 to 8 hours.

Prednisone. Adult dose 50 to 80 mg the first day. Each day, the dose is decreased by 10 mg. The pediatric dose is 1 mg per kg (2.2 lb) of body weight the first day, tapered every 4 days by halving the dose. Administer with food or with an antacid, if possible. Corticosteroids should always be taken with the understanding that a rare side effect is serious deterioration of the head ("ball" of the ball-and-socket joint) of the femur, the long bone of the thigh.

For Relief from Mild Asthma

In addition to drugs under "For Relief from Severe Asthma":

Ipratropium bromide (Atrovent) metered-dose inhaler. Adult dose two puffs every 4 to 6 hours as needed. Do not exceed 12 puffs in 24 hours. Do not use in children less than 12 years of age.

Beclomethasone dipropionate (Vanceril) metered-dose inhaler. Adult dose 2 puffs every 4 to 6 hours, not to exceed 20 puffs in 24 hours; pediatric dose (6 to 12 years of age) 1 or 2 puffs every 6 hours, not to exceed 10 puffs in 24 hours. Rinse the mouth after each use.

Zafirlukast (Accolate). Adult dose 20 mg tablet twice a day taken 1 hour before or 2 hours following meals. Do not use in children less than 12 years of age.

For Treatment of Chest Pain (Angina)

Nitroglycerin ¹⁄₁₅₀ grain (0.4 mg) or lingual aerosol (0.4 mg metered dose per spray). Adult dose one tablet dissolved under the tongue, or one spray under the tongue, for treatment of angina. This may be repeated every 10 minutes for two additional doses.

Side effects: dizziness (low blood pressure), headache. If a person uses nitroglycerin and becomes faint, he should lie down with his legs elevated until his skin color returns to normal and he feels better (usually, in a minute or two). If chest pain or weakness persist, this may indicate a heart attack (see page 45).

For Treatment of Congestive Heart Failure

Furosemide (Lasix) diuretic (promotes urination). Adult dose 1 to 4 tablets (20 to 80 mg) each day for the fluid retention associated with heart failure. Diuretics should not be used for fluid retention not associated with heart failure (such as that from high altitude) or for weight reduction.

Digoxin (Lanoxin). Adult dose 0.125 to 0.25 mg each day.

For Treatment of Seizures (Epilepsy)

Diphenylhydantoin (Dilantin). Adult dose 300 to 400 mg per day; pediatric dose 2.5 mg per kg (2.2 lb) of body weight twice a day.

Phenobarbital. Adult dose 60 to 120 mg three times per day; pediatric dose 1 to 1.5 mg per kg (2.2 lb) of body weight three times a day.

Carbamazepine (Tegretol). Adult dose 400 to 1,200 mg a day in two to three divided doses; pediatric dose 10 to 20 mg per kg (2.2 lb) of body weight each day in two to three divided doses.

For Relief from Pain

Acetylsalicylic acid (aspirin). Adult dose 650 mg (10 grains) every 4 to 6 hours; pediatric dose 60 mg (1 grain) per year of age (not to exceed 600 mg) every 4 to 6 hours.

Side effect: stomach irritation. Do not administer to a person with an ulcer or upset stomach. Take with food or an antacid, if possible. Enteric coated aspirin (such as Ecotrin) helps prevent stomach irritation and should be used whenever possible. To avoid Reye's syndrome (postviral encephalopathy and liver failure), do not use aspirin to control fever in a child under the age of 17.

Acetaminophen (Tylenol). Adult dose 500 to 1,000 mg every 4 to 6 hours; pediatric dose: up to 1 year, 60 mg; 1 to 3 years, 60 to 120 mg; 3 to 6 years, 120 mg; 6 to 12 years, 240 mg.

Codeine. Adult dose 30 to 60 mg every 6 to 8 hours; pediatric dose 0.5 to 1 mg per kg (2.2 lb) of body weight.

Side effects: Codeine is a narcotic and has side effects of drowsiness and alteration of mental status. In addition, it may cause constipation.

Acetaminophen (Tylenol) 325 mg with codeine 30 mg. Adult dose one to two tablets every 4 to 6 hours.

Bromfenac sodium (Duract). Adult dose 25 mg every 6 to 8 hours. This is a potent new nonsteroidal anti-inflammatory drug that should not be used for more than 10 consecutive days.

For Relief from Fever

Acetylsalicylic acid (aspirin). Same as "For Relief from Pain." To avoid Reye's syndrome (postviral encephalopathy and liver failure), do not use aspirin to control fever in a child under the age of 17.

Acetaminophen (Tylenol). Same as "For Relief from Pain."

Ibuprofen (Motrin, Advil, Nuprin). Adult dose 400 to 600 mg every 4 to 6 hours; pediatric dose 5 to 10 mg per kg (2.2 lb) of body weight, not to exceed 400 mg.

For Relief from Muscle Aches or Minor Arthritis

Acetylsalicylic acid (aspirin). Same as "For Relief from Pain."
Acetaminophen (Tylenol). Same as "For Relief from Pain."

Nonsteroidal anti-inflammatory drugs ("NSAIDs" should not be taken on an empty stomach; side effects are abdominal pain and diarrhea):

Ibuprofen (Motrin, Advil, Nuprin). Adult dose 400 to 800 mg every 6 to 8 hours.

Ketoprofen (Orudis KT, Actron). Adult dose 12.5 to 50 mg every 6 to 8 hours.

Naproxen (Naprosyn, Aleve). Adult dose 220 to 500 mg every 6 to 12 hours.

Naproxen sodium (Naprelan). Adult dose 375 or 500 mg sustained release every 24 hours.

Ketorolac (Toradol). Adult dose 10 mg every 8 to 12 hours; do not exceed 3 days' consecutive use.

For Relief from Itching

Diphenhydramine (Benadryl). Same as "For Relief from a Mild Allergic Reaction."

Hydroxyzine (Atarax). Adult dose 25 to 50 mg every 8 hours; pediatric dose: up to 6 years, 10 mg every 8 hours; 6 to 12 years, 10 to 25 mg every 8 hours.

For Relief from Toothache

Benzocaine-phenol-alcohol (Anbesol, Numzit). For topical application to the gums.

Oil of cloves. For topical application to the gums.

For Relief from Motion Sickness

Dimenhydrinate (Dramamine). Adult dose 50 mg every 4 to 6 hours; pediatric dose (8 to 12 years of age) 25 mg every 4 to 6 hours.

Side effect: drowsiness.

Meclizine (Antivert, Bonine). Adult dose 25 to 50 mg one to two times per day. Do not give this drug to children under the age of 12.

Side effect: drowsiness.

Cyclizine (Marezine). Adult dose 25 mg; pediatric dose 12.5 mg for age 9 to 12.

Scopolamine (Transderm Scōp Transdermal Therapeutic System). Adult dose: Apply one patch (1.5 mg scopolamine) on the hairless area behind the ear. A single patch is good for 3 days. Take care to wash the hands carefully after application of the patch, to avoid getting any medication in the eyes. Not approved for children under the age of 12.

Side effects: blurred vision, dry mouth, decreased sweating, difficulty with urination, propensity to heat illness, altered mental status. A diver who uses this preparation should be alert to the danger of heat illness while out of the water encased in a constrictive (heat-retaining) wet suit.

Astemizole (Hismanal). Adult dose 10 mg every 24 hours. Although not approved for this purpose, astemizole appears to prevent motion sickness as a side effect by suppressing the vestibular (inner-ear) system. People with impaired liver function or who are taking ketoconazole, itraconazole, erythromycin, clarithromycin, or troleandomycin should not take this drug.

For Relief from Nausea and Vomiting

Prochlorperazine (Compazine). Adult dose 5 to 10 mg by mouth every 8 to 12 hours (by suppository 25 mg twice daily). Do not give this drug to children under the age of 12.

Side effects: neck spasms, difficulty in swallowing and talking (inability to control the tongue), difficulty with eye movement, and muscle stiffness. These side effects may occur in combination ("dystonic reaction"). If any of these occur, discontinue use of the drug and administer diphenhydramine (Benadryl) 50 mg every 6 hours for four doses. If a child has a dystonic reaction, the dose of diphenhydramine (Benadryl) to alleviate the side effects is 1 mg per kg (2.2 lb) of body weight. Be certain that the victim is capable of purposeful swallowing.

Promethazine (Phenergan). Adult dose 25 mg every 6 to 8 hours (by suppository 12.5 to 25 mg every 12 hours); pediatric dose 0.25 to 0.5 mg per kg (2.2 lb) of body weight by mouth or per rectum (suppository).

Side effects: similar to those with prochlorperazine.

Trimethobenzamide (Tigan). Adult dose 250 mg by mouth or 200 mg by suppository every 6 to 8 hours.

Side effects: similar to those with prochlorperazine.

Cyclizine hydrochloride (Marezine). Adult dose 25 to 50 mg every 6 to 8 hours.

For Relief from Diarrhea

Loperamide (Imodium or Pepto Diarrhea Control caplets). Adult dose two pills (2 mg each) initially, followed by one pill after each loose bowel movement, not to exceed eight pills. With uncomplicated (no fever or blood in stools) watery diarrhea, this drug can be given to children age 2 years and older. The dose in children is 0.2 per kg (2.2 lb) of body weight every 6 hours. The liquid preparation contains 1 mg per 5 tsp (5 ml).

Diphenoxylate (Lomotil). Adult dose two tablets two to four times per day. Do not give this drug to children under the age of 18.

Bismuth subsalicylate (Pepto-Bismol). Adult dose 2 tbsp (30 ml) or 2 tablets every 30 to 60 minutes, not to exceed 8 to 10 doses; pediatric dose: 3 to 6 years, 1 tsp (5 ml) or ½ tablet; 6 to 10 years, 2 tsp (10 ml) or 1 tablet; 10 to 14 years, 4 tsp (20 ml) or 1½ tablets; may repeat dose in children every 1 hour, not to exceed four doses. This drug should not be given to people who are sensitive to aspirin-containing products.

Side effect: black discoloration of the tongue and bowel movements.

Kaolin-pectin (Kaopectate). Adult dose 4 to 8 tbsp (60 to 120 ml) after each loose bowel movement; pediatric dose: 3 to 6 years, 1 to 2 tbsp (15 to 30 ml); 6 to 12 years, 2 to 4 tbsp (30 to 60 ml); older than 12 years, 4 tbsp (60 ml) after each loose bowel movement. This drug is of limited value; it does not shorten the course of diarrheal illness, and acts only to add a little consistency to stools.

For Relief from Constipation

Mineral oil. Adult dose 1 to 2 tbsp (15 to 30 ml); pediatric (older than 5 years) dose 1 to 2 tsp (5 to 10 ml). This drug is a mild laxative.

Docusate sodium (Colace). Adult dose 50 to 100 mg twice a day; pediatric dose 0.3 mg per kg (2.2 lb) of body weight once or twice a day. The dose should be adjusted to the response. This drug is a stool softener.

Docusate sodium (stool softener) with casanthranol (laxative) (Peri-Colace). Adult dose one capsule once or twice a day.

Docusate sodium (stool softener) 5 ml microenema. Adult dose 200 mg (one enema) once a day as necessary.

Docusate calcium (stool softener) (Surfak Stool Softener Gel Cap). Adult dose 240 mg once or twice a day.

Senna extract (Senokot). Two tablets a day at bedtime. This drug is a mild laxative.

Milk of Magnesia. Adult dose 1 to 2 tbsp (15 to 30 ml) at bedtime. This drug is a mild laxative.

Lactulose syrup, USP (Duphalac). Adult dose 1 to 2 tbsp (15 to 30 ml) daily. This drug is a mild laxative.

Bisacodyl (Dulcolax). Adult dose two 5 mg tablets or one 10 mg suppository. This drug is a moderate laxative. A child age 6 to 12 years may take one 5 mg tablet.

Cascara sagrada 150 mg; aloe 100 mg (Nature's Remedy) (laxative). Adult dose two tablets a day.

Psyllium mucilloid (Metamucil). Adult dose one to two packets per day dissolved in water. This natural psyllium fiber product increases the bulk of the stool, and should be ingested with at least a quart (liter) of liquid.

For Relief from Ulcer Pain

Mylanta II. Adult dose 2 tbsp (30 ml) or two tablets (chewed) 1 and 3 hours after meals, at bedtime, and as needed. This is a mixture of aluminum hydroxide, magnesium hydroxide, and simethicone.

Rolaids. Adult dose 1 to 2 tablets (chewed) after meals as necessary. These contain dihydroxy-aluminum sodium carbonate. Because of the relatively high sodium content, these should not be used routinely by people with congestive heart failure (see page 41).

Cimetidine (Tagamet). Adult dose 300 mg three times a day with meals and at bedtime. This H2RA (antagonist to histamine H2 receptor) drug decreases the secretion of gastric acid.

Ranitidine hydrochloride (Zantac). Adult dose 75 to 150 mg two times a day. This H2RA drug decreases the secretion of gastric acid.

Famotidine (Pepcid). Adult dose 20 mg twice a day or 40 mg at bedtime for 4 weeks to treat an active duodenal ulcer, then 20 mg at bedtime for 2 to 4 weeks for suppression therapy to diminish the secretion of gastric acid. This H2RA drug decreases the secretion of gastric acid.

Propantheline bromide (Pro-Banthine). Adult dose 7.5 to 15 mg three times a day before meals and at bedtime. This drug is used to control gastric acid secretion and to reduce bowel activity (decrease cramping).

Sucralfate (Carafate). Adult dose one tablet (gram) 1 hour before meals and at bedtime. This drug binds to the ulcer crater, and therefore requires the presence of acid to work properly. Thus, antacids should not be ingested within 30 minutes before or after the ingestion of sucralfate.

Omeprazole (Prilosec). Adult dose one capsule (20 mg) a day given 30 minutes before a meal. This PPI (proton [acid] pump inhibitor) drug diminishes gastric acid secretion.

For Relief from Indigestion or Gas Pains

Antacid (such as Mylanta II). Same as "For Relief from Ulcer Pain."

Simethicone (Mylicon-80). Adult dose one to two tablets (chewed) after meals and at bedtime.

For Relief from Heartburn (Reflux Esophagitis)

Antacid (such as Mylanta II). Same as "For Relief from Ulcer Pain."

Ranitidine hydrochloride (Zantac). Adult dose 75 mg every 12 hours as needed. This H2RA (antagonist to histamine H2 receptor) drug decreases the secretion of gastric acid.

Cimetidine (Tagamet HB). Adult dose 200 mg (two 100 mg tablets) 30 to 60 minutes before a meal, not to exceed twice in a 24-hour period. This H2RA drug decreases the secretion of gastric acid.

Famotidine (Pepcid). Adult dose 20 mg tablet twice a day for up to 6 weeks.

Gaviscon or Gaviscon II. Adult dose one to two tablets (chewed) or one to two tbsp (15 to 30 ml) (liquid preparation) after each meal and at bedtime. This is a mixture of aluminum hydroxide, magnesium trisilicate, sodium bicarbonate, and alginic acid.

Metoclopramide hydrochloride (Reglan). Adult dose 10 mg up to four times a day, 30 minutes before meals and at bedtime.

Side effects: rarely, neck spasms, difficulty in swallowing and talking (inability to control the tongue), difficulty with eye movement, and muscle stiffness. These side effects may occur in combination ("dystonic reaction"). If any of these occur, discontinue use of the drug and administer diphenhydramine (Benadryl) 50 mg every 6 hours for four doses. Be certain that the victim is capable of purposeful swallowing.

For Relief from Nasal Congestion

Pseudoephedrine (Sudafed). Adult dose 30 to 60 mg every 6 to 8 hours; pediatric dose 1 mg per kg (2.2 lb) of body weight.

Phenylephrine hydrochloride 0.25% nasal spray (Neo-Synephrine ¼%). Adult dose two to three drops or sprays twice a day; pediatric dose (older than 6 years) use 0.125% two drops twice a day. Do not use this drug for more than 3 consecutive days, to avoid "rebound" swelling of the nasal passages from chemical irritation and sensitization to the medicine.

Oxymetazoline hydrochloride 0.05% (Afrin). Adult dose two to three drops or sprays twice a day; pediatric dose (older than 6 years) use two 0.025% (half-strength) drops twice a day. Do not use this drug for more than 3 consecutive days, to avoid "rebound" swelling of the nasal passages from chemical irritation and sensitization to the medicine.

For Relief from Cough

Glyceryl guaiacolate (Robitussin) expectorant. Adult dose 1 tsp (5 ml) every 3 to 4 hours; pediatric dose ½ tsp (2.5 ml) every 3 to 4 hours.
Robitussin-AC: plus codeine (cough suppressant).
Robitussin-DAC: plus codeine, pseudoephedrine (decongestant).
Robitussin-PE: plus pseudoephedrine.
Robitussin-DM: plus dextromethorphan (cough suppressant).
Codeine. Adult dose 15 to 30 mg every 4 to 6 hours. This is a potent cough suppressant.
CoTylenol Liquid Cold Formula. Adult dose 2 tbsp (30 ml) every 6 hours; pediatric dose (6 to 12 years) ½ to 1 tbsp (7.5 to 15 ml) every 6 hours. Two tbsp (30 ml) contains dextromethorphan hydrobromide 30 mg (for cough), acetaminophen 650 mg (for fever, aches), chlorpheniramine maleate (antihistamine) 4 mg, and pseudoephedrine hydrochloride (decongestant) 60 mg.
Dextromethorphan hydrobromide–guaifenesin (Vicks Cough Syrup). Adult dose 2 to 3 tsp (10 to 15 ml) every 4 to 6 hours; pediatric dose; 2 to 6 years, 1 tsp (5 ml) every 6 hours; 6 to 12 years, 1 to 2 tsp (5 to 10 ml) every 6 hours.
Dextromethorphan hydrobromide–guaifenesin–phenylpropanolamine (Naldecon cough syrup). Adult dose 1 tsp (5 ml) every 4 hours; pediatric dose ½ tsp (2.5 ml) every 4 hours.

For Relief from Sore Throat

Benzocaine-hexylresorcinol (Sucrets Antiseptic Throat Lozenges).
Benzocaine-cetylpyridinium (Cēpacol Lozenges, Vicks Lozenges).

Cold Formulas

Contac. Phenylpropanolamine (decongestant), chlorpheniramine (antihistamine).
Contac Severe Cold Formula. Pseudoephedrine (decongestant), chlorpheniramine, acetaminophen (for fever, aches), dextromethorphan (for cough).
Chlor-Trimeton. Chlorpheniramine.
Chlor-Trimeton Decongestant. Chlorpheniramine, pseudoephedrine.
Coricidin. Chlorpheniramine, aspirin.

Coricidin "D". Phenylpropanolamine, chlorpheniramine, aspirin.
CoAdvil. Ibuprofen (for fever, aches), pseudoephedrine.
CoTylenol. See "For Relief from Cough."
Dristan. Phenylephrine (decongestant), chlorpheniramine, aspirin, caffeine.
Dristan Time Capsule. Phenylephrine, chlorpheniramine.
TheraFlu. Acetaminophen, pseudoephedrine, chlorpheniramine.

Skin Medications

Antiseptic Ointments

Apply thinly to the skin twice a day.

Bacitracin antiseptic ointment.
Bacitracin–polymyxin B sulfate (Polysporin) ointment.
Mupirocin (Bactroban) 2% ointment.
Mupirocin (Bactroban) calcium cream.
Bacitracin–polymyxin B sulfate–neomycin (Neosporin, Triple Antibiotic, or Mycitracin) ointment.
Neomycin-gramicidin (Spectrocin) ointment.
Neomycin (Myciguent) ointment.
Povidone iodine 0.5% (Betadine First Aid) cream.
Silver sulfadiazine (Silvadene) cream. Soothing antiseptic cream for burns; apply to the skin once or twice a day. Do not use in children younger than 2 years. Avoid use on the face.
Benzalkonium chloride (Zephiran) antiseptic solution (1:750 dilution in water). May be used full strength to clean unbroken skin, but should be diluted 1:2 or 1:3 with water to swab an open wound or animal bite (to kill rabies virus).
Hexachlorophene scrub (pHisoHex). Use as a scrubbing soap on cuts, scrapes, and infected skin. Do not use on children under 1 year of age.
Povidone iodine (Betadine) antiseptic solution. Use in a 1:10 dilution with water to gently scrub cuts and scrapes.

Anti-Itch, Anti-Sting

Campho-phenique. Topical anti-itch gel medication consisting of camphorated phenol in mineral oil.

Campho-phenique Maximum Strength ointment or Neosporin Plus ointment or Mycitracin Plus ointment. Topical anti-itch and antiseptic medication consisting of lidocaine hydrochloride, bacitracin zinc, neomycin sulfate, and polymyxin B sulfate.

Lidocaine hydrochloride 2.5% anesthetic ointment. Use for relief from pain due to scrapes; apply to the skin and leave in place for 10 minutes prior to scrubbing. Do not apply if the area to be covered is greater than 5% of the total body surface area (an area approximately four to five times the size of the victim's palm).

Benzalkonium chloride 0.13%; lidocaine hydrochloride 2.5% (Bactine solution). Very mild antiseptic-anesthetic combination available over the counter. May be used to swab animal bites if Zephiran is not available.

Calamine lotion. Apply thinly as a drying agent two to three times a day to skin affected with poison ivy, oak, or sumac.

Phenolated (1%) calamine lotion. Apply thinly as a drying agent two to three times a day to skin affected with poison ivy, oak, or sumac.

Calamine–pramoxine hydrochloride 1% (Caladryl). Apply thinly as a drying agent two to three times a day to skin affected with poison ivy, oak, or sumac.

Itch Balm Plus (hydrocortisone acetate 0.5%, diphenhydramine 2%, tetracaine 1%) skin balm. For topical application to skin lesions caused by insect and worm bites; poison oak, ivy, sumac, and other plant irritations; marine stings; and so on. Apply four times a day for no more than 4 days; do not use in children under the age of 2 years.

Pramoxine (Prax, PrameGel, Itch-X spray). Topical anti-itch medication for skin rashes due to plant allergy, insect bites, or sunburn. Apply two to three times a day.

Antifungal Cream, Lotion, and Powder

Apply to the skin two to three times a day for athlete's foot or jock itch.

Tolnaftate 1% (Tinactin, Aftate)
Clotrimazole 1% (Lotrimin, Mycelex)
Zinc undecylenate (Desenex)
Miconazole nitrate 2% (Micatin)
Nizoral cream. Apply thinly once or twice a day to treat yeast or fungal infection.
Nizoral. 400 mg one oral dose for tinea versicolor (harmless yeast overgrowth on the skin); induce mild sweating 2 to 4 hours after dose; don't shower for 8 hours after dose (the drug is excreted in sweat).

Spectizole cream. Apply thinly once or twice a day to treat yeast or fungal infection.

Anti-Mites

Lindane (Kwell) 1% lotion. Apply to entire skin, leave on for 8 hours, then shower for treatment of scabies.

Permethrin 5% cream (Elimite). Apply to entire skin, leave on for 8 hours, then shower for treatment of scabies; appears to be safe in pregnant women and children over 2 months of age.

Permethrin 1% creme rinse (Nix). Apply to washed and towel-dried hair, leave on for 10 minutes, then rinse thoroughly and comb out nits for treatment of head lice.

Topical Steroids

Hydrocortisone 1% cream, 2.5% cream (Hytone). Safe for infants, face, peri-anal area, skin folds.

Triamcinolone 0.1% ointment. Often mixed with Eucerin cream 1:1; moisturizer increases penetration—too potent for face, genitalia, or infants.

For Sleep

Diphenhydramine (Benadryl, Sominex, Nytol). Adult dose 50 mg at bedtime.

Triazolam (Halcion). Adult dose 0.125 to 0.25 mg at bedtime. This is short-acting and may be a better choice at high altitude.

　　Side effects: short-term memory loss, bad dreams.

Zolpidem tartrate (Ambien). Adult dose 5 to 10 mg at bedtime. There have been rare reports of hallucinations in people who took higher doses; elders may be prone to such a reaction.

Temazepam (Restoril). Adult dose 15 to 30 mg at bedtime.

Flurazepam (Dalmane). Adult dose 15 to 30 mg at bedtime.

Melatonin. The hormone melatonin is endogenously produced by humans in the pineal gland from the precursor tryptophan. Melatonin levels in the blood increase and are highest during normal hours of sleep, decreasing toward morning.

　　Sold over the counter, melatonin is considered a "dietary supplement," and thus does not come under the scrutiny of the Food and

Drug Administration. The science supporting its use to induce sleep, decrease wakefulness during sleep, and decrease jet lag is preliminary and suggests that it might be beneficial, without any obvious adverse effects. The doses cited range from 1 mg to 5 mg administered orally 1 to 2 hours before going to bed.

Insect Repellents

Choose a product with one or more of these four active ingredients: N, N-diethyl-3-methylbenzamide (DEET); butyl 3,4-dihydro-2,2-dimethyl-4-oxo-2H-pyran-6-carboxylate (Indalone); 2-ethyl-1,3-hexanediol (EHD; Rutgers 612); dimethyl phthalate (DMP).

Good choices include: *Ben's 100* (100% DEET), *Cutter spray* (18% DEET, 12% DMP), *Cutter stick* (33% DEET), *Cutter cream* (52% DEET, 13% DMP), *Muskol spray* (25% DEET), *Muskol lotion* (100% DEET), *OFF spray* (25% DEET), *Deep Woods OFF cream* (30% DEET), *Deep Woods OFF liquid maximum strength* (100% DEET), *6–12 Plus spray* (25% EHD, 5% DEET), and *Repel spray* (40% DEET). *Sawyer Products' Gold* (16.6% DEET plus MGK 264 synergist) is an effective lotion that can be applied to skin to repel ticks, mosquitoes, gnats, flies, and fleas. *Sawyer Controlled Release Deet Formula* is advertised to provide 24-hour protection and to minimize absorption of DEET by using an encapsulating protein to keep the chemical off the skin.

Do not use repeated applications or concentrations of DEET greater than 15% on children under the age of 6 years. In adults, 75 to 100% DEET may cause skin rash or rare serious neurological reactions.

Permanone is 0.5% permethrin. This is for spray application to clothing and is an excellent tick repellent.

Sunscreens

SPF: stands for "sunscreen protection factor." Higher numbers indicate greater protection.

Butyl methoxybenzoylmethane 3% plus padimate O 7%: Photoplex.

Para-aminobenzoic acid (PABA)–alcohol: PreSun (SPF 4, 8, or 12).

Padimate O–oxybenzone: Chap Stick Sunblock (SPF 15), Coppertone Supershade (SPF 15), Block Out (SPF 10 or 15), Ban de Soleil (SPF 15), Eclipse (SPF 10 or 15), Sundown (SPF 15).

Padimate O: Ban de Soleil (SPF 2, 4, 6, or 8), Eclipse (SPF 5), Sea and Ski (SPF 2, 4, or 6), Sundown (SPF 4 or 8).

Padimate O–aloe: Hawaiian tropic (SPF 4, 6, or 8).

Water-resistant preparations: BullFrog 15 or 3, PreSun 29, Sawyer Products Bonding Base 45, Sundown 30, Vaseline 14, Aloegater 40.

Side effects of sunscreens: skin irritation, yellow discoloration of skin and clothing, allergic reactions. People sensitive to PABA should use a non-PABA product, such as Piz-Buin or Uval.

Antibiotics

Amoxicillin. Adult dose 250 to 500 mg every 8 hours; pediatric dose 10 to 15 mg per kg (2.2 lb) of body weight every 8 hours (three times a day).

Amoxicillin-clavulanate (Augmentin). Adult dose 500 to 875 mg two times a day; pediatric dose 25 to 45 mg per kg (2.2 lb) of body weight in two divided doses per day. For otitis media in children, use the higher dose.

Ampicillin. Same dose as phenoxymethyl penicillin (see below).

Azithromycin (Zithromax). Adult dose 500 mg day one, then 250 mg per day for 4 additional days; pediatric dose 10 mg per kg (2.2 lb) of body weight day one, then 5 mg/kg body weight for 4 additional days.

Cefadroxil (Duricef). Adult dose 500 mg to 1 g twice a day. For pharyngitis, to eradicate the Group A streptococcus, an acceptable dose is 1 g once a day for 10 days. Pediatric dose: for skin infections 30 mg per kg (2.2 lb) of body weight per day in two divided doses; for pharyngitis, administer in a single dose or two divided doses for 10 days.

Cefixime. Adult dose 400 mg per day; pediatric dose 8 mg per kg (2.2 lb) of body weight once per day; no refrigeration needed—discard 14 days after the dry powder is reconstituted with water.

Cefuroxime axetil. Adult dose 500 mg twice a day; pediatric dose 30 mg per kg (2.2 lb) of body weight in two divided doses a day.

Cefpodoxime (Vantin). Adult dose 200 to 400 mg twice a day for pneumonia.

Cephalexin (Keflex). Adult dose 250 mg every 4 to 6 hours or 500 mg every 12 hours; pediatric dose the same as for phenoxymethyl penicillin. *Avoid use* in a person with penicillin allergy, because 5 to 10% of those allergic to penicillin are also allergic to cephalosporins.

Ciprofloxacin (Cipro). Adult dose 500 mg twice a day for 3 days to treat infectious diarrhea. This drug should not be given to pregnant women or children under the age of 18.

Clarithromycin (Biaxin). Adult dose 500 mg twice a day; pediatric dose 15 mg per kg (2.2 lb) of body weight in two divided doses per day.

Dicloxacillin. Same dose as phenoxymethyl penicillin (below).

Doxycycline (Vibramycin). Adult dose 100 mg twice a day for treatment, or once a day for prevention, of infectious diarrhea. Do not give to pregnant women or children up to the age of 7, because this drug may cause permanent dark discoloration of the teeth.

Erythromycin. Same dose as phenoxymethyl penicillin (see below). Common side effects are stomach upset and diarrhea. This drug is the first alternative to penicillin in penicillin-allergic individuals.

Fleroxacin. Adult dose 400 mg once a day for 3 days for the treatment of infectious diarrhea.

Levofloxacin. Adult dose 250 to 500 mg once a day.

Metronidazole (Flagyl). Adult dose 250 mg three times a day. *Do not drink alcohol when taking this medication and for 3 days afterward; the interaction would cause severe abdominal pain, nausea, and vomiting.*

Noroxin. Adult dose 400 mg every 12 hours.

Ofloxacin. Adult dose 300 to 400 mg every 12 hours.

Phenoxymethyl penicillin (Penicillin Vee K). Adult dose 250 to 500 mg every 4 to 6 hours; pediatric dose: 2 to 6 years, 125 mg every 6 to 8 hours; 6 to 10 years, 250 mg every 6 to 8 hours. For pharyngitis, to eradicate the Group A streptococcus, an acceptable adult dose is 1 g twice a day for 10 days.

Sparfloxacin (Zagam). Adult dose 400 mg day one, then 200 mg each day.

Sulfisoxazole (Gantrisin). Pediatric dose 50 mg per kg (2.2 lb) of body weight based upon the erythromycin component in four divided doses a day.

Tetracycline. Adult dose 500 mg four times a day. Do not give to pregnant women or children up to the age of 7, because this drug may cause permanent dark discoloration of the teeth.

Trimethoprim-sulfamethoxazole (Bactrim or Septra DS [double strength]). Adult dose one pill (80 mg trimethoprim with 400 mg sulfamethoxazole) twice a day for infectious diarrhea or bladder infection; one pill once a day for prevention of traveler's diarrhea. The pediatric dose for an ear infection or severe infectious diarrhea (caused by *Shigella* bacteria) is 1 tsp (5 ml) of the pediatric suspension per 10 kg (22 lb) of body weight every 12 hours (twice a day), not to exceed 4 tsp (20 ml) (the adult dose) per dose. More precisely, the pediatric dose is 4 mg/kg/dose TMP with 20 mg/kg/dose SMX.

Trovafloxacin (Trovan). Adult dose 200 mg once a day for ten days to treat acute sinusitis.

Appendix Two

CONVERSION TABLES

Fahrenheit/Centigrade (Celsius) Temperature Conversion

To convert degrees Fahrenheit (F) into degrees Centigrade (C, or Celsius), subtract 32, then multiply by 5, then divide by 9. To convert degrees C into degrees F, multiply by 9, then divide by 5, then add 32. For extrapolation into "subzero" (below 0° F) range, be aware that 1 Fahrenheit degree represents the temperature change of $\frac{5}{9}$ of a Centigrade degree, or 1 Centigrade degree represents 1.8 times the temperature change of a Fahrenheit degree. For example, to obtain the Centigrade number equivalent to 0° F, subtract 32 from 0° (which yields −32), then multiply by $\frac{5}{9}$, which yields −17.8 Centigrade. However, recall that when most people use the phrase *17 below*, they are referring to below 0 on the Fahrenheit scale.

DEGREES CENTIGRADE	DEGREES FAHRENHEIT
−17.8	0
−17	1.4
−16	3.2
−15	5.0
−14	6.8
−13	8.6
−12	10.4
−11	12.2
−10	14.0
−9	15.8
−8	17.6
−7	19.4
−6	21.2
−5	23.0
−4	24.8
−3	26.6
−2	28.4
−1	30.2
0	32.0
1	33.8
2	35.6

DEGREES CENTIGRADE	DEGREES FAHRENHEIT
3	37.4
4	39.2
5	41.0
6	42.8
7	44.6
8	46.4
9	48.2
10	50.0
11	52.0
12	53.6
13	55.4
14	57.2
15	59.0
16	60.8
17	62.6
18	64.4
19	66.2
20	68.0
21	69.8
22	71.6
23	73.4
24	75.2
25	77.0
26	78.8
27	80.6
28	82.4
29	84.2
30	86.0
31	87.8
32	89.6
33	91.4
34	93.2
35	95.0
36	96.8
37	98.6
38	100.4
39	102.2
40	104.0
41	105.8
42	107.6

DEGREES CENTIGRADE	DEGREES FAHRENHEIT
43	110.0
44	111.2
45	113.0
46	114.8
47	116.6
48	118.4
49	120.2
50	122.0
100	212.0

Measures of Length

UNIT	U.S. EQUIVALENT	METRIC EQUIVALENT
inch	1"	0.0254 m; 2.54 cm
foot	12"; .333 yd	0.3048 m; 30.48 cm
yard	3'; 36"	0.914 m
fathom	6'; 72"	1.83 m
rod	16.5'; 5.5 yd	5.029 m
mile	5,280'; 1,760 yd	1,608.64 m; 1.609 km
millimeter	0.03937"	0.001 m
centimeter	0.3937"	0.01 m
decimeter	3.937"	0.1 m
meter	39.37"; 3.28'	1 m
decameter	10.93 yd	10 m
hectometer	328.08'; 109.36 yd	100 m
kilometer	0.6214 miles	1,000 m

Measures of Volume (Capacity)

UNIT	U.S. EQUIVALENT	METRIC EQUIVALENT
minim	1/60 fluidram	0.061610 ml
drop	0.017 fluid oz	0.5 ml
fluidram	60 minims	3.696 ml
teaspoon	0.170 fl oz	5 ml
tablespoon	3 tsp; 0.51 fl oz	15 ml
fluid ounce	8 fluidrams	29.573 ml
gill	4 fl oz	118.291 ml
cup	8 fl oz; 16 tbsp	236.58 ml

UNIT	U.S. EQUIVALENT	METRIC EQUIVALENT
pint	2 cups	0.473 liter
quart	2 pints; ¼ gallon	0.946 liter
gallon	4 quarts	3.785 liters
barrel	31.5 gallons	119.23 liters
hogshead	2 barrels; 63 gallons	238.46 liters
milliliter	0.034 fl oz	0.001 liter
centiliter	0.338 fl oz	0.01 liter
deciliter	3.38 fl oz	0.1 liter
liter	1.05 quarts	1 liter; 1,000 ml
kiloliter	1,050 quarts; 262.5 gallons	1,000 liters

Measures of Weight

UNIT	U.S. EQUIVALENT	METRIC EQUIVALENT
grain	0.002083 oz (apothecary)	0.0648 g; 64.8 mg
gram	0.04 oz; 0.002 lb	1 g
ounce (avoirdupois)	437 grains	28.349 g
pound (avoirdupois)	16 oz; 7,000 grains	0.453 kg; 454 g
ton (short)	2,000 lb	0.907 metric ton

Appendix Three

Guidelines for Prevention of Diseases Transmitted via Human Blood and Other Body Fluids

Hepatitis and acquired immunodeficiency syndrome (AIDS) are diseases transmitted by viruses, which are themselves transmitted in human blood and other body fluids. AIDS, caused by the human immunodeficiency virus, has become a scourge of Asia and sub-Saharan Africa, largely through indiscriminate sexual contact, although transmission of the virus occurs more reliably when a contaminated blood product or needle-sharing is involved. Hepatitis viruses are most commonly transmitted via blood or feces (contaminated water and food). Other germs, such as influenza virus, are spread in respiratory secretions, while the agents of other diseases, such as the spirochetes of syphilis and bacteria of gonorrhea, are found in fluids transmitted during sexual intercourse.

Human fluids commonly encountered by laypeople during medical or recreational activities that would be considered high risk for the transmission of disease include blood, semen, vaginal secretions, saliva, and any fluid contaminated by blood, feces, and urine. Not all fluids are of equal risk, depending upon the infectious agent. For instance, feces, nasal secretions, respiratory secretions, sweat, tears, urine, and vomitus do not appear to appreciably transmit the human immunodeficiency virus, but it is usually very difficult to tell if these fluids are contaminated with blood. Therefore, it is safest to assume that any body fluid can transmit disease, and to avoid unprotected contact with any moist human body substance.

In order to minimize the transmission of infectious disease, a medical rescuer should:

- Be careful with sharp objects, such as knives and needles. Obtain all available useful immunizations (including hepatitis; see page 397).
- Use personal protective equipment, such as disposable latex or hypoalergenic gloves, goggles (eyeshields, glasses, ski goggles), pocket mask or barrier shield (for rescue breathing), and gown or overclothing. In cold weather, thin glove liners can be worn under disposable gloves.
- After any victim contact, even if gloves are worn, wash your hands thoroughly with soap and water. If a glove breaks during contact with a victim, remove it and wash your hands immediately.
- Unbroken skin is very protective. However, if broken or unbroken skin is exposed to a victim's body fluid, it should be washed immediately with

soap and water. If soap and water are not available, use waterless antiseptic hand cleanser, plain water, or snow.

- Carry materials contaminated by body fluids in clearly labeled nonpermeable containers, such as heavy plastic bags.
- If equipment (such as a litter) has been contaminated by a body fluid and must be reused, it should be cleaned by washing with soap and water, then scrubbing with a minimum 1:10 dilution of household bleach (sodium hypochlorite) in water. Alternative minimum dilutions (in water) for disinfection include 0.3% hydrogen peroxide, 25% ethyl alcohol, 35% isopropyl alcohol, 0.5% Lysol, and 0.25% povidone iodine (Betadine). Wear gloves while cleaning the equipment. Eyeglasses can be washed with soap and water.

The purpose of educating you about precautions is not to discourage you from helping another in need. Rather, it is to support the notion that with just a moment of thought and the initiation of proper precautions, needless transmission of infectious diseases can be prevented, and a medical rescue proceed without harm to the rescuer.

GLOSSARY

abdomen: the part of the body between the chest and the pelvis

abrasion: a scraped area of skin

abscess: a localized collection of pus, usually surrounded by inflamed tissue

acclimatize: to adapt to a new altitude, climate, environment, or situation

acidotic: in a state of abnormally reduced alkalinity; overwhelmed by acid; related to decreased pH

acute: sudden in onset

airway: passage for air into the lungs, including the mouth, nose, pharynx, larynx, trachea, and bronchi

alkaline: having the properties of a base; related to high pH

allergy: exaggerated reaction (sneezing, runny nose, itching, skin rash, difficulty in breathing) to substances that do not affect other individuals

alveoli: microscopic air spaces in the lung where oxygen is exchanged for carbon dioxide

ambulatory: able to walk

amnesia: loss of memory

amniotic fluid: liquid that surrounds unborn child within the membranes inside the uterus

amputate: to cut from the body

analgesia: relief from pain

anaphylaxis: hypersensitivity to substances following prior exposure, resulting in a severe allergic reaction

anemia: deficiency in red blood cells

anesthesia: loss of sensation

aneurysm: abnormally dilated blood vessel

angina pectoris: episodic chest pain caused by insufficient oxygen supply to the heart

antibiotic: drug used to kill bacteria

antibody: body substance, produced by specialized cells, that combines with and neutralizes foreign substances or toxins

antiemetic: drug used to control nausea and vomiting

antihistamine: drug used to inactivate histamine

anti-inflammatory: drug used to prevent or correct inflammation

antiseptic: substance that limits or stops the growth of microscopic germs

antivenin: drug used to inactivate the effects of animal or insect venom

anus: posterior opening from the intestine to the outside world

aorta: the large artery that carries oxygenated blood from the heart to be distributed to the body

appendectomy: surgical removal of the appendix

appendicitis: inflammation of the appendix

appendix: wormlike appendage of the bowel, located in the right lower quadrant of the abdomen

aqueous: mixed with or related to water

argasid: related to soft ticks

arrest: sudden stop

arterial: pertaining to an artery

artery: muscular- and elastic-walled blood vessel that carries oxygenated blood from the heart to the body

arthritis: inflammation of the joints

arthropod: invertebrate animal with jointed limbs belonging to the phylum Arthropoda: insect, spider, or crustacean

aspirate: to draw by suction; to inhale into the lungs

asthma: labored breathing caused by narrowing of the smaller air passages (past the bronchi) in the lungs, associated with shortness of breath, wheezing, cyanosis, and coughing

atherosclerosis: hardening of the arteries

aura: a sensation of lights or sounds that occurs prior to a migraine headache or seizure

barotitis: disorder of the ear due to increased or decreased atmospheric pressure

bile: green fluid produced by the liver and stored in the gallbladder, where it is released into the duodenum to aid in the digestion and absorption of fats

bilirubin: a pigment formed from the destruction of red blood cells

blister: fluid-filled elevation of the epidermis

borrelial: related to microorganisms of the genus *Borrelia*, which transmit diseases such as Lyme disease

bowel: intestine

brain stem: part of the central nervous system between the spinal cord and brain, which controls certain critical functions, such as breathing

breech: buttocks first, as in breech birth

bronchitis: inflammation of the bronchial tree

bronchodilator: drug used to relax and widen the bronchi

bronchus: main passageway from the trachea to the smaller air passages in the lungs

bruise: injury that does not break the skin, with rupture of small blood vessels that causes blue or purplish discoloration

bursa: fluid-filled sac that allows smooth motion of muscles or tendons over a bone or joint

bursitis: inflammation of a bursa

buttocks: the seat of the body; the rump

calorie: the amount of energy necessary to raise the temperature of 1 g of water by 1° C; 1 food calorie ("kilocalorie") is equal to 1,000 energy calories

cancer: malignant tumor; uncontrolled growth of cells that invade normal body tissues for no reason and serve no purpose

canker sore: small, painful ulcer of the mouth

cannula: small tube for insertion of fluid or air

capillary: microscopic blood vessel that connects an artery to a vein

carbonaceous: rich in carbon; black like soot

carbon dioxide: gas that combines with water to form carbonic acid; formed by the combustion and decomposition of organic substances

cardiac: pertaining to the heart

cardiopulmonary: pertaining to the heart and lungs

carotid artery: chief artery that travels up the neck and carries blood to the head and brain

cartilage: elastic tissue that is transformed into bone

cartilaginous: composed of cartilage

cataract: opacity in the lens of the eye

caustic: corrosive; capable of destroying by chemical action

central nervous system: the brain and spinal cord

cerebral: pertaining to the brain

cervical: pertaining to the neck

chilblain: inflammation, swelling, and blistering of the skin caused by exposure to cold

cholecystitis: inflammation of the gallbladder

chronic: of long duration

colic: acute pain caused by spasm, obstruction, or twisting of a hollow organ

colitis: inflammation of the colon

colon: the large intestine

coma: a state of profound unconsciousness

comatose: in a coma

comminuted: in multiple pieces; shattered

compound fracture: broken bone accompanied by torn skin

conjunctiva: membrane that covers the insides of the eyelids and extends over the whites of the eyes

convulsion: seizure; abnormal involuntary contraction or series of contractions of the muscles

COPD: chronic obstructive pulmonary disease, caused by scarred lung tissue

core: center; involving the abdomen and chest organs

cornea: the transparent covering of the eyeball over the iris and pupil that allows light to enter the eye

corticosteroid: one of a number of hormones produced by the adrenal glands

costochondritis: inflammation of the cartilage that attaches the ribs to the sternum

CPR: cardiopulmonary resuscitation, with artificial breathing and chest compressions

cravat: triangular cloth bandage folded into a longitudinal strap

crepitus: a crackling sound or feeling

culture: to grow in a prepared laboratory medium

cyanosis: blue or purple discoloration of the skin due to inadequate oxygen in the blood

cyst: an abnormal sac containing gas, fluid, or solid material

debridement: surgical removal of torn, contaminated, or devitalized tissue

decompression: loss of pressure; contributes to diving-related bends

dehydration: depletion of body fluids

dermatitis: inflammation of the skin

dermis: layer of skin just underneath the epidermis that contains sensitive nerve endings, blood vessels, and hair follicles

diagnose: to identify a disease

diaphragm: muscular wall that separates the chest from the abdomen

dilatation: stretching to normal or beyond normal dimensions

dinoflagellate: marine plankton

discharge: liquid released from an organ or tissue surface

dislocation: displacement of bones at a joint

disseminated: spread over a wide area

distal: at the end of; in the area farthest from the center of the body

diuretic: medicine that promotes urination

diverticulitis: inflammation of a diverticulum

diverticulum: small outpouching from a hollow organ (such as the large intestine)

dressing: bandage; covering for a wound

duodenum: first part of the small intestine

ectopic: at a remote site; in the wrong place

edema: swelling caused by the accumulation of fluid

electrolyte: soluble inorganic chemical (such as sodium or potassium) found in body fluids

embolism: sudden obstruction of a blood vessel by an embolus

embolus: abnormal particle (such as a blood clot or air bubble) circulating in the bloodstream

encephalopathy: disease of the brain that often results in abnormal mentation

endemic: native to

endotracheal: through the trachea

envenom: to poison with venom

epidermis: outermost layer of the skin

epigastrium: area lying over the stomach; central upper area of the abdomen

epiglottis: soft tissue pillar in the throat that covers the vocal cords and keeps food and liquid from entering the trachea during swallowing

epiglottitis: inflammation of the epiglottis

epilepsy: disorder associated with disturbed electrical discharges in the central nervous system that cause convulsions

erythema: redness

esophageal reflux: return of food and acid from the stomach into the esophagus; major cause of heartburn

esophagitis: inflammation of the esophagus

esophagus: muscular tube from the pharynx to the stomach

eustachian tube: a tube of bone and cartilage that connects the middle ear with the upper throat and allows equalization of pressure on both sides of the eardrum

exhale: to breathe out

expectoration: sputum, phlegm, or mucus; the act of spitting out saliva or mucus from the air passages via the mouth

extend: lengthen; reach out

extremity: arm and hand (upper extremity) or leg and foot (lower extremity)

facial: pertaining to the face

fallopian tube: small tube that conducts the egg from the ovary to the uterus

fascia: tough, fibrous tissue that surrounds muscle bundles

fasciitis: inflammation of the fascia

feces: solid human bodily waste discharged through the anus

feculent: pertaining to or resembling feces

femoral artery: large artery that carries blood to the leg

femur: large bone of the thigh

fibrillation: unsynchronized quivering

flagellate: possessing a flagellum

flagellum: whiplike organelle (tail) for locomotion

flail chest: series of detached ribs that cannot move properly to assist with breathing

flatulence: the presence of excessive gas in the bowel

flatus: gas generated in the digestive tract and discharged via the anus

flex: bend; fold

follicle: skin cavity in which a root of hair lies

fracture: to break; a broken object

frostbite: freezing of the tissues

gallbladder: muscular, hollow organ that stores bile produced by the liver

gangrene: tissue death due to loss of blood supply; may be caused by injury or infection

gastroenteritis: inflammation or irritation of the stomach and/or intestine

gastrointestinal: pertaining to the stomach and intestine; digestive system

gauge: the diameter of a hypodermic needle expressed as a standard number

genitals: external organs of reproduction

gland: a specialized group of cells that either selectively removes substances from the blood, concentrates or alters substances in the blood, and/or creates and releases special substances into the blood

glaucoma: disease of the eye associated with increased pressure within the eyeball

glucose: type of sugar used by the body for energy

gonorrhea: sexually transmitted disease caused by the bacterium *Neisseria gonorrhoeae*

graft (skin): piece of skin taken from one area of the body to cover a defect or burn in another area

grain: a measure of weight equal to 0.0648 g

gram: a measure of weight equal to 15.432 grains

grand mal seizure: convulsion manifested by violent generalized muscle contractions, clouded consciousness, and a period of confusion after the event

hallucinate: to see visions or experience lack of reality

hallucination: imaginary perception

heartburn: burning discomfort behind the sternum related to irritation or spasm of the lower portion of the esophagus

Heimlich maneuver: technique for removal of a foreign object caught in the upper airway

helminth: intestinal worm-shaped parasite

hemoglobin: iron-containing, oxygen-carrying pigment in red blood cells

hemorrhage: bleeding

hemorrhoid: dilated vein found at the anal margin

hepatitis: inflammation of the liver

hernia: protrusion of part or all of an organ through a wall of the space in which it is normally contained

hiatal hernia: protrusion of part of the stomach through the diaphragm

histamine: chemical compound that plays a major role in allergic reactions

hives: raised red skin wheals associated with allergic reactions

hormone: chemical substance formed in the body that is carried in the bloodstream to affect another part of the body; an example is thyroid hormone, produced by the thyroid gland in the neck, which affects growth, temperature regulation, metabolic rate, and other body functions

hydrate: to cause to take up water

hyper- (prefix): excessive

hyperbaric: pertaining to increased atmospheric pressure

hyperextension: accentuated extension or straightening of a limb

hypertension: elevated blood pressure

hyperthermia: elevated core body temperature

hypertrophy: enlargement of; excessive size

hyphema: collection of blood in the chamber of the eye between the lens and the cornea (anterior chamber)

hypo- (prefix): insufficient; underneath

hypodermic: under the skin

hypoglycemia: low blood sugar

hypothermia: low core body temperature

ileum: the last (and longest) segment of the small intestine

ileus: profoundly decreased physiologic activity (motility) of the bowel, characterized by dilatation, abdominal pain, and vomiting

iliac: pertaining to the ilium

ilium: the upper bone that forms the side of the pelvis

immobilize: to prevent freedom of movement

immune: not susceptible to

immunity: condition of being able to resist a certain entity or disease

immunization: the process of developing immunity; often refers to an injection

impetiginize: to involve with impetigo

impetigo: contagious skin disease caused by *Staphylococcus* or *Streptococcus* bacteria, characterized by weeping, crusting, and areas of pus formation

incarcerate: to confine; to entrap

infarction: area of tissue death caused by obstruction of blood circulation

inflammation: response to cell injury that involves dilatation of small blood vessels, redness, warmth, pain, and migration of white blood (pus) cells to the region; part of the healing process that removes noxious substances and damaged tissue; can be destructive as a primary disease process

infrared: light that lies outside of the visible spectrum, with wavelengths longer than those of red light

inhale: to breathe in

inspiration: the act of breathing in

intestine: the digestive tube that passes from the stomach to the anus; the small intestine (bowel) consists of the duodenum, jejunum, and ileum; the large intestine (bowel) consists of the cecum (with attached appendix), colon (ascending, transverse, descending, and sigmoid), and rectum

intoxication: state of poisoning

intravenous: into a vein

irrigate: to rinse

ischemic: in a condition of lowered blood flow; lacking sufficient oxygen to sustain function

-itis (suffix): inflammation of

jaundice: yellow pigmentation of the tissues and body fluids

jejunum: the segment of the small intestine that follows the duodenum and precedes the ileum

ketoacidosis: condition of excessive ketones in the bloodstream, associated with increased systemic acidity; a life-threatening condition of diabetics

ketone: acid by-product of metabolism

kg (abbreviation): kilogram

kilo- (prefix): one thousand of something

kilocalorie: 1 food calorie, or 1,000 energy calories; the energy necessary to raise the temperature of 1 kg of water by 1° C

kilogram: 1,000 g; 2.2 lb

lacerate: to tear or cut roughly

lateral: away from the midline; outer

larynx: the portion of the trachea that contains the vocal cords; the voice box

lb (abbreviation): pound

lethargy: drowsiness or aversion to activity, caused by disease

ligament: fibrous connective tissue that attaches bone to bone

liter: volume of water that weighs 1 kg; 1.0567 quarts

localized: confined to a specific area

lumbar: pertaining to the lower back

lymph: amber nutrient fluid that contains white blood cells; it circulates in lymphatic system and is involved with injuries, infections, and cancers

lymphatic: related to lymph glands, cells, or fluid; small vessel that transports lymph fluid

lymph node: collection of lymph cells that function as a gland; node (colloquial)

mandible: lower bone of the jaw

manipulate: to move mechanically, usually with the hands

melena: dark-colored, tarry stools (feces), due to the presence of blood altered by intestinal fluids

meningitis: inflammation of the covering of the brain and upper spinal cord

mental status: condition of alertness and comprehension

metabolism: the energy-producing and energy-utilizing processes that occur in the human body

mg (abbreviation): milligram

micron: measure of length equal to one one-millionth of a meter

microorganism: small life form that requires a microscope to be seen

migraine: recurrent severe headaches generally accompanied by an aura (classic migraine), nausea, vomiting, and dizziness

milli- (prefix): one one-thousandth

milligram: $\frac{1}{1,000}$ of a gram

milliliter: $\frac{1}{1,000}$ of a liter

ml (abbreviation): milliliter

mononucleosis: infectious disease characterized by an abnormal increase in monocytes (a type of white blood cell) in the blood, weakness, fever, sore throat, and enlargement of the spleen and lymph nodes in the neck

mottled: covered with colored spots or blotches

mucus: slippery secretion created by mucous glands associated with mucous membranes (such as those that line the nose, throat, and mouth) for lubrication and some protection against bacteria

myocardial: pertaining to the heart muscle

myoglobin: iron-containing, oxygen-carrying pigment present in muscle tissue

nanometer: one one-billionth of a meter

narcosis: altered mental status ranging from confusion to coma

nebulize: to reduce to a fine spray

neurological: pertaining to the nervous system

nm (abbreviation): nanometer

nonsteroidal: not containing steroids

organ: part of the body with a specific function

otitis: inflammation or infection of the ear

ounce: measure of weight equal to 28.35 g; $\frac{1}{16}$ lb

ovulation: release of an egg from the ovary

oxygen: colorless, odorless gas necessary for combustion and life

oxygenate: to supply with oxygen

oz (abbreviation): ounce

ozone: triatomic form of oxygen (O_3) that is formed by electric discharge through air

pallor: pale skin color

palpate: feel with the hands

palpation: the act of feeling with the hands

palpitation: abnormal beating of the heart felt by the victim

pancreas: gland that produces and secretes digestive enzymes (juices) and the insulin hormone

pancreatitis: inflammation of the pancreas

paroxysmal: sudden

pediatric: pertaining to children

pelvic: related to the pelvis

pelvis: strong, basin-shaped bone structure that provides support for the spine, hips, and legs

peptic: related to digestive fluids

peristalsis: natural contractions of the muscular walls of the bowel that move bowel contents forward

peritoneum: lining of the abdominal organs and cavity

peritonitis: inflammation of the peritoneum

petit mal seizure: form of epilepsy characterized by brief periods of confusion without major abnormal muscle activity

pharyngitis: inflammation of the pharynx; sore throat

pharynx: throat

phlegm: mucus secreted in the respiratory passages

photophobia: aversion to light

photosensitivity: sensitivity to light, particularly to ultraviolet radiation

placenta: organ implanted within the uterus that supports an unborn child, which is attached by the umbilical cord

plankton: microscopic plant life found in natural bodies of water

plantar: on the bottom

pleura: lining that covers the lungs and the inside of the chest cavity

pleural space: a small space between the pleura that covers the lung and that which lines the inside of the chest wall; normally, this space is minuscule (cannot be seen) because it is filled with negative pressure, which allows the lung to expand with the chest wall

pleuritis: inflammation of the pleura

pneumonia: infection of the lung characterized by fever, cough, shortness of breath, and the production of purulent or bloody sputum

pneumothorax: collapsed lung with air in the pleural space

potable: drinkable (preferably, disinfected)

prognosis: projected outcome

prone: lying flat with the face down

prophylactic: for the purpose of prophylaxis

prophylaxis: measures designed to maintain health and to prevent disease

protozoan: microscopic unicellular or acellular animal

proximal: closer to starting point or center; nearest to central part of the body

pubic: pertaining to the region of the pubis

pubis: the lowermost and anterior bone of the pelvis

pulmonary: pertaining to the lungs

punctate: like a dot or small mark

pupil: contractile round opening in the center of the iris of the eye through which light is transmitted to the lens

purulent: foul

pus: white, yellow-green, or beige creamy fluid that is formed by decomposing tissue, white blood cells, and tissue fluids

quadrant: one of the four quarters into which a region can be divided

radial artery: the main artery that travels through the wrist to supply the hand

radiation: emission of energy in the form of waves or particles

radiation of pain: pain that travels from one region to another, such as from the hand to the shoulder

rebound tenderness: pain in the abdomen that is worse upon release of pressure than it is upon creation of pressure (compression); often indicates peritonitis

recompression: the method whereby increased atmospheric pressure is used to treat victims of air embolism or decompression sickness (diving-related disorders)

reflux: backward flow

reflux esophagitis (heartburn): inflammation of the esophagus caused by backward flow of acid from the stomach

renal: related to the kidney

respiratory: pertaining to the organs of breathing or the act of breathing

resuscitate: to revive from death or unconsciousness

retina: the posterior inside surface of the eye, which receives a light image refracted through the cornea and lens, and transmits it to the brain via the optic nerve

saline: salty (solution); normal saline (liquid compatible with most human tissues) is 0.9% sodium chloride in water

saturate: to soak; to dissolve to the highest possible concentration

seizure: epileptic convulsion

serum: the fluid component of blood after the cells are removed

shock: a clinical state manifested by profound depression of all body functions, caused by insufficient blood and nutrient supply to the tissues; signs and symptoms include low blood pressure, cool and clammy skin, altered mental status, and collapse

silica: silicon dioxide

soft tissue: body tissue that is not composed of bone or cartilage; generally refers to skin, muscle, and fat; generally excludes internal organs

spasm: involuntary muscular contraction

sphincter: muscular ring that serves as a junction between two tubes, such as the esophageal sphincter (between the esophagus and stomach)

spirochete: curled or spiraled microorganism capable of causing infectious disease

sprain: incomplete stretching or tearing of ligaments

sputum: phlegm composed of saliva and discharges from the respiratory passages

status: unchanging situation, such as status asthmaticus (severe, unchanging asthma), or status epilepticus (nonceasing convulsions)

sterile: uncontaminated by infectious agents

sternocleidomastoid: prominent neck muscle that connects the mandible to the collarbone and sternum

sternum: breastbone

steroids: hormones, vitamins, body constituents, and drugs with a specific chemical structure

strain: incomplete stretching or tearing of tendons or muscles

stridor: harsh vibrating noise heard in the upper airway during breathing; commonly associated with an outflow obstruction during exhalation; may be inspiratory

sub- (prefix): underneath

subconjunctival: under the conjunctivae

subcutaneous: under the skin

sublingual: under the tongue

supine: lying flat with the face up

supraventricular: above the level of the ventricles (lower chambers) of the heart

suture: to sew with surgical thread or nylon; the thread or nylon used to sew a wound closed

symphysis: a barely movable junction of two bone surfaces connected by a fibrous cartilage pad

syndrome: a collection of signs and symptoms that, taken together, constitute a particular disease or abnormality

synthesize: to create or compose

syringe: device used to inject fluids into or remove them from the body

systemic: affecting the entire body

tachycardia: rapid heart rate (beat)

tendon: fibrous tissue that attaches muscle to bone

tension pneumothorax: collapsed lung under pressure from air in the pleural space

tetanus: an infectious disease caused by the bacterium *Clostridium tetani*, characterized by severe muscle contractions and inability to open the mouth (lockjaw); the bacterium that causes tetanus

thermoregulatory: in control of temperature

thrombophlebitis: an inflammation of the veins that causes the formation of blood clots

tissue: a group of cells that combine in the body to serve a specific function

tourniquet: a device used to control blood flow by impeding or preventing circulation

toxin: poisonous substance

trachea: main passageway for air from the pharynx to the bronchi

tracheostomy: surgical opening created in the neck into the trachea to allow breathing when the upper airway is obstructed

trauma: mechanical injury

traumatic: related to mechanical injury

triage: sorting of patients by priority

tubal: related to a tube

tumor: abnormal growth of tissue that arises in the body without purpose; may be benign (noncancerous) or malignant (cancerous)

tympanic membrane: eardrum

ulcer: erosion; open sore

ultrasonic: beyond the normal range of sound waves

ultraviolet: light outside of the violet end of the visible spectrum with a wavelength shorter than that of visible light

unconscious: unaware; unarousable

ureter: muscular tube that carries urine from the kidney to the bladder

urethra: passage that carries urine from the bladder to the external opening in the genital region

urticaria: itchy, patchy, raised, and red skin rash, often associated with allergy

uterus: muscular reproductive female organ in which a child develops; womb

vaccinate: to inject a special preparation for the purpose of achieving immunity from disease

vaginitis: irritation of the vagina

varicose: abnormally swollen or dilated

vascular: pertaining to the blood vessels

vein: blood vessel that carries blood from the body back to the heart

venom: poison secreted from venom glands in animals and insects; usually introduced into the victim with a bite or sting

venous: pertaining to the veins

ventricle: one of two large chambers of the heart

vertebra: one of the bony segments that form the spinal column (backbone)

vertigo: dizziness; sensation of whirling motion

vessel: container; a blood vessel may be an artery, vein, or capillary

vitreous: gelatinous fluid within the eye

wheezing: labored breathing, usually noted on expiration, associated with lung disorders characterized by airway narrowing, such as asthma

INDEX

ABOUT THE AUTHOR

Dr. Paul S. Auerbach is Clinical Professor of Surgery in the Division of Emergency Medicine at Stanford University and Chief Operating Officer for MedAmerica in Oakland, California. A founder and past president of the Wilderness Medical Society, Dr. Auerbach serves as an advisor to the Divers Alert Network, National Ski Patrol System, and Institute for Preventative Sports Medicine and participates as a consultant or committee member in many other scientific, medical, and outdoor education-recreation organizations, such as the United States Army Research Institute of Environmental Medicine, Healthwise, and Sea Studios. He was the first editor of the journal *Wilderness and Environmental Medicine* (formerly *Journal of Wilderness Medicine*), is editor of *Wilderness Medicine,* the definitive textbook for medical professionals, medical editor for *Dive Training* magazine, and author of *A Medical Guide to Hazardous Marine Life, Diving the Rainbow Reefs,* and *An Ocean of Colors.* Dr. Auerbach is a recipient of the Education Award from the Wilderness Medical Society and the DAN America Award from the Divers Alert Network. He lives in Los Altos, California.